Recent Results in Cancer Research

Volume 218

Series Editor

Prof. Dr. med. Heike Allgayer, MD, Ph.D,
Full Professor and Director,
Department of Experimental Surgery—Cancer Metastasis,
Medical Faculty Mannheim, Ruprecht Karls University, Heidelberg, Germany

More information about this series at http://www.springer.com/series/392

Axel W. Bauer • Ralf-Dieter Hofheinz •
Jochen S. Utikal
Editors

Ethical Challenges in Cancer Diagnosis and Therapy

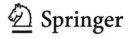 Springer

Editors
Axel W. Bauer
History, Philosophy and Ethics in Medicine
University Medical Centre Mannheim
Mannheim, Baden-Württemberg, Germany

Ralf-Dieter Hofheinz
Outpatient Department
Interdisciplinary Tumour Centre
University Medical Centre Mannheim
Mannheim, Baden-Württemberg, Germany

Jochen S. Utikal
Skin Cancer Unit, German Cancer Research
Center (DKFZ)
University Medical Centre Mannheim
Mannheim, Baden-Württemberg, Germany

ISSN 0080-0015   ISSN 2197-6767   (electronic)
Recent Results in Cancer Research
ISBN 978-3-030-63751-4   ISBN 978-3-030-63749-1   (eBook)
https://doi.org/10.1007/978-3-030-63749-1

This Springer imprint is published by the registered company Springer Nature Switzerland AG
The registered company address is: Gewerbestrasse 11, 6330 Cham, Switzerland

Introduction

Cancer: A Deadly Threat

About one in every four people in Western industrialized countries die of cancer. In Germany, 238,345 of the 954,874 deaths in 2018, or 24.96 %, were attributed to cancer. In 2000, a total of 838,797 deaths included 210,738 caused by cancer, which is 25.12% (Statista Research Department 2020; Radtke 2020). These numbers have remained frustratingly consistent for at least the last 20 years. With the advent of successful ground-breaking therapies, the picture might be expected to look different. While the case fatality rate (CFR) following a diagnosis of cancer has declined, this is also due to a considerable increase in the number of these diagnoses. In 2018, around 18.1 million new cancer cases and 9.6 million cancer deaths were seen worldwide. The number of cancer cases had increased by 4 million since 2012, but the number of cancer deaths only increased by 1.4 million (Bray et al. 2018). Statistically, this reduced the CFR from 58.2 to 53.0%.

As recently as the beginning of the twentieth century, while medicine was celebrating triumphs over cancer, doctors were also suffering bitter disappointments. The introduction of scientific methods into everyday medicine proved considerably more arduous than the profession's leading representatives, or even the public, had hoped and expected. In 1900, the weekly journal *Deutsche Medicinische Wochenschrift* published statistics, according to which malignant tumours in England and Wales had increased from 2.5 to 4.5% of all causes of death between 1880 and 1896, a relative increase of more than 80% (Reiche 1900). Prussian Medical Adviser Robert Behla (1850–1921), author of an international oncological bibliography published in 1901, wrote that the medical mind had made progress with the problem of cancer and that although eyes had grown tired under the microscope, research would not rest until it had wrested its secrets from nature (Behla 1901, XXIV–XXV; Bauer 1989).

Cancer Research and Therapy: Financial, Bureaucratic and Ethical Obstacles Today

About 120 years later, one of the main problems for experimental cancer research is funding. Financial resources are limited, leading to tough competition with other research areas—a highly relevant contemporary example being the current COVID-19 research. To obtain research funding, scientists are subject to strong informal or formal pressure to publish their results as frequently as possible, and in highly reputable journals with a high impact factor (IF). Increasingly, this may also lead to unfair, mostly anonymous, accusations from competitors, resulting for example in unjustified exclusion from publication in high impact journals or from research funding. In the current, in part, 'management-dictated' environment, scientists with non-mainstream, critical views and perspectives, who are not going with the flow, have a particularly hard time obtaining research funds or getting published in highly ranked publications.

Extension of scientists' contracts is directly linked to their research success, as measured in (ideally, 'top') publications (hence the dictum 'publish or perish') and to successful grant applications (also increasingly linked to their track records in top publications). An increasing number of academic institutions request their scientists to publish at IFs above 5—publications with lower IFs are sometimes not even counted when it comes to tenure decisions, or to budget allocation amongst faculty members. With the researcher's livelihood increasingly dependent on successful, or even spectacular, research results, this pressure can lead to 'polished' or even falsified research results. There have been cases of false experimental research results which have led to human clinical trials that were ultimately negative, or even caused harm to patients. The dependency of research on the impact factor and grant money leads to excessive pressure on science. Frequency of citation (a crucial numerator in the calculation of the IF of a journal) depends not only on the reputation of a journal or a working group, but above all on the number of scientists who are interested in the topic, which affects citation numbers. This results in, for example, rare tumour entities or childhood cancers being represented poorly in journals with a high impact factor, since the chance of citation is lower.

Other ethical problems of experimental research involve the use of human clinical material. In the past, biobanks have been created without the informed consent of the donors. Tumour cell lines were established that were still in use long after the donor's death. A famous example is the HeLa cervical cancer cell line that was named after its donor Henrietta Lacks (1920–1951). Amazingly, she was never asked for her consent for cell lines to be established from her tumour tissue. Moreover, according to her biographer (Skloot 2010), extra biopsies were even removed during her surgical procedure for the exclusive purpose of establishing cell lines. This certainly would not comply with today's ethical biobanking standards. With regard to tumour cell lines used in current cancer research, there are repeated incidences of cell lines that are contaminated or mixed up, and/or do not originate from the original tumour entity the researcher has been assuming (Lichter et al.

2010). This can result in publication of false data of which the authors are not even aware, and to subsequent clinical trials with negative results.

The transition from experimental research to clinical research and clinical trials is mainly dominated by pharmaceutical companies. They decide which target or tumour entity should be further evaluated, depending, among other criteria, on its potential future profits. Rare tumour entities are thus of less interest, and hardly any therapies are approved by the EMA or FDA for the treatment of the majority of these rare cancers, due to lack of clinical studies. One of the great problems of clinical research—not only in oncology, of course—is financing the increasingly expensive studies. The possibilities of initiating so-called investigator-sponsored trials (ISTs) independently of commercial funding are very limited. In Germany, for example, sponsors of independently funded studies include the German Research Foundation (DFG), the Federal Ministry of Education and Research (BMBF) and German Cancer Aid. The amount of finance these institutions are able to provide is still not sufficient to support the high number of translational-clinical studies necessary in the current era of personalized medicine.

During recent years, legal frameworks have led to an enormous increase in costs when such studies are carried out. The funding framework for publicly funded studies is usually very limited. It is thus no longer possible to take part in ISTs, especially for smaller study centres. There is enormous competition worldwide from studies initiated by the pharmaceutical industry, which are usually much better endowed. As a result, ISTs in which the reality of care is better represented, and which address open questions of care much more efficiently from the practitioner's point of view, are difficult to finance and to implement. Given this situation, the question is whether and to what extent the scientific community can still participate in the development of clinical-oncological studies in which important therapeutic questions such as (i) multimodal settings (e.g., radiation therapy: yes/no?), (ii) vulnerable patient groups (e.g., treating the elderly and/or infirm, children) or (iii) therapy escalation (can the same effectiveness be achieved with a lower dose?) are being addressed.

Another complex set of ethical problems is the fact that the increasingly cost-effective and more widely available molecular characterization of tumours and the associated identification of potentially effective molecularly targeted therapies, do not harmonize with current approval practices. This has direct consequences for doctor–patient interaction. Let us take a patient with a malignant melanoma and a BRAF mutation as an example. Here, a combination of BRAF and MEK inhibitor can be prescribed, at the health insurance company's expense, in accordance with the approval regime. However, this therapy is initially inaccessible to a patient with biliary tract cancer showing a BRAF mutation. The molecular characterization of tumours is now anchored in routine clinical practice in many places, and patients rightly demand the best possible molecular characterization and therapy. This means doctors are often able to offer a potentially effective therapy based on the analysis of the tumour that is not covered by the health insurance company and requires an application for 'off-label use' which may not be approved. While it is good news that the EMA recently approved the first 'tumour-agnostic therapy' for patients with tumours and a NTRK fusion, molecular characterization already provides us with many therapeutic options that may have approvals for individual tumour entities, but not for all tumours with a dedicated molecular target, regardless of the location of the malignancy. Nowhere is the speed of approvals keeping pace with the therapeutic possibilities.

Nowadays, doctors are called upon to comply with an increasing amount of documentation and bureaucratic requirements, for example in the context of certi-fication, or classification into diagnosis-related groups (DRGs). This fact is cited by many doctors as the main reason for poor job satisfaction. The scope of doctors' activities has changed dramatically without the corresponding preparation being solidly anchored in medical training. The same applies to the increasing digitization of work processes in medicine. The increase in the privatization of hospitals and the increasing economic pressure in the health care system also contribute to a con-tinuously changing professional practice which has noticeably changed the role of doctors—a move towards the health sector being seen as service providers. Last but not least, the increasingly discussed 'burnout pandemic' amongst doctors working in the field of oncology is a consequence of these circumstances.

A final critical consideration: in the context of the current COVID-19 pandemic, Prof. Christian Drosten, an eminent German virologist and director of the Institute of Virology at the Charité Hospital in Berlin, has identified a new battleground in the fight for medical resources: "Something has to change in science, too: In Germany, for example, medical research is very cancer-oriented. Infectious diseases are—and we are not only noticing this now—extremely important in medicine. We need a lot more research there. Antibiotic resistance is the next big problem. This also applies to us in high-performance medicine. We see revenge when we neglect areas of activity that don't seem to affect us" (World Health Summit 2020). Is Drosten right, will a new era of dispute over resources arise within biomedical research and will we see a re-setting of priorities in patient treatment during the 2020s, such as a further reduction in the financial support given to cancer research and therapy (already observed in 2020) to the benefit of research into COVID-19 or future viruses? We believe and hope Drosten is not right. If we compare the number of those who die from cancer and those who die from COVID-19 every day, there is little to support this hypothesis. Even during a pandemic, we must not lose sight of reality; for the benefit of these many patients we must maintain a balance, keeping in mind the top killer diseases that demand the attention of the scientific and clinical community every day.

Ethical Challenges in Cancer Diagnosis and Therapy

This book presents 18 different perspectives on the challenges to be faced by research, diagnosis and treatment of cancer during the 2020s. This includes a look at history as well as a critical consideration of epidemiological and biometric aspects. Questions about the benefits and harm of preventive measures require not only scientific, but also ethical and legal reflection. The role of the public media in the dissemination of supposed oncological knowledge must be viewed just as critically as the recruitment of patients for controlled clinical trials. Opinion leaders and the media should continuously keep in mind that they are talking about seriously ill people who should not be under any illusions about the supposedly sensational success of new treatments. After all, the perspective of the patient and their multi-faceted suffering brings with it serious ethical problems, the unsuccessful handling of which can sometimes lead, among others, to thoughts of suicide, challenges to family relationships and 'collateral' diseases for cancer patients and their relatives.

Our authors contribute a holistic span of specialist expertise, from cell biology to law to the history of science and medicine. Through their international perspectives and culture-specific approaches, they enrich our view on cancer and the many unresolved problems and dilemmas associated with it. The editors would like to thank the authors who, through their contributions, have been selflessly involved in the conception and realization of this book. The work could not have come about without their generous cooperation. We would also like to thank our colleague Prof. Heike Allgayer, MD, Ph.D., for suggesting this volume and for including it in her *Recent Results in Cancer Research* series. Meike Stoeck, Sylvana Freyberg, Corinna Hauser, Banu Dhayalan, Sudhany Karthick and Sindhu Sundararajan from *Springer Nature* were always at hand to clear obstacles out of the way.

Mannheim/Heidelberg, Germany   Axel W. Bauer
May 2021   Ralf-Dieter Hofheinz
                                                                       Jochen S. Utikal

References

Bauer AW (1989) Naturwissenschaftliche Medizin der Jahrhundertwende. Fiktion und Realität um 1900. Dtsch Med Wschr 114:1676–1679

Behla R (1901) Die Carcinomlitteratur. Eine Zusammenstellung der in- und ausländischen Krebsschriften bis 1900. Schoetz, Berlin

Bray F, Ferlay J, Soerjomataram I et al (2018) Global cancer statistics 2018: GLOBOCAN estimates of incidence and mortality worldwide for 36 cancers in 185 countries. Cancer J Clin 68(6):394–424

Lichter P, Allgayer H, Bartsch H et al (2010) Obligation for cell line authentication: appeal for concerted action. Int J Cancer 126(1):1

Radtke R (2020) Jährliche Todesfälle aufgrund von Krebs und anderen Neubildungen in Deutschland in den Jahren 2000 bis 2018. https://de.statista.com/statistik/daten/studie/172573/umfrage/krebstote-in-deutschland/. Accessed 20 Sept 2020

Reiche F (1900) Beiträge zur Statistik des Carcinoms. Dtsch. med. Wschr. 26:120–121

Skloot R (2010) The immortal life of Henrietta lacks. Crown Publishers, New York

Statista Research Department (2020) Anzahl der Sterbefälle in Deutschland von 1991 bis 2019. https://de.statista.com/statistik/daten/studie/156902/umfrage/sterbefaelle-in-deutschland/. Accessed 20 Setp 2020

World Health Summit (2020) Drosten: "Deutschland hat nichts besser gemacht als andere Länder, nur früher". Focus online, 23 Sept 2020 https://www.focus.de/gesundheit/coronavirus/auf-world-health-summit-drosten-deutschland-hat-nichts-besser-gemacht-als-andere-laender-nur-frueher_id_12463048.html. Accessed 23 Sept 2020

Contents

'The King of Diseases': An Essay on the Special Attention Paid to Cancer Patients and How It Came About

1

Wolfgang U. Eckart

1.1 Introduction

A new book on the history of cancer, first published in 2011 under the title *The Emperor of All Maladies—A Biography of Cancer* (Mukherjee 2011), has enjoyed successful publication in Germany since January 2012, and has been highly praised in the media. The author, Siddhartha Mukherjee, tells the story of the disease, the suffering it has caused and the attempts by researchers to counteract this 'scourge of humanity'. In the US, the book has sold more than 300,000 copies, worldwide nearly one million. *Time* magazine listed it among the 100 best non-fiction works of the last 100 years and it won the prestigious Pulitzer Prize in 2011.

Siddhartha Mukherjee was born in New Delhi, India, and studied at the elite universities of Stanford, Oxford and Harvard. He researches at Columbia University in New York. *The Emperor of All Maladies* is a title evidently chosen also for reasons of marketing; it reminds the reader of today of another big hit, although one in the genre of film: *The Lion King*, Walt Disney's (1901–1966) most successful cartoon film since *Mickey Mouse*. Mickey Mouse and his companion Donald Duck have been in the minds of all young people (and those who have stayed young) ever since their film debut some 90 years ago, while *The Lion King* has been enthralling young and old since 1994 as a moving feature-length cartoon film.

Both these anthropomorphic characters win viewers' hearts. In contrast, however, to the harmless mouse with humanoid features and very human everyday problems, *The Lion King* is a reminder of the old film theme of the permanent struggle of good versus evil. Simba, the newborn son of the old Lion King, Mufasa, is supposed to follow his father as a good ruler, but is soon confronted with

W. U. Eckart (✉)
Institute for History and Ethics in Medicine, Heidelberg University,
Reinhard-Hoppe-Straße 15, 69118 Heidelberg, Germany
e-mail: Wolfgang.eckart@histmed.uni.heidelberg.de

© Springer Nature Switzerland AG 2021
A. W. Bauer et al. (eds.), *Ethical Challenges in Cancer Diagnosis and Therapy*,
Recent Results in Cancer Research 218,
https://doi.org/10.1007/978-3-030-63749-1_1

Mufasa's younger brother, the malicious, indeed devilishly dictatorial character Scar, who is competing with him for domination of the animal world. Good is, in the end, victorious over evil and rules in the form of Simba wisely and benevolently, leading the animal world back to peace and plenty.

But let us return to our author, whose anthropomorphic biography of a disease has no happy ending; indeed, it basically fulfils all the conditions for a tragedy, although the hope of a cure does at least shine through a little. Humanity has lived with cancer for over 5000 years, and has been succumbing to it for just as long. And yet, cancer is regarded as a 'modern' malaise, because no other illness has shaped our time to such an extent. The names given to it are quite indicative: 'the king of all diseases', or an 'insatiable monster, hungrier than the guillotine'. In its perfidious perfection, its adaptability, its resistance, cancer takes on human attributes in Mukherjee's tale. His story is a biography: it is the story of suffering, of obsessive research, of brilliant ideas, of perseverance, but also of pride, arrogance and countless mistakes.

Siddhartha Mukherjee dedicates himself to the subject with the precision of a cellular biologist with historical ambitions and with the passion of a biographer. He tells us fascinating stories: of the Persian Queen Atossa and how her Greek slave may have cured her of breast cancer; of patients in the nineteenth century; of the first radiation treatments and the chemotherapies they had to undergo; and again and again he tells of his own patients. *The Emperor of All Maladies* gives us a fascinating glimpse of the future of cancer treatment and delivers a brilliant new perspective on the way doctors, scientists, philosophers and lay people have understood the body in sickness and in health for thousands of years.

There is no doubt that Mukherjee has fittingly described this disease, its almost human and demonic aspects, how it corresponds to our vision of the worst illnesses and sicknesses that can possibly happen to us, especially since the fears awakened by acquired immunodeficiency syndrome (AIDS) from the 1980 onward seem to have ebbed somewhat in today's society. But the book throws up a number of questions which I would like to discuss in the following sections of this chapter. Is it true, for instance, that humanity has regarded cancer as the *Emperor of All Maladies* for thousands of years, or is this perhaps an ahistorical projection of modern perspectives onto the past? Could it not be that cancer has only more recently acquired such significance in human perception? If so, what were the conditions leading to this new evaluation?

There is no doubt that we see descriptions of cancer in medical sources spanning thousands of years, or at least descriptions of mostly horrible courses of illness, which we dare to identify as owing to the symptoms described. I am deliberately being very cautious here, for we medical historians have very good reason to be extremely careful with diagnoses *ex post*. Not every 'cancerous swelling' of the female breast, for example, will have been a mammary carcinoma. Certainly, we meet the term—*karkínos, karkínoma,* cancer—in ancient texts, and this is the designation for hard-to-treat local illnesses, thus 'malignant' in this sense, generally swellings, tumours then, and ulcers or abscesses. But the terms tumour and ulcer or abscess are collective concepts covering many things; from ancient times to early modern times, they had nothing of the precision associated with them today (Eckart 2005: 448–452). Galen, in the second century CE, chose the image of Cancer, the zodiacal crab, because he thought there was an exterior resemblance of the tumour thus named—particularly that of the female breast—with the animal's appearance. These early forms of cancer are all of humoral-pathological origin, and result from an excess of gall, which is why treatment consisted at first of the usual evacuating methods (emetica, laxatives, blood-letting).

Later, however, after failure of these methods, the cauterizing iron and the knife dominate; cancerous tumours are thus cut out or burnt away. These are certainly ultimative, indeed heroic measures, although the patients are hardly likely to have survived them for long. But we must make one thing clear at this point: in the spectrum of diseases described from ancient times through the Arabic and Western Middle Ages and the early modern period until well into the nineteenth century, cancer remains a remarkable exception, and for this reason worthy of description—it is by no means the rule. It certainly cannot be called the *Emperor of Diseases*. The undoubted King or Emperor of maladies in Europe since ancient times is surely the epidemic, the pest, the plague. Although 'plague' is the most common term used, we must understand it as referring to a plethora of infectious diseases, among which the plague *proprie dictu* certainly played a leading, but not the only, role.

Severe epidemics of smallpox, flu, typhus and measles, too, were part and parcel of the misery, as were pandemics (referring to Eurasia of the time). Thanks to palaeobacterial evidence, we now know that the Black Death, the great plague of the fourteenth century in Asia and Europe, corresponded quite exactly to the modern bubonic plague; it has been possible genetically to show the existence of modern types of *Yersinia pestis*. Apart from these dramatic epidemics, we may assume the fairly constant prevalence of deadly infectious diseases, indeed, they seem to have been almost ubiquitous in the past. They were just as effective in limiting the life expectancy of humans who had survived the extreme risks of birth and early childhood as were wars, natural disasters, economic crises, bad harvests and famine. The list is long: tuberculosis, typhus, pneumonia, malaria, syphilis and many another servant of the Grim Reaper. In the nineteenth century, we find, along with the White Death of tuberculosis, which was primarily a disease of the urban proletariat, cholera as the great leveller, the hitherto unknown sickness from the East, the Asiatic Hydra, a monster that befell Western Europe in 1832, swallowing millions of lives. The first wave ebbed away, but individual centres flared up repeatedly, until the Hamburg cholera catastrophe of 1892. In 1869, the German journalist Karl Gutzkow (1811–1878) recalled listening to the Berlin lectures of the philosopher Georg Wilhelm Friedrich Hegel (1770–1831) and the outbreak of 1832, which he barely survived:

> Cholera, 'the Asian visitor' as it was known, the 'pest', as it was called from the pulpits, came to Europe for the first time. It was the very image of horror for humanity. It seemed to come riding, on a worn-out Cossack nag, holding the seven plagues as a seven-headed cudgel in its hand, this Asiatic poisoner, throwing the germ of death into every well, every stream, every bit of food. A haggard, pale creature with tousled hair—filth on her clothing —the personified—emesis! (Eckart 2011).

When, in 1911, news came of the plague breaking out in China again, the horror of the pest of past centuries was already fading. Death, the Grim Reaper whirling about the Manchurian steppe in the Far East, did cause some surprise and horror in Europe, but it had lost much of its potency.

1.2 Socio-Biological Transitional Phenomena

Two socio-biological phenomena, however, were to have a decisive influence on the clearly measurable and both epidemiologically and popularly growing perception of cancer and neoplastic illnesses on the spectrum of chronic and degenerative diseases. It was only in the last decades of the twentieth century that historians of society and culture identified these epidemiological and demographic transitions, thanks to the French Annales school. What exactly are these transitions, changes into other epidemiological paradigms? How have they affected the prevalence and perception of cancer?

Let us start with the epidemiological transition. This describes chronological changes in the frequency of illnesses and causes of death in a particular society, and in their dependence on changing sociocultural determinants (economy, wars, climate, nutrition, habitual phenomena, etc.). Thus, from the end of the eighteenth century until the beginning of the twentieth, we observe a change in the frequency of certain illnesses, or in causes of death within large populations in modern states. This change in the structure of morbidity is characterized by the replacement of infectious diseases by chronic-degenerative illnesses as the most frequent cause of death. With the decline of infectious diseases, the chronic-degenerative illnesses become more visible again in the coordinate system of epidemiologists, even though the absolute numbers of these illnesses did not increase. But these numbers, too, are subject to long-term changes, such as industrial methods of production and the associated increased exposure to pollutants. Hans Christian Andersen's (1805–1875) *Little Match Girl* (1845) died as a result of the early capitalist truck system, because she had to live by selling the quantity of matches assigned to her, out in the ice and snow, and she froze to death.

At the same time, chronic-degenerative diseases, such as silicosis, lung cancer and cancer through arsenic exposure, were on the increase, owing to exposure to toxic pollutants. Habitual changes are also relevant, that is, changes in living habits caused by industrialization and urbanization, and deviance through poverty: for example, the increase in liver degeneration and cancer of the liver was caused, at least in part, by cheap industrial alcohol (think of absinthe addiction), with many a worker substituting a cheap flask of brandy or gin for their midday bread.

The demographic transition was closely associated with the epidemiological one. The decisive results of the epidemiological transition can be seen mainly in the increase in average life expectancy of the members of observed groups or societies. The epidemiological transition is a process that can constantly be observed, since it is precisely these changes in average life expectancy that cause changes in population structure (with reference to age), and consequently a change in disease patterns. This process not only had a decisive influence on the increased perception of chronic-degenerative diseases, including malignant neoplasms, it also affected the absolute increase in such illnesses in a population growing ever older. Longer lives means higher rates of survival, which conditions the effect of such neoplasmic illnesses as cancer of the prostate or colon, which have not yet developed at a younger age, or at least have not yet appeared in a pathophenomenological sense.

The ideal curve of population development shows how, right up to the present day, this has continually changed in parallel with the epidemiological phenomena of transition. Decreasing mortality and the increase in life expectancy associated with this are mutually dependent. I will not go into the role of decreasing birth rates here, because this extremely complex aspect would distract from my argument. If we examine these phenomena of epidemiological and demographic transition with reference to the German Empire, taking the examples of mortality rates in cases of infectious diseases and cancers, it will become clear how these processes continually operate in individual societies of great industrial and urban complexity, albeit slowly and with disturbances to their course. How fast such transitional phenomena occur in detail, for example, changes in living habits, can be shown by looking at the changes in mortality rates for bronchial carcinoma in the years from 1950 to 2010. Here it becomes clear how significant changes in consumption of cancer-causing agents in association with gender express the gender bias in the epidemiological transition, something that has been neglected for too long.

Using these kinds of graphics and numbers, the rise of the *Emperor of All Maladies*, to return to the title of Siddhartha Mukherjee's book, can be clearly seen from about 1900, although only from the limited perspective of the developed countries. Something that Mukherjee does not deal with is the relativity of such findings, which is immediately apparent from a glance at the rest of the chronic-degenerative diseases, which have profited just as much from the demographic transition as has cancer. The skewed relations become even clearer if we take the global perspective into consideration as it appeared around 1900, but is now dramatically showing itself at the beginning of the twenty-first century in the course of a process *à la longue durée*, because we now have the corresponding numerical and statistical material to hand.

The image presented by Siddhartha Mukherjee of cancer as *Emperor of All Maladies* now changes very dramatically indeed. The case of the Federal Republic of Germany alone clearly shows cancer in the form of bronchial carcinoma in fourth place on the spectrum of causes of death in 2007; in 2008, it is in seventh place globally. It also becomes clear that infectious diseases in highly developed countries such as Germany no longer play any role in the upper echelons of the mortality spectrum, but from a global perspective they play a considerable role. This is especially clear when one also considers the role of infectious diseases in rather camouflaged designations such as 'bronchial diseases'. The entire global picture of the demographic transition has also been strongly distorted over the past few decades by the dramatic processes of industrialization and adaptation in countries such as China and India. The true killers and 'emperors of maladies' in the less developed nations are still the infectious diseases resulting from poverty and distributional problems, and not cancer.

But what has taken the place of the old monster, plague, in the form of Death trampling down and harvesting people? Was this epidemiological transition which we have just discussed from the historian's point of view perceived at all in its time, or is it just a phenomenon of historiography, not perceived in history itself? Not at all, as a brief look at the year 1900 shows. Let us imagine we are unnoticed onlookers in the conference hall of the Prussian Ministry of Culture. It is 6 p.m. on Sunday, 18 February. The dying rays of the sun are filtering through the windows of the hall. There is a last murmuring and coughing, then stillness. Ernst von Leyden (1832–1910), the great internist, director of the first Medical Clinic of the Charité Hospital in Berlin, is speaking. Just a few hours before, he has founded the first German Committee for Cancer Research. "The result, then", says the internist, "is that cancer is on its way to becoming an endemic disease, affecting all classes … May we hope to create a cure by working together? Such a hope must be negated from the start, for this task is insoluble at this time. But what we have succeeded in doing in the case of other illnesses, to find some prophylaxis by studying their spread, their causes, and their morbidity, that does lie within the bounds of the possible." (Eckart 2000).

1.3   Cancer Research and Propaganda in National Socialist Germany

Cancer research occupied an outstanding position during the period of Nazi rule (Eckart 2012, 2010: 219–240). This is also true of state research funding under the aegis of the German Research Council (GRC, in German DFG). While it had been something of a poor relation with regard to funding during the 1920 and early 1930, cancer research under the Nazi dictatorship advanced to first place among the research areas funded by the GRC. Repeated complaints of fragmentation in German cancer research, an area of medical research that had been weakened more than any other by the painfully tangible losses caused by the dismissal and exile of Jewish researchers, led to a unique centralization (*Reichsausschuss für Krebsbekämpfung* or Imperial Commission for Combatting Cancer) and financial support for cancer research in the years between 1936 and 1945. Cancer research became more or less the chief scientific activity in the medical research financed by the GRC.

The course of the war and the collapse of the Nazi dictatorship, but also the over-ambitious expectations and hopes of a centralized state cancer research programme led to the failure of the Imperial Commission. The Munich pathologist and president of the Imperial Commission for Combatting Cancer, Maximilian Borst (1869–1946), was called in. In close cooperation with the GRC, Borst developed an ambitious research programme. It was thought that this programme, certainly unique internationally at the time in its application of centralized research guidance and funding, could be realized by combining efforts in several disciplines, and supra-regional research groups were set up and working teams assigned to them to deal with the centre in the 'struggle against cancer'. Berlin had to "become a centre of this struggle", Minister of Propaganda Joseph Goebbels (1897–1945) wrote in the *Völkischer Beobachter*. In January 1939, the party newspaper printed an extensive interview with Maximilian Borst on the subject of "Cancer—the world's enemy number one", in which "Germany's leading authority in the matter of combatting cancer" explained in black-and-white terms the health care policy of the cancer research programme, which had been set up in "close cooperation with the Reich Propaganda Ministry (Dr Thomalla, Ministry Director Gutterer)" and the *Reichsärzteführung* (the Nazi state doctors' organization).

The clear effort to attain parity with the international 'modern' state of cancer research is striking. New fields of research were being more strongly considered even in Germany, such as papilloma virus research, emphasized particularly in the US in the 1930 (Borst, Haagen, Seeger), research into the influence of sex hormones in carcinogenesis (Druckrey, Heubner) or research into the chemistry of growth substances and carcinogenic substances (Wieland, Butenandt, Kaufmann).

A cancer 'training programme', ideologically part of Nazi health guidance, but financially part of the cancer programme funding, was planned for the leading medical associations in the hope that broader patient education could be achieved. "Although this is not a research task, it should be the job of the leading men in cancer research to enforce this training in the medical associations. We should also remember to have the National Socialist associations, such as the Women's Association, the SA, the SD, and so forth to help in educating patients." The cancer research programme was accompanied by flamboyant articles in the *Völkischer Beobachter*, which used the occasion of a visit by Goebbels to the Virchow Hospital in Berlin on 24 November 1938 to point to "the provision of a large sum of money for researching the disease of cancer".

The readers of the *Völkischer Beobachter* were, of course, not informed of the internal difficulties besetting the ambitious cancer programmes of the GRC and the Reich Research Council. Conflicts occurred repeatedly, and within the framework of Nazi cancer research, particular significance was certainly attached to the carcinogenic effects of tobacco consumption. It may be doubted that any real success was attained here, however. "The Führer does not drink alcohol and does not smoke", Baldur von Schirach (1907–1974), head of the Hitler Youth from 1931 to 1940, told the German people, with an admonishing forefinger, as it were, in his biographical propaganda work of 1932, *Hitler, wie ihn keiner kennt* (*Hitler as nobody knows him*), intended to do battle with alcohol and tobacco abuse. The 'chosen people', however, were recalcitrant and not only smoked away the equivalent of several KdF (Volkswagen) cars every day, but also damaged their lungs and circulatory systems in ways that seemed to belie their 'chosen' status. Indeed, the fact that even the SA[1] contributed to this vice with sponsored cigarette brands such as Alarm, Trommler or Sturm was doubtless counterproductive.

---

[1]The Sturmabteilung (SA; German Abbreviation; literally "Storm Detachment", was the Nazi Party's original paramilitary wing. It played a significant role in Adolf Hitler's rise to power in the 1920s and 1930s. Its main purposes were providing protection for Nazi rallies and assemblies; disrupting the meetings of opposing political parties; fighting against the paramilitary units of opposing parties, especially the „Roter Frontkämpferbund" of the German Communist Party (KPD).

At least the Nazi anti-smoking campaign was backed up by scientific research results that proved the connection between smoking and lung cancer for the first time (Franz Hermann Müller), even identifying so-called passive smoking as carcinogenic. The aggressive poster and newspaper campaign against all types of tobacco consumption initiated from 1939 could not really be avoided, at least in the pre-war period, by any *Volksgenosse* (a citizen in the jargon of Nazism). Entire universities (Jena, for instance) were radically declared to be smoke-free institutions —after all, by this time they had had plenty of practice excluding entire groups of persons—and non-smoking sections were established in the German Reichsbahn trains, in public buildings, post offices and party bureaus; the drastic increase in tobacco taxes had the same intention. But measurable successes were lacking; and especially after 1939 the proportion of smokers among men continued to rise.

To refuse tobacco rations to soldiers at war would have been so unpopular that the regime hesitated to carry out such a step. As for women ("German women do not smoke!"), tobacco consumption had dropped, but whether this was owing to the campaign or more to the dramatically worsening war economy is unclear. Another question that needs clarification is whether this propaganda was really produced under the aegis of the Nazi dictatorship and whether 'good' science was actually practised in successful cancer research. The struggle against cancer, in particular cancer caused by smoking, after all, also served the long-term purpose of creating a Utopia of a racially hygienic *Volk*, as did most of the health campaigns of the regime; it was all about protecting this *Volk* from pollution and contamination by luxuries such as tobacco, the vices of 'inferior races'. The toxic effects of smoking and drinking, or of carcinogenic substances in the world of work (asbestos, mercury, lead, arsenic) were set alongside other 'racially destructive' foreign bodies, Jews, gypsies, homosexuals, 'antisocial elements' and the mentally ill. Social responsibility had no part in the anti-smoking campaigns of the Nazi regime.

Of course, it must be conceded that cancer research under National Socialism— for reasons of both research strategy and ideology with regard to the health of the 'ethnic body'—experienced enormous advancements and is an example of the state funding of this period. In the end, however, the course of the war and the collapse of the Nazi dictatorship, together with exaggerated expectations of what centralized state cancer research could accomplish, led to the collapse of the Imperial Commission for Combatting Cancer.

1.4 Noticing Cancer in the Cold War

Doubtless the anti-smoking campaign of the Nazis, expressly orientated towards cancer prevention, brought cancer into the public consciousness in a way that no other measure had ever done. Was this a typically German thing? Hardly—the march of chronic-degenerative diseases deserves to be called international from the 1930 onwards, as shown by an American poster of the early 1930. Cancer was not only marching forward within international research on its genesis, aetiology, therapy and epidemiology, but also in public consciousness worldwide. The military term 'marching', which I have deliberately chosen, was to have a critical influence on the perception of cancer in the decades following Hiroshima and Nagasaki. Metaphors of battle had been used primarily for infectious diseases and for great epidemics and plagues since the nineteenth century. But their main representatives had disappeared, at least in the developed countries of the Northern hemisphere, from people's consciousness.

Naturally, the classical great plagues had not disappeared entirely from the world —they are still with us!—but they did not signify any longer in the consciousness of people in Europe and North America, with the possible exception of the Asian flu in 1957 and 1958 and the Hong Kong flu between 1968 and 1970, each of which claimed some two million lives. On the contrary, quite different things were now present in the consciousness of people, things that had come about after the two great hot wars and had to do with war, but this time a cold war—the war that was anticipated but had to be prevented through fear of it, between the communist bloc led by the Soviet Union on one side, and the Western allies led by the US, on the other. A central aspect of this period of world history was the build-up of nuclear weapons, together with the euphoric feeling of a new paradise offered by nuclear energy. It is not surprising, then, that in the public perception, the metaphorical transition of military battlefield terminology from infectious diseases to cancer should also be conditioned by images of the Nuclear or Atomic Age.

Atomic bombs and atomic artillery showed up in picture form nearly every week in the press. Their opposites in this time of technological threat were the technical and euphemistic images of 'good' bombs and artillery in the fight against cancer. But the old metaphors of degeneration were still there in the minds of the reading public—particularly the German reading public—so the Cologne *Stadtrundschau* headlines in the year 1952 hit the nail on the head as far as this public was concerned: "The 'Radium Cannon' Against Degenerated Tissue". In 1964, the new 'cobalt bomb' was introduced, and at the same time a 'cannon of humanity' could be presented at the Cologne University Clinic. The highly mechanized irradiation of cancer between the 1950 and 1970 is at the same time both an expression of the quest for the perfect symbiosis of machine and man—just as in early space exploration, taking place at this time, and in cybernetics and robotics—and an expression of the attempted balance of nuclear energy and nuclear war. Both were signs of the times and strongly influenced the optimistic perception of a new weapon in the fight against the world's enemy, cancer.

However, in the US the boom in complex technical irradiation against cancer had already begun in the 1930. This was due as much to a widespread celebration of technology and its possibilities as to a widespread desire for new technomorphic ways to treat cancer using X-rays and radioactive materials, as well as the trend towards modernity, which had received strong impulses (pun intended) from the enthusiasm for electricity of the first half of the twentieth century. Thus, the series of high-voltage X-ray plants produced for treating cancer (Eckart and Bröer 1995), between 1 and finally 15 MV power, had started in the early 1930, following experimentation. German industry, in particular Siemens, AEG and the Hamburg enterprise C.H.F. Müller, had also become strongly involved. By 1955, the loss of personnel and resources to the war effort and reservations about cooperation on the part of the victorious power, the US, in the immediate post-war period had been overcome. Radium and cobalt cannons, betatrons, linear accelerators (Linacs) and telecobalt apparatus flooded Western markets. This development is ongoing, as exemplified by the presentation in October 2012 of a 670-tonne gantry in the German Cancer Research Centre (DKFZ) in Heidelberg.

1.5 Environmental Discourses

One final aspect that has probably significantly influenced public perception of cancer since the 1970 is the greatly increased environmental and anti-nuclear discourse. Public interest has been awakened in carcinogenic environmental poisons and excessive radioactive contamination. The triggers and amplifiers of this were especially the disasters.

Since the accident with dioxin in Seveso on 10 July 1976, the name of the Italian town has been synonymous with one of the greatest environmental catastrophes in Europe. The dioxin set free there and its oxidation products are carcinogenic, and since Seveso there has been almost continuous discussion of the carcinogenicity of dioxin. The new discourse of carcinogenic radioactive contamination of the civilian population by products of nuclear fission, which was important in the early phase of the Cold War, cannot now be separated from the catastrophe at Chernobyl on 26 April 1986. In the three countries hardest hit, expert testimony states that there will probably be some 9,000 additional fatal cancer and leukaemia cases owing to the increased exposure to radiation. For the whole of Europe, a conservative estimate is that there will be around 16,000 cases of thyroid cancer and some 25,000 other additional cancers by 2065. The radioisotope caesium 137, with a half-life of 30.17 years, is responsible. It will continue to contaminate our forest floors, and thus particularly wild mushrooms and wild pigs, for another 4–5 years (Bauer and Ho 2015). However that may be, Chernobyl's carcinogenicity had been somewhat forgotten, when, on 14 March 2011, Japan and the world were shaken by the Fukushima nuclear catastrophe. The emission of substances set free there was probably only 10–20% of that of Chernobyl, but the long-term effects cannot be estimated. It is clear, however, that Chernobyl and Fukushima together are going to increase the number of cases of cancer well into the hundreds of thousands, possibly even millions, over the next few decades.

1.6 Aids / Hiv

The increasing attention paid to cancer throughout the twentieth century seemed to have produced a result that apparently reversed the effects of the epidemiological transition for a few decades. In the early 1980, the appearance of AIDS and its triggering agent, the human immunodeficiency virus HIV, recalled the old plagues to the collective memory. A flood of fashionable publications bringing up the anxious and profitable question of whether the old plagues were returning had the publishers' cash registers ringing. The question can be answered just as rapidly as it was posed: the old plagues have never gone away, with the exception of smallpox. They have only been pushed out of the limelight, because changes in the spectrum of disease, dependant on the economic and cultural phases of development, occur with as much variation as this development itself. In the long-term view, the epidemiological transition cannot be reversed globally, unless some catastrophe were to set us back to the conditions of past centuries. This means that chronic-degenerative diseases, including cancer, will continue to attract increasing public attention if they are addressed by the media. Nonetheless, global development medicine must continue to look primarily at diseases in connection with resource availability, and these are basically dietary and infectious illnesses. It is water and nutritional security, the improvement of working and reproductive conditions, birth control, and the containment of local and regional epidemics that are in the front line here, not the fight against cancer.

1.7 Individual Medicine and Predictive Medicine

The catchphrase for the newest development in medicine is *individual medicine* (synonyms: personalized, stratified, tailored medicine). *Predictive medicine* is a part of this individualized medicine. All of this, in turn, is part of a broader development which might best be described by the concept of precision medicine. The approaches named are based primarily on the realization that individuals have quite different risks of falling ill, that there are also various different sub-groups of comparable diseases, and that medications or other treatments can have quite different effects in different patients. These approaches also have in common that individual differences in the genetic patterns (variations of the DNA sequences) of the patients are to be taken more into consideration when choosing a treatment than has hitherto been the case. Against this background, sub-groups of patients can be identified and given more exact prognoses and therapeutic interventions.

This is especially true of the area of carcinomas. Clinical research currently assumes that, with around 500,000 new cancer diagnoses annually in Germany, a reasonable concept can be developed in this personalized medicine for almost one in ten patients, independently of tumour type. In this way, a therapeutic concept that is significantly more exact than the average can be developed. The aim of individualized medicine, then, is the precise, optimized treatment of defined patient groups. Among its current core areas are: predictive genetic diagnostics, individual pharmacogenetics, prognosis of tumour course based on molecular biology, and the adaptation of strategies of treatment and medicines to the molecularly or genetically determined subtype of a disease, e.g., a tumour illness. The moral challenge for society lies in providing goal-orientated financing and so making the advantages of individual precision medicine accessible to the largest possible number of patients.

1.8 Self-Help and Cancer

In the Federal Republic of Germany, self-help groups began to develop in the late 1960 in connection with various emancipatory movements. These groups—voluntary, self-organized associations of the people concerned or their relatives, who work on social or health problems—have appeared in the most varied areas: psychological-therapeutic self-help groups, medical self-help groups, self-help groups for the expansion of consciousness, life organization groups, work-orientated groups, self-help study groups in the educational sector, citizens' initiatives, and so on.

Self-help groups in the area of health are special only as regards their goals, not in principle. According to the fundamental precepts of compulsory health insurance (CHI) umbrella organizations, these groups are[2]:

> [V]oluntary associations of people on a supra-regional basis, whose activities are directed toward the combined effort to overcome diseases or psychological problems or both, that affect the people concerned or their relatives. Their goal is to change their personal circumstances of life, and often to attempt to influence their social and political surroundings. In regular, usually weekly, meetings they emphasise equality, shared discussions, and mutual help. The goals of self-help groups are orientated primarily toward their members. In this way, they are different to other forms of 'civil action'.

The self-help group movement has undoubtedly now become international, but its character has changed. Its civil and social habitus has been replaced by forms of a fashionable, collective subculture which has been arriving in Europe since the end of the twentieth century, with enormous acculturative pressure, from the US. A weak, yet telling indicator is the market for self-help books, as a recent contribution to the US self-help culture states:

> In the final third of the twentieth century, 'the tremendous growth in self-help publishing … in self-improvement culture' really took off—something which must be linked to post-modernism itself—to the way 'postmodern subjectivity constructs self-reflexive subjects-in-process.' Arguably at least, 'in the literatures of self-improvement … that crisis of subjecthood is not articulated but enacted—demonstrated in ever-expanding self-help book sales'. (McGee 2012: 188; Eckart 2005: 448–452).

It is obvious that massive economic interests lie behind this individual phenomenon. In 2006 alone, the turnover of the US 'self-improvement market' was around US$9.6 billion. Self-help as an element of a 'self-improvement culture', the discovery of 'autonomous self-existence', are positively valued phenomena in our

---

[2]The German Health Care System (=https://www.bundesgesundheitsministerium.de/fileadmin/Dateien/5_Publikationen/Gesundheit/Broschueren/200629_BMG_Das_deutsche_Gesundheitssystem_EN.pdf, 12 March 2021).

culture, but they also stand for depoliticization and replace social subsidiarity and responsibility with a group-subjective welfare that, in the end, aims at individual help, serving that autonomous 'self'. The state has withdrawn from its role as direct welfare instance, if it ever was such. It does appear again in the form of the German Parity Association for Social Welfare and Charity (*Deutscher Paritätischer Wohlfahrtsverband*), which claims the privilege of officially benefiting the public (a legal status in Germany), and finances itself not only through voluntary contributions, but also from compulsory contributions to health insurance and from other public funds.

Of course, it is true that the combination of expert knowledge, individual experience, mutual support and information on everyday coping strategies, together with increased sensitivity to one's own health, makes self-help in the healthcare system quite interesting, for various reasons, not least economic ones. In hospital care, this is true of the increasing cooperation between self-help groups and privatized hospitals. In the health market, this is particularly true of the explosion of dietary supplements para-relevant to health—from vitamin tablets through green tea extracts to polyphenol-rich red wine from the Madiran region, especially popular among patients with cancer of the prostate (generally men who like to drink red wine in any case).

Cancer self-help groups are now coordinated by the *Haus der Krebs-Selbsthilfe* (House of Cancer Self-Help) in Bonn. This institution, which has rapidly become the central seat of leading public benefit aid organizations, is dedicated to supporting cancer patients with various forms of the disease across the country. The *Stiftung Deutsche Krebshilfe* (Foundation for German Cancer Aid), with an income in 2007 of €100.4 million, furthers these self-help initiatives so as to constantly improve the network of support for cancer patients in Germany. Since 2013 this institution has comprised nine supra-regional associations. Project coordination expenditure financed from contributions amounted to €55,250 in 2015.

1.9   Conclusion

This chapter has looked at the long history of the perception of cancer, which has continued to change over the years. This constitutes a new research area for historians of medicine. Some aspects force themselves on us, bringing us back to Siddhartha Mukherjee's book *The Emperor of All Maladies*. Cancer is probably as old as the world of plants and animals itself, thus as old as, indeed older than, humanity. In our mass perception, however, it has played an increasing role among the chronic-degenerative diseases only since the start of the twentieth century, initially as a result of the epidemiological and demographic transition. While comparative studies of countries and systems are needed, the German example successfully shows how, in the 1930 and early 1940, state health propaganda took up this change in the disease spectrum and—under the sign of dictatorship—moved towards effective political anti-cancer agitation. Public interest, recognizable primarily in the literary topos of cancer, was drawn away from the old external enemy, the great popular plagues that were seeing initial therapeutic successes (tuberculosis, syphilis, small-pox), and increasingly towards the internal enemy, the 'degenerate' tissues of cancer. In parallel with the epidemiological and demographic transitions, a metaphorical transition took place, especially with regard to militarism in language. The tumour illnesses were declared the new 'world enemy', despite the continuing dominance of other, non-carcinomous chronic-degenerative pathophenomena.

This process was amplified by the changes and technological euphoria of the Cold War, in which images of a destructive, yet simultaneously hope-bearing nuclear technology began to resemble, and to an extent, overlap each other. Research has hitherto paid little attention to this cultural and historical process of change, which appears crucial for the presence of cancer perception and the hopes of a cure from the close symbiosis of man and machine. The same is true of the attention being paid to environmentally conditioned tumour illnesses, influenced since the 1970 by the ecological and anti-nuclear movements and by dramatic environmental and natural disasters. For a short time in the 1980, the explosive appearance of the new pandemic AIDS/HIV seemed to have revised or even reversed perspectives on the spectrum of disease. However, this baseless supposition of a change in perspective does not appear to have been very permanent.

References

Bauer AW, Ho AD (2015) Tschernobyl 1986—Katastrophenhilfe als Mittel der Entspan-nungspolitik. Wie Knochenmarktransplantationen durch amerikanische Hämatologen zur Annäherung zwischen Ost und West beitrugen. Medizinhistorische Mitteilungen 34:195–209

Eckart WU, Bröer R (1995) Die Behandlung des Brustkrebses — Aspekte der Therapiegeschichte von der Antike bis ins 20. Jahrhundert. Eine Ausstellung anlässlich der Festveranstaltung 100 Jahre Endokrine Therapie des Mammakarzinoms, Heidelberg, Juni 1995. Zeneka, Plankstadt

Eckart WU (ed) (2000) 100 years of organized cancer research—100 Jahre organisierte Krebsforschung. Thieme, Stuttgart

Eckart WU (2005) Krebs. In: Steger F (ed) Jagow Bv. Literatur und Medizin. Ein Lexikon. Vandenhoeck & Ruprecht, Göttingen, pp 448–452

Eckart WU (2010) Instrumentelle Modernität und das Diktat der Politik: Medizinische Forschungsförderung durch die Notgemeinschaft/Deutsche Forschungsgemeinschaft 1920–1970. In: Orth K, Oberkrome W (eds) Die Deutsche Forschungsgemeinschaft 1920–1970. Forschungsförderung im Spannungsfeld von Wissenschaft und Politik (= Beiträge zur Geschichte der Deutschen Forschungsgemeinschaft, 4). Steiner, Stuttgart, pp. 219—240

Eckart WU (2011) Illustrierte Geschichte der Medizin—Von der französischen Revolution bis zur Gegenwart, 2nd edn. Springer, Berlin

Eckart WU (2012) Medizin in der NS-Diktatur—Ideologie, Praxis. Folgen, Böhlau, Köln, Wien

McGee M (2012) Self-Help. In: Makeover culture in American Life. Oxford Scholarship Online, May 2012. https://doi.org/10.1093/acp%DCrof:os0/9780195171242.001.0001, p 188

Mukherjee S (2011) The emperor of all Maladies. A Biography of Cancer, Fourth Estate, London

One in Four Dies of Cancer. Questions About the Epidemiology of Malignant Tumours

2

Christel Weiss

2.1 Introduction

Some years ago, in 2000, the former city mayor of New York Rudolph M. Giuliani underwent treatment for his prostate cancer. After having been cured he stated: "My chance of surviving prostate cancer—and thank God, I was cured of it—in the United States? Eighty-two per cent. My chance of surviving prostate cancer in England? Only 44 per cent under socialized medicine" (Dobbs 2007). Trusting these numbers, Giuliani's chances of surviving seemed to be nearly twice as high in the United States as in England.

Most definitely, Giuliani intended to claim that health care in the USA was superior to health care in Great Britain. In 2000, when Giuliani became ill, according to the National Cancer Institute new cases of prostate cancer have been observed in about 180 out of 100,000 male citizens in the USA. In the same period, only 49 out of 100,000 British men were diagnosed with prostate cancer. 28 of them died within five years (Gigerenzer et al. 2008). Actually, this means a 5-year-survival rate of only 21/49 = 43% (perhaps Giuliani made a slight calculation error when stating 44% instead of 43%, but this was not the biggest one).

Yet this comparison is meaningless because the populations in the USA and in England differ dramatically in how the cancer diagnosis has been made. In the USA, prostate screening using prostate-specific antigens (PSA) had been introduced some years before Giuliani suffered from his cancer. Therefore, most prostate cancers under US American men had been detected by screening. In contrast, in England most prostate cancers were discovered through clinical symptoms. The mortality rates however that relate to the total population of men are about the

C. Weiss (✉)
Medical Statistics and Biomathematics, Medical Faculty Mannheim,
Heidelberg University, Theodor-Kutzer-Ufer 1-3, 68167 Mannheim, Germany
e-mail: christel.weiss@medma.uni-heidelberg.de

© Springer Nature Switzerland AG 2021
A. W. Bauer et al. (eds.), *Ethical Challenges in Cancer Diagnosis and Therapy*,
Recent Results in Cancer Research 218,
https://doi.org/10.1007/978-3-030-63749-1_2

same: 26 prostate cancer deaths per 100,000 men in the USA versus 27 in Britain (Shibata and Whittemore 2001). Therefore, the screening program in the USA does not seem to offer any major advantages.

This example very clearly demonstrates, how non-transparent framing of information creates misunderstandings and confusions which may lead to serious consequences for health—for individuals as well as for a total population.

2.2 Diagnostic and Screening Tests

2.2.1 Characteristics

Diagnostic and screening tests are done in order to obtain information concerning the health status of an individual. The indications for ordering such a test are mainly (1) to establish a diagnosis in a patient with clinical symptoms, i.e. by performing a mammogram on a woman with a palpable breast mass or (2) to screen for a certain disease in asymptotic people, i.e. a PSA test (prostate-specific antigen) in an apparently healthy man. In both situations, a positive test result usually leads to a change of clinical strategy and mostly to the initiation of a therapy, i.e. to a prostatectomy following a positive test result for PSA. In contrast, a negative test result implies that the relevant disease may be ruled out.

There are several ways of quantifying the usefulness of a diagnostic test. Most important is the diagnostic accuracy: The test should be able to discriminate between sick and healthy people. To assess the accuracy, the test results have to be compared with a so-called gold standard—a diagnostic procedure which (at least theoretically) is 100% accurate and defines correctly the presence or absence of the disease for each individual. Typical gold standards are surgical or pathological specimen, blood culture for bacteremia or X-rays. The diagnostic test compared to the gold standard is less accurate, but easier to perform, safer or cheaper.

The probability that people with the disease get a positive test result is the **sensitivity**, whereas the percentage of healthy people who are correctly categorized as negative is called the **specificity**. These are essential criteria as they quantify the goodness of the test. Therefore, in studies of diagnostic tests or screenings these characteristics (or derived measures such as likelihood ratios or odds) are most often reported. Ideally, both values should be close to 100%.

False positive findings (positive test results for individuals who actually do not suffer from the disease) mostly have a deleterious effect. They may lead to severe psychological stress and to an overtreatment which is unnecessary, bothersome and costly. On the other hand, false negative results which occur when an existing disease remains undetected may lull the patient into a deceptive sense of safety. Valuable time may pass without treatment or, in the case of infectious diseases, time in which other people can be infected. Thus, false test results—whether positive or negative—should be avoided as far as possible. However, in nearly all circumstances the probability to obtain a false result is more than 0. This means that a doctor cannot trust the result of a diagnostic test by 100%. Instead, he has to consider that a given test result could be wrong.

Diagnostic tests or screenings are instruments that provide a basis for revising disease probabilities. A clinician and his patient are interested in how they can rely upon a diagnostic finding. When a patient is confronted with a positive finding: What is the likelihood that the disease is really present? In the case of a negative result: What is the probability that the tested person is healthy? **Predictive values** quantify the extent to which a test result predicts the presence or absence of a disease, respectively. In clinical practice, these probabilities are even more important than sensitivity and specificity.

The positive predictive value is the proportion of patients with the disease among all those people with a positive test result. This value depends considerably on the prevalence, that is the probability of the presence of the disease. These associations will be illustrated by means of mammography as an example. Firstly, we consider a high-risk population with a given prevalence of 10%. Assuming a sensitivity of 90% and a specificity of 95% and a population of 10,000 participating women we expect the frequencies presented in Table 2.1 (left side). It is easy to estimate the positive predictive value in this group as 900 / 1,350 = 66.7%.

Accordingly, the negative predictive value is the proportion of tested individuals without the disease among all negative test results. In our example, the negative predictive value is estimated as 8,550 / 8,650 = 98.8%. This means: a negative test result is highly reliable indicating that the tested woman has no carcinoma. A positive test result however cannot be considered as a trustworthy diagnosis. In only two of three positive findings, a carcinoma is present.

The situation is quite different in a group of women undergoing mammography screening. Under these circumstances, only four of thousand women are assumed to have a carcinoma which is equivalent to a prevalence of 0.4% (Kerlikowske 1997). Given a sensitivity of 90% and a specificity of 95% (as mentioned above), we expect 36 correct positive and 498 false positive test results for 10,000 participants which yields to a positive predictive value of only 36/534 = 6.7%. Obviously, the majority of positive findings (14 out of 15) are incorrect. In the case of a negative finding, however, you can rely with a very high probability that a carcinoma can be ruled out.

Table 2.1 Expected frequencies for mammography testing assuming a sensitivity of 90%, a specificity of 95% and a prevalence of 10% (left side) or 0.4% (right side), respectively

	With cancer	without cancer	Total		With cancer	without cancer	total
Positive result	900	450	1,350	Positive result	36	498	534
Negative result	100	8,550	8,650	Negative result	4	9,462	9,466
	1,000	9,000	10,000		40	9,960	10,000

Many patients and doctors alike are not aware that the predictive value of a diagnostic test depends on the prevalence. They confuse "sensitivity" with "positive predictive value" and think that—given a sensitivity of 90%—a positive test result is correct with 90%. Analogously, they confuse "specificity" with "negative predictive value". However, this way of thinking is incorrect and misleading.

It is a misconception assuming that a positive test result is synonymous to "disease present" or that a negative result equals "tested person is healthy". More than that, it is unreasonable to believe that high values for sensitivity and specificity guarantee reliable test results. In the case of low prevalence, as is common in screenings, the positive predictive value may be rather low whereas in a risk group with a fairly high prevalence one can rather rely on a positive test result. This fact is quite important to be considered when interpreting a test result.

2.2.2 Pitfalls and Bias

In the previous section, it has been shown that it may be challenging to draw an appropriate conclusion from a positive test result, especially in screenings where prevalence is low. In this special situation, a clinician should know if the person being tested belongs to a certain risk group and—if applicable—which prevalence may be assumed. As this fact is not commonly known, benefits of screening processes often are overestimated. Furthermore, bias occurring in studies of screening tests may contribute to this overestimation. Several selection and information biases are typical when investigating screening outcomes.

Lead time bias is an information bias which is caused by the early detection of tumours in screenings before clinical symptoms appear. This procedure advances the time of diagnosis and thus pretends a longer survival time for the screened patients compared to a controlled group without screening. The "lead time" is defined as the interval between diagnosis by screening and the appearance of clinical symptoms. However, longer survival time does not mean longer life! Lead time does not affect date of death. Hence, early detection is of no relevant benefit, if no effective therapy is available. Quite the opposite may happen: When lead time is spent for inefficient interventions, this could be (because of side effects) very uncomfortable for the patient. Individuals in the screening group know of their disease some time longer. The total life span however is the same, with or without screening. When defining the survival time as the period between time of diagnosis and patient's death, it is not fair to compare the survival times of the screening group with those of a control group whose participants have not been screened: It may be assumed that in the control group the survival times are much shorter because the diagnosis is made later. Thus, lead time bias in clinical studies tends to an overoptimistic evaluation of the screening's benefit.

Another information bias, the **length time bias**, is associated with the fact that mainly slow-growing tumours are detected by screening. A less aggressive form of a cancer usually has a longer asymptotic phase than an aggressive tumour and thus a larger chance to be detected trough screening. On the other hand, a slow-growing tumour has a more favorable prognosis than a fast growing one: Affected patients are more likely to be cured and may live a long time after screening until they die of other reasons. Patients in the control group however only become visible through clinical symptoms: Many of them have aggressive cancers and die shortly after diagnosis. Thus, length time bias may lead to the perception that screening leads to better outcomes regarding the survival rates.

Overdiagnosis can be regarded as the most extreme form of a length time bias. It is associated with the detection of an insignificant disease where actually no treatment is needed. Part of this bias is caused by technological progress which leads to more sensitive screening skills which result in the detection of cancers that will never progress and will never affect the patient's lifetime. Consequences of this bias may be unnecessary treatment (i.e. surgery, other invasive treatments, radiation therapy or chemotherapy), anxiety and harm to the screening participants as well as high costs in health care. Overdiagnosis should not be confused with a false positive detection. With an overdiagnosis, a cancer is diagnosed correctly (even if it harmless for the patient), whereas a false positive test result is regarded as an abnormality which does not meet the pathologic definition of a cancer.

Furthermore, in observation studies **selection bias** must be feared because of baseline imbalances, i.e. when two populations are compared under different framework conditions. One special type is the **volunteer bias** (or self-selection bias) which may be inherent in a study where a group of individuals participating in a screening program is compared with a control group whose subjects are recruited from the general population which does not undergo screening. However, there is cause for concern that the volunteers tend to be healthier, to have a higher socio-economic status or to be more compliant with therapy. Thus, the spectrum of disease may be different in both groups and better outcomes in the screening group are not necessarily concerning the screening's benefits. Other types of biases are the **performance bias** and the **detection bias**, which arise from differences in the care of groups being compared or from systematically different measurements of the outcomes, respectively. Each of these biases makes it impossible to conclude that one program is more or less effective than the other one.

An unknown bias may rise to a major problem, because a biased study loses validity. **How to deal with biases?** Selection bias may be prevented by a randomized trial because this study design ensures a similar spectrum of disease in screened and unscreened patients. Hence, in order to judge the clinical relevance of a study, it should be paid attention how subjects have been recruited. Given a non-randomized design, conclusions must be drawn in a very careful way. On the other hand, randomized studies where subjects are randomly attributed into the screening or no-screening group are not easy to conduct because of ethical and organizational reasons.

Lead time and length time biases are inherent to screenings and cannot be completely avoided by randomization. They may lead to an overestimation of survival time or survival rate of the screening group which then erroneously are regarded as a screening benefit. Researchers, authors and readers of relevant publications should know that it is likely to occur when discussing or interpreting the results.

2.3 Morbidity and Mortality

2.3.1 Measures of Risk

A risk is simply defined as the probability of the occurrence of an undesired event (i.e. disease or death). Typical risks in clinical or epidemiological research are the incidence (rate of appearance of new cases over time), the mortality and the case fatality rate (number of cause-specific deaths over time related to a total population or to diseased people, respectively).

Assessing and comparing risks (done by an appropriate statistical analysis) make it possible to ensure the association between a specific factor and a relevant outcome (i.e. emergence of disease or death). In risk studies, for instance, the association between an etiological factor and a certain disease is investigated, whereas clinical trials or studies of screening tests deal with the benefits of a treatment or a screening intervention. How to assess these risks in a trial? Looking at a study population during a certain observation period (i.e. one year), we denote:

N size of the study population.
C number of patients diagnosed with a certain cancer (or another disease).
D number of patients who die due to this cancer.

These numbers allow to assess the following disease-specific risks:
    incidence:C / N.
    mortality: D / N.
    case fatality rate:D / C.

From these formulas, the following relationships can be derived:
    mortality = incidence · case fatality rate.
    case fatality rate = mortality / incidence.

The difference $(C–D)$ quantifies the number of patients diagnosed with cancer who survive until the end of the observation period. Thus, survival rate can be calculated as.
    survival rate:$(C–D) / C = 1$—case fatality rate.

It is important to note that mortality is related to the total size of the study population (N) which is independent from screening results. As the number of individuals who die during the observation period (D) can be determined exactly, also the mortality (D/N) can be estimated accurately. However, the number of patients with positive screening results (C) depends on the screening procedure. Thus, the case fatality rate as well as the survival rate may be affected by lead time or length time bias.

2.3.2   Comparing Risks

When comparing groups (i.e. persons who undergo screening with persons who do not), there are several options in reporting risks. The simplest one is just to present the absolute risks and the resulting difference.

This will be illustrated using an example of randomized clinical trials which evaluated the benefits of mammography screening (Kerlikowske 1997). About 500,000 women were involved in this trial, half of them underwent regular screening. For women aged 50 to 69 years, breast cancer-related mortality over 10 years revealed to be about 3 per mil in the screening group and 4 per mil in the control group. Obviously, the mortality rate is smaller in the screening group. On the other hand, this result emerges clearly that screening alone cannot prevent death by breast cancer.

The difference of the two risks is the **absolute risk reduction**, which is 1 per mil. What does this difference mean? The number of deaths in the no-screening group could be diminished by 1 per mil (from 4 to 3 per mil) if all members underwent screening. Another way of interpretation: In the no-screening group 1 from 4 per mil is attributable to the fact that women did not undergo screening. Therefore, the absolute risk difference is also called the **attributable risk**. Actually, this number is rather low and suggests, that the benefit of screening is not very high. However, it should be taken into account that also the basic risks are rather low. Even in the best case, the absolute risk reduction cannot be more than 4 per mil (if there were no breast cancer deaths in the screening group at all).

Another way of comparing the mortality rates is given by the **relative risk** which reveals to be $4/3 = 1.33$. From this number, it may be concluded that mortality in the no-screening group is about 33% higher than in the group with the screened women. Although numerically correct, the relative risk obscures the fact that the basic risks on their own are rather low.

The **relative risk reduction** is the absolute risk reduction in relation to the risk in the no-screening group. In the mammography study, it is assessed as $(4–3)/4$, which is 25 per cent. This means: The mortality rate in the no-screening group could be decreased by 25 per cent, if all women in this group changed their mind and underwent screening. In other words: one in four dies of cancer.

A convenient concept to estimate the effectiveness of screening is the **number needed to screen** (NNS). It quantifies the number of individuals to be screened in order to prevent exactly one cancer related death. The NNS is calculated as the reciprocal value of the absolute risk reduction. Thus, in the example above the NNS is about 1,000 indicating that one thousand women have to be screened regularly over a period of 10 years in order to reduce the number of breast cancer related deaths in one additional woman (4 will die without and 3 will die despite screening). The majority of women derive no utility from the screening procedure because they wouldn't die of breast cancer—neither with nor without screening. The NNS is a measure of efficacy which illustrates the effort which is required in attempting to save one life.

On the other hand, it has to be taken into consideration that lots of women who undergo screening regularly (every two years) will be burdened with at least one

Table 2.2 Comparing mortality rates (Kerlikowske 1997)

	Results determined	Best possible results
Absolute risk no-screening group	4 / 1000	4 / 1000
Absolute risk screening group	3 / 1000	0
Relative risk	1.33 (4/3)	Infinite (4/0)
Absolute risk reduction	0.001	0.004
Relative risk reduction	25%	100%
NNS	1,000	250

false positive test result. When women participate in a 10-year program of biennial mammography, the chances of false results multiply. Given a specificity of 95%, the probability to obtain five negative test results for a healthy woman can be assessed by $0{,}95^5$ which equals 77%. Thus, 23% of all women (nearly one in four) who never develop a breast cancer during ten years' observation time will have at least one false positive test result—compared to one of thousand women, who benefits.

In Table 2.2, risk measures are listed together with the values being expected under the best-case scenario (if screening could prevent each death of breast cancer). Even in this most optimistic case 250 women would be needed to prevent one woman from breast cancer-related death. Comparing the obtained results with the best optimistic results may help to judge the true benefit of a screening procedure.

The numbers presented in Table 2.2 can easily be calculated on the base of the absolute mortalities which are 3 and 4 per mil. Resulting from a large-scale randomized trial, they are objective and traceable. Nevertheless, the inherent information in these measures are somewhat different. Imagine a woman who refuses to be screened. Telling her "With mammography you can reduce your individual risk of dying of breast cancer in next ten years by 0.1 per cent" or "Perhaps you are the one out of thousand women who will profit by screening" might not convince her. Phrases like "Your individual risk of dying by breast cancer is 33% higher" or "Screening can reduce your personal risk by 25%" sound much more impressive. The 0.1% refers to the total population of women who do not undergo screening, whereas the 25% refer to the small subgroup of women who die of breast cancer without having been screened. Anyway, relative risks are likely to cause confusion! This is particularly important when the incidence of disease events or deaths is low.

2.4 Cancer Screening

2.4.1 Cancer Epidemiology

Despite the variety of cancer screening programs established worldwide, the number of global deaths due to cancer has increased form 5.7 million in 1990 up to 9.1 million in 2016 (Ritchie 2019). In Germany, 197,000 and 238,000 cancer-related deaths have been counted indicating an increase of more than 20% from 1990 to 2016. The leading cancer types in 2016 (referring to Germany) are tracheal, bronchus and lung cancer (47,000 deaths), followed by colon and rectum cancer (30,000) and breast cancer (19,000). For some cancer types, the number of deaths remained virtually stable (i.e. breast cancer, colon and rectum cancer), for other types the number increased (i.e. prostate cancer from 9,000 to 16,000), whereas for other cancer types, this number diminished (i.e. stomach cancer from 18,000 to 13,000).

However, these numbers do not account for changes in population size, age structure and rising life expectancy. The majority of cancer deaths occur in people over 70 years. Thus, the growing incidence of a variety of cancers after the second world war, especially in industrial countries, may be partly attributed to a fact that is actually gratifying: namely to extended lifespans (Torre et al. 2016). Worldwide, in 1990 34% patients who died from cancer belonged to this age group; this fraction was 46% in 2015. This fact explains why highly developed countries continue to have high incidence rates compared to less highly developed countries (Torre et al. 2016). Referred to Germany, 55% (in 1991) and 65% (in 2015) of all cancer deaths concern people older than 70 years (Ritchie 2019). According to Robert Alan Weinberg (*1942), a pioneer in cancer research, the leading risk factor for developing cancer is age. In Weinberg's opinion, everybody would get cancer, sooner or later, if he or she lived long enough (Johnson 2010). However, the age-related pattern of cancer—although well-documented in many publications—is rather complex.

Yet age is not the unique factor to be considered since rising incidence can be observed across all age categories, including children. It is well known that some lifestyle and environmental factors such as tobacco smoking, drinking alcohol, obesity or air pollution play an important role. Furthermore, mutant alleles accumulation in some populations is considered as an aetiology due to heritability of many cancers (You and Henneberg 2018). On the other hand, there are some cancer types (i.c. testicular cancer or leucemia) with early life incidence peaks for unknown reasons. Other types, i.e. some ovarian or stomach cancers, are associated with inherited predispositions.

Lifestyle factors are modifiable to a certain degree. However, it is not easy for exposed people to change their behaviour in order to reduce their personal risk. For genetic factors, it seems to be illusory for an individual concerned trying to prevent the development of cancer.

However, all these factors cannot fully account for the observed growing incidence of cancer. New diagnostic techniques and screening tests also contribute to this phenomenon. Without these features, many tumours would have never been detected. No doubt, it is beneficial to detect a tumour in an early stage if an efficient therapy is available which is able to prevent the progression of the cancer. On the other hand, in cases of over-diagnosis screenings are unnecessary and potentially harmful, because they may produce more damages than benefits—for the individual as well as for the healthcare system.

To illustrate these phenomena, incidence and mortality rates will be considered for two wide-spread cancer types, namely breast and prostate cancer.

2.4.2 Breast Cancer and Mammography

At the very beginning of her article, actually in the first sentence of the abstract, Kerlokowske proclaims: "Mammography has been shown to reduce mortality from breast cancer about 25 to 30%" (Kerlokowske 1997). This sounds great! Many physicians who read this phrase are likely to think that this percentage refers to all their middle-aged women. Moreover, lots of women who are confronted with this information feel personally addressed. They suppose that this percentage refers to people like themselves. Yet it only refers to the baseline of people who do not participate in screening and die of cancer. The absolute risk of dying by breast cancer is only 3–4 pro mils. This information however cannot be found in the abstract.

What about the case fatality rates? Actually, they are not given in Kerlikowske's article. In the recently published paper by Katalinic et al. (2019) annual incidence and mortality rates are presented, separately for several age groups and cancer stages before and after the implementation of mammography screening program in Germany. Data refer to the time periods 2003/2004 and 2013/14, respectively. We consider the group of 60–69 aged women (which is the largest one).

Looking at Table 2.3, it becomes obvious that global incidence rises with screening (from 320.8 to 381.1 per 100,000 women). This is not astonishing because screening is intended to detect extremely small tumours at a very early stage which would remain undetected without screening. However, this higher incidence is by no means a screening's success, but profoundly biased by a lead-time bias.

Table 2.3 Breast cancer incidences and mortalities (per 100,000) and case fatality rates (in %) for 60–69 aged women before and after implementation of mammography screening in Germany (Katalinic et al. 2019). Percentages in parentheses refer to the populations before or after screening implementation

Stage	Before screening implementation	After screening implementation	Difference (after—before)
DCIS	17.4 (5.4%)	46.1 (12.1%)	+ 28.7
Stage I	118.5 (36.9%)	171.9 (45.1%)	+ 53.4
Stage II	111.9 (34.9%)	109.7 (28.8%)	−2.2
Stage III	47.5 (14.8%)	34.1 (8.9%)	−13.4
Stage IV	25.5 (7.9%)	19.3 (5.1%)	−6.2
Total incidence	320.8 (100%)	381.1 (100%)	+ 60.3
Mortality	79.9	62.9	−17.0
Case fatality rate	24.9%	16.5%	−8.4%

Katalinic et al. (2019) indicated mortality rates of 79.9 and 62.9 per 100,000 women per year for 60–69 aged women. Hence, the breast-related mortality is reduced by mammography by 0.017% (absolute risk reduction) or about 21% (relative risk reduction).

What about the case fatality rates? They are estimated as they ratio of mortality and incidence (see Sect. 2.3.1) and result in 24.9 and 16.5% for unscreened and screened women, respectively. They correspond to annual survival rates of 75.1 and 83.5%. Apparently, the case fatality rate of 24.9% before mammography implantation can be reduced by 8.4% due to screening meaning a relative risk reduction of 34%. Thus, the comparison of the case fatality rates seems to be much more conspicuous than the comparison of the mortality rates (17 per 100,000). However, case fatality rates are based on incidences and are therefore biased by lead-time and length–time bias. On the contrary, mortality rates are based on the number of deaths (instead of number of detected cancers) and are therefore not biased.

In the 1990 years, reports have been published indicating mammography benefits also for younger women aged 40 to 49 years (Curpen et al. 1995; Smart et al. 1993). The authors claim improved survival for women who underwent mammography. However, using these survival statistics mammography benefits may be overestimated because of bias.

In summary, the unanswered question is whether early detection and subsequent therapies results in improved patient outcomes (Zahl et al. 2011; Gøtzsche et al. 2012). Breast cancer is a heterogenous disease with some cancers growing very rapidly and others never causing clinical symptoms. Mammography enhances the chance particularly for the latter ones to be detected. If we knew more about the natural history of the various types of breast cancer tumours, it might be possible to eliminate lead time and length biases that are inherent in results from screening studies, even in a randomized study design (Bleyer and Welch 2012). Since this will probably not be the case in the near future, mortality rates (which are not affected by lead time or length time biases) should be preferred to case fatality or survival rates.

2.4.3 Prostate Cancer and PSA Screening

Back to Mr. Giuliani: Drawing a comparison between prostate cancer-related survival rates was not fair because of several reasons. As mentioned above, in the context of screening survival rates seem to be non-valid metrics. Actually, in the USA most prostate cancers are diagnosed by screening for PSA, whereas in the UK the majority of patients detect their prostate cancer by clinical symptoms. It may be assumed that among American men many non-progressive or slowly progressing cancers have been found which would have never caused any inconveniences during men's life if they had been undiscovered. Thus, the incidence in the USA is influenced by a lead-time and a length–time bias which in turn affect the case fatality and the survival rate. This fact explains why the 5-year-incidence in USA was much higher than in England (180 versus 49 per 100,000 men). In order to judge which country was doing better it makes sense to look at the 5-year-mortality rates which hardly differ: 26 (United States) and 27 per 100,000 (Shibata and Whittemore 2001).

Recently, it has been shown that for 100,000 US-American men receiving PSA screening in 1997, almost 5,000 additional men underwent prostate biopsy, nearly 1,600 underwent prostate cancer treatment whereas only a minority of about 60 fewer men died from prostate cancer-related death (Howrey et al. 2013). No relationship between PSA screening and the mortality from other causes could be found. Another study worth taking a closer look at is the eighteen-year follow-up of the Göteborg Randomized Population-based Prostate Cancer Screening Trial (Hugosson et al. 2018). Looking at Table 2.4, it becomes obvious that incidence is higher in the screening arm (due to a length time bias), whereas case fatality rate and prostate cancer mortality is lower in the screening arm. Median times from randomization to diagnosis were 8.6 versus 10.3 years (illustrating the lead time bias).

However, the overall mortality rates are nearly identical in both arms. This metrics suggests that PSA screening reduces mortality due to the prostate cancer but does not affect the overall mortality. Among the attendees, 35% had been screened positive at least once and 32% of them underwent a biopsy—although the incidence in this subgroup was only half.

Another aspect regarding the study design is noteworthy. It was designed as a randomized trial. However, not each of the 9,950 men attributed to the screening group was willing to attend screening regularly. Out of them, 23% had no screening at all; from the remaining 7,647 men it is only known that they attended at least one screening. This illustrates the difficulties which may be inherent when conducting a randomized trial. The divergent overall mortality rates of the attendees and non-attendees (23.1% vs. 46.9%) are rather impressive. However, they might be distorted by a volunteer bias and are therefore meaningless.

Table 2.4 Prostate cancer cases and deaths and derived metrics in the Göteborg Randomized Trial (Hugosson et al. 2018)

	Control	Screening all	Screening attendees	Screening non-attendees
Total group size	9,949	9,950	7,647	2,303
PC cases	962	1,396	1,272	124
Deaths				
- From PC	122	79	51	28
- From other causes	2,735	2,765	1,712	1,053
- Total number	2,857	2,844	1,763	1,081
Incidence (%)	9.7	14.0	16.6	5.4
Case fatality rate (%)	12.7	5.7	4.0	22.5
PC-related mortality (%)	1.2	0.8	0.7	1.2
Overall mortality (%)	28.7	28.6	23.1	46.9

PC = prostate cancer

2.5   Conclusion

"Cancer screening saves lives". It is a message we're all familiar with, disseminated by screening initiatives. This phenomena is not new: During the 1950s and 1960s, it was commonly thought among physicians that finding a disease at a very early stage would lead to more efficient treatment, to prolonged survival time and to improved quality of life. Under these circumstances, it may be alluring to believe into the power of screenings—especially since many doctors and medical scientists promise benefits such as reduced mortality rates or increased life spans. Today, it is commonly known among researchers: It is not that simple. Certainty is an illusion.

Although screening may help to detect a cancer disease at a very early stage and to improve survival by initiation of timely treatment, the claim that screening by itself saves lives is difficult to support. The apparent welfares are by far not as high as is often assumed. The overoptimistic expectations are created by false information and nontransparent risk communication. Even scientific journals report evidence that suggests big benefits combined with small harms of screening interventions. Screening advocates often cite disease detection rates as proof that screening can work. This is mainly due to the progress in medical technology. Nowadays, many cancers are diagnosed which in former times would have remained undetected until the person died of other causes. However, there is not much evidence that early detection of a tumour is associated with cure or reduced mortality. Other endpoints frequently reported in screening studies are compliance rates, survival rates, case fatality rates or compliance (Black et al. 2002). However, these endpoints are misleading information. They may be distorted by bias and therefore are not sufficient to demonstrate the effectiveness of screenings. It is important to be aware that various types of bias (i.e. lead time or length time bias) may contribute to the apparent survival benefits.

The inability to assess risks is common to healthy people, sick patients, physicians, journalists and politicians. Thus, many medical doctors are unaware that higher survival rates by cancer screening do not automatically imply longer life. They believe in progress in cancer research, which in reality is much smaller than inadmissible conclusions from publications would suggest. This has serious consequences for health: practicing physicians think that screenings contribute to diminished mortality rates by cancer and will advise their patients inadequately in the good faith doing the best for them. Trusting their doctor, people are convinced that screenings reduce their individual risk of developing cancer or even think that they can be saved from the death by participating in screenings.

According to Mayer (2004), there are some relevant criteria which should be fulfilled to ensure that a screening test is valid and purposeful. (1) The disease must be relatively common in the screened population. It is unreasonable, for instance, to screen 20-year-old men for prostate cancer. (2) Furthermore, the disease itself must be detectable at an early stage with good chances of recovery. (3) The screening test should be accurate, that is, it should have a high sensitivity in order to detect disease in patients who are in the pre-symptomatic phase. The test should have a high specificity as well to be able to exclude disease in healthy persons. Both criteria are important. (4) Practical considerations refer to the costs and the feasibility in practice. If the test procedure is connected with a high level of discomfort, it will not be accepted by the public. (5) Most important there must be a treatment available which will result in a markedly improved outcome, i.e. longer survival time. Otherwise, diagnosis at an early stage is not helpful.

However, all these criteria do not solve the dilemma of overdiagnosis. When a cancer has been detected by a screening procedure and confirmed by a pathologist, it cannot be predicted whether this cancer will progress rapidly or slowly or whether it will remain stable or even regress. Nevertheless, such a diagnosis makes the patient feel like a ticking time bomb. Thus, a (over-)treatment will be started from which nobody knows if it is really necessary or not.

What can be done? Statistical thinking is indispensable in order to adequately assess the results of a trial. Dealing with risks may be difficult, even for clinical experts. Thus, it is extremely important to teach statistical thinking in medical education and training students and physicians in this discipline.

The best way to examine the benefits of screening is to conduct a randomized controlled trial, because random assignment of participants to the screened and unscreened groups is regarded as an excellent tool for removing the distorting effects of selection bias. Furthermore, all-cause mortality should be presented. This is the only reliable endpoint in screening studies because it is unaffected by lead time or length time bias. Unless these types of bias are avoided, the results of a screening trial cannot provide valid information (Porzsolt et al. 2016).

One of the most troubling challenges is our own cognitive limitations occurring when established thoughts become resistant to disconfirming information. Constructive scepticism is needed in order to critically assess benefits in medical care and to use diagnostic and therapeutic techniques efficiently.

References

Black WS, Haggstrom DA, Welch HG (2002) All-cause mortality in randomized trials of cancer screening. J National Cancer Institute 94:167–173

Bleyer A, Welch HG (2012) Effect of three decades of screening mammography on breast cancer incidence. N Engl J Med 367:1998–2005

Curpen BN, Sickles EA, Sollitto RA, Ominsky SH, Galvin HB, Frankel SD (1995) The comparative value of mammographic screening for women 40–49 years old versus women 50–64 years old. AJR Am J Roentgenol 164:1099–1103

Dobbs M (2007) Rudy wrong on cancer survival chances. Retrieved from https://voices.washingtonpost.com/fact-checker/2007/10/rudy_miscalculates_cancer_surv.html

Gigerenzer G, Gaissmaier W, Kurz-Milcke E, Schwartz LM, Woloshin S (2008) Helping doctors and patients make sense of health statistics. AssocPsycholSci 82:53–94

Gøtzsche PC, Jørgensen KJ, Zahl PH, Mæhlen J (2012) Why mammography screening has not lived up to expectations from the randomized trials. Cancer Causes Control 23:15–21

Howrey BT, Kuo YF, Lin YL, Goodwin JS (2013) The impact of PSA screening on prostate cancer mortality and overdiagnosis of prostate cancer in the United States. J Gerontology 68 (1):56–61

Hugosson J, Godtman RA, Carlsson SV, Aus G, Bergdahl AG, Lodding P, Pihl CG, Stranne J, Holmber E, Lilja H (2018) Eighteen-year follow-up of the Göteborg randomized population-based prostate cancer screening trial: effect of the sociodemographic variables on participation, prostate cancer and mortality. Scandinavian J Urology 52(1):27–37

Johnson G (2010) Unearthing prehistoric tumors, and debate. The New York Times. Retrieved from https://www.nytimes.com/2010/12/28/health/28cancer.html

Katalinic A, Eisemann N, Kraywinkel K, Noftz MR, Hübner J (2019) Breast cancer incidence and mortality before and after implementation of the German mammography screening program. Int J Cancer. https://doi.org/10.1002/ijc.32767

Kerlikowske K (1997) Efficacy of screening mammography among women aged 40 to 49 years and 50 to 69 years: comparison of relative and absolute benefit. J National Cancer Inst Monographs. 22:79–86

Mayer D (2004) Chapter 26: Screening tests. In: Essential Evidence-Based Medicine. Cambridge University Press

Porzsolt F, Wambo GMK, Rösch MC, Weiß C (2016) Prävention muss effizienter werden. Dtsch Med Wochenschr 141(09):651–653

Ritchie H (2019): How many people in the world die from cancer? https://ourworldindata.org/how-many-people-in-the-world-die-from-cancer

Shibata A, Whittemore AS (2001) Re: Prostate cancer incidence and mortality in the United States and in the United Kingdom. J Natl Cancer Inst 92:1109–1110

Smart CR, Hartmann WH, Beahrs OH, Garfinkel L (1993) Insights into breast cancer screening of younger women. Evidence from the 14-year follow-up of the Breast Cancer Detection Demonstration Project. Cancer 72 (4Suppl):1449–56

Torre LA, Siegel RL, Ward EM, Jemal A (2016) Global cancer incidence and mortality rate and trends—an update. Cancer Epidemiol Biomark Prev 25(1):16–27

You W, Henneberg M (2018) Cancer incidence increasing globally. The role of relaxed natural selection. Evolutionary applications 11(2): 140–152

Zahl PH, Gøtzsche PC, Mæhlen J (2011) Natural history of breast cancer detected in the Swedish mammography screening programme: a cohort study. Lancet Oncology 12:1118–1124

HPV Vaccination in Bangladesh: Ethical Views

3

Marium Salwa and Tarek Abdullah Al-Munim

Mass-level vaccination for preventing diseases is certainly a massive boost for the general public. For developing countries, the value for vaccinations cannot be underestimated. This has certainly been one of the reasons for the increased life expectancy and improvement of the quality of life, resulting in better productivity and increased economic and social prosperity for families and societies. Vaccines, in Bangladesh, are considered as an almost guaranteed protection from diseases. Institutionalized vaccination programs have been an effective practice in the healthcare services for Bangladeshi masses. Polio and smallpox vaccination programs are just two of such examples which have seen effective eradication of these deadly and debilitating diseases. This has increased the trust on such programs, making it a popular and effective method of running vaccination programs in Bangladesh. Many vaccination programs have started off as demonstration projects that have later on become part of a nationwide immunization program. As much as the benefits of the vaccination programs are well-recorded, the ethics of administration of it is not focused highly. Rather the focus tends to be on the most efficient method to get it done. This should be addressed given the program itself decides for the public what goes into their bodies. Furthermore, in many cases the vaccination is administered to children and infants who have no say in the process. To illustrate this dilemma, this chapter is looking into one case that relates to the human papilloma virus (HPV) vaccination program in Bangladesh.

HPV infection is a global concern. More than a half-million cancers—including cervical, vulvar, anal, penile, and oropharyngeal cancer—and over 250,000 deaths are attributed annually to HPV infection (Bruni et al. 2016). Globally, cervical

M. Salwa (✉)
Bangabandhu Sheikh Mujib Medical University, Shahbag, Dhaka-1000, Bangladesh
e-mail: mariumsalwa@gmail.com

T. A. Al-Munim
Independent Consultant, House #238, Road #5, Mohammadi Housing Society,
Mohammadpur, Dhaka-1207, Bangladesh

© Springer Nature Switzerland AG 2021
A. W. Bauer et al. (eds.), *Ethical Challenges in Cancer Diagnosis and Therapy*,
Recent Results in Cancer Research 218,
https://doi.org/10.1007/978-3-030-63749-1_3

cancer is the fourth leading female cancer and the second most common cancer among women aged 15 to 44 years (WHO 2019). Copenhagen consensus center reveals that 10,000 women deaths are caused by cervical cancer every year. In 2016, the human papillomavirus (HPV) vaccine was introduced in Bangladesh by a two-year demonstration project. Governed by the Ministry of Health and Family Welfare of Bangladesh and with financial support from the Global Alliance for Vaccines and Immunization (GAVI, the Vaccine Alliance), the bivalent preparation of the HPV vaccine (Cervarix) has been administered to 5th grader school-going girls as well as girls who were not attending schools aged between 10 and 12 years residing in five selected areas of Gazipur District, located close to the capital city— Dhaka. For better efficiency and to manage costs better, the program was conducted under the Expanded Program of Immunization (EPI), which allowed the HPV vaccination program to utilize the existing resources of the EPI, letting it easy access to schools, and ride on the already established trust on the EPI program, thereby making the acceptance and cooperation from the public and the students easier. National scale-up of the HPV vaccination program is planned after the HPV demonstration program is evaluated and deemed successful.

On the day of the vaccination, a health education session was conducted among the vaccine candidates. Candidates were made aware about the vaccine and its importance in preventing cervical cancer as part of this health education. However, what is noteworthy is that information about HPV infection, its route of transmission and the cofactors related to its spread along with other cervical cancer prevention strategies were left out of this health education. If it were such that HPV on its own was the most dominant factor behind cervical cancer, then this would be understandable as giving as much information to the recipient as may deem to be needed. However, data may indicate otherwise as the following breakdown of HPV, its effect on cervical cancer and other cofactors of cervical cancer illustrates.

HPV is one of the aetiological causes of cervical cancer. HPV 16 and 18 serotypes, especially, are responsible for about 70% of cervical cancer worldwide (WHO 2019). However, infection with HPV does not necessarily result in cervical cancer. There are some established cofactors (modifiable risk factors) for progression of cervical HPV infection to cancer in the long run, such as early age of first sexual intercourse, multiple sexual partners, tobacco use, immune suppression such as co-infection with human immunodeficiency virus (HIV), high parity, long-term hormonal contraceptive use, and poor nutritional status (Bruni et al. 2016; WHO 2019). HPV infection, therefore, can be prevented primarily through vaccination and interventions targeting these modifiable risk factors.

Discussions about sexual health may not be an easy talk to take with 5th graders or girls within the similar age bracket in Bangladesh. However, given the fact that sexual contact is the main route of transmission of the vaccine-preventable HPV serotypes, such withholding of information when HPV is actually being discussed and a vaccine is actually being administered, not even with the teachers and parents of the recipients, raises questions on whether this withholding of information is beneficial for the actual prevention of the cancer that the vaccination is intended for. Given this may the first discussion on a female-specific health concern that these girls will be facing, it will have a lasting impression on the person's ideas and knowledge of what are the foundations of cervical cancer in general. The outcome of such a discussion that only takes care of the correlation between HPV and cervical cancer without the role that modifiable risk factors involving male partners play may lead to a false understanding that cervical cancer is female specific from the cause to the illness without any male having any role to play. The other risk lies in providing the same education to non-school going girls in the similar age bracket as 5th graders. As much as in a school environment, there may be opportunities to clarify misconceptions or provide additional information when sought, a one off education on HPV and cervical cancer without discussing other contributing factors may only help establish a wrong perception that this is a female centric disease. In an already male-biased society, this may have a lasting impact on the morale and confidence of the female recipient who is not part of the education system.

Another aspect of notable concern is that while the education connecting HPV and cervical cancer is relevant, so is the method by which a person can get themselves tested for HPV. Among secondary prevention methods of cervical cancer, cervical screening tests show great promise, especially the Papanicolaou test (Pap test), visual inspection with acetic acid (VIA) test, HPV DNA test or the HPV determination test (Navarro-Illana et al. 2014; Sherris et al. 2009). Not providing information about other cervical cancer prevention strategies, particularly cervical screening, poses ethical questions. Vaccination cannot replace the role of screening. Besides, the effectiveness of HPV vaccination is higher where there is a strong screening system. As vaccines only prevent 70% of cervical cancers, surveillance via screening must be continued. There is a risk that such over-emphasis on HPV vaccination may divert the recipients' attention from the perceived importance of screening. It is anticipated that some vaccinated girls may forego the recommended screening in the adult life due to this false sense of security, a situation that may paradoxically result in a higher incidence of cervical cancer if less than 70% of the population is screened (Harper et al. 2010). In Bangladesh, even though cervical screening programs began in 2004, the coverage rate remains very poor and is limited to opportunistic tests (Basu et al. 2010). In this situation, tailored information to advertise vaccination would further reduce the importance of screening in population mindset.

Furthermore, the vaccine currently provided under the program only covers two serotypes of HPV (16, 18) out of about 20 possible high-risk cancer-causing serotypes (Clifford et al. 2005). Over 80% borderline lesions and 70 percent cervical intra epithelial neoplasia are unrelated to HPV-16 or HPV-18 and thus cannot be prevented by vaccination (Raffle 2007). There is also an ethical dilemma regarding the actual efficacy of the vaccine (Lippman et al. 2007). Communications around the HPV vaccination program convey the impression that cervical cancer is hundred percent preventable with vaccination. The program communication also does not disclose adequate information about the durability of protection with the HPV vaccination and the need for possible booster immunization. This arise ethical concerns about the lack of accountability of the vaccination implementers that may put the risk of failing public trust regarding preventive health services.

As much as the above are ethical dilemmas which demand attention, the counterargument to providing full information can also be put forward. For the utilitarian benefit, it could be argued that full information about HPV might arise sociocultural controversies and hinder vaccine uptake. Highlighting the anti-cancer role of the HPV vaccine over its true role in preventing sexually transmitted HPV infection is demonstrated in higher vaccination coverage in several low- and middle-income countries (Gallagher et al. 2018). The counterargument, while may have partial merit, accurate and complete information is proven to be effective against rumor and misinformation which at the age of the vaccine recipient is of critical importance since this is when information tends to form the foundations of future knowledge and at times-engrained bias. About STIs, full information may be necessary to avoid marginalizing any specific gender, in social settings that have historically victimized females for many STI issues (Nack 2002). Also, due to the lack of public discourse and the sensitivities around making STI-related information readily available, there is little opportunity to command people's full, undivided attention on multiple occasions; therefore, it is only convenient to provide full information when the opportunity arises, in order to avoid presenting only partial information that can produce a false sense of safety when no such guarantees exist. In fact, revealing the nature of HPV transmission, even though it may raise feelings of stigma and shame, is proven to reduce the stress (Waller et al. 2007). Also, the success of the measles rubella (MR) campaign in increasing MR vaccination coverage in Bangladesh demonstrates that good social mobilization in which the recipient can learn about the disease in question can result in high vaccine uptake (Uddin 2016).

In the vaccination program, every girl is taken separately for vaccination to an empty classroom or a secluded corner for privacy and to minimize anxiety. For every recipient vaccinated, vaccination cards are issued which is preserved by the school authorities. For the target recipients who may have been missed due to absenteeism, they can get vaccinated from a nearby school if it is in schedule or from the community EPI center. Adolescent girls of the same age who do not attend schools can get the vaccine from community-based routine, fixed, and outreach vaccination sites, thereby ensuring that the probability of not being vaccinated despite being of the age stipulated is as low as possible.

While the above method of moving forward with the vaccination may seem straight forward, a few key issues have glaring ethical issues that need to be addressed. Obtaining consent from adolescents or their guardians before giving vaccination is considered as a major ethical dilemma regarding HPV vaccination. Adolescence is a unique life stage that bridges childhood and adulthood. WHO stresses on special attention to pay for obtaining informed consent when administering vaccination for this age group (Paxman 1987). Many HPV vaccination programs around the world use an implied consent procedure from guardians (Zimmerman 2006). In Bangladesh, written guideline or procedure is absent on ensuring the obtaining of guardian's consent or the assent of the adolescents for vaccination. Presence of girls at school in vaccination day is regarded as implied consent from their guardians. The assent of the girls, which is considered important for vaccination according to WHO (2014), is not covered under the procedures.

Further, the regimented way in which the vaccination program is administered in schools, all selected girls feel obliged to accept it, either due to peer pressure or to please schoolteachers. They have no opportunity to take an informed and independent decision regarding the matter. This creates an ethical dilemma, given that no choice is available to the recipients or their guardians when deciding whether to take the vaccine. Besides, involving guardians in the discussion at the time of vaccination enhances communication about cervical cancer prevention and the role of the HPV vaccine (Sussman 2007), which is ignored in the current vaccination program. Furthermore, the HPV vaccination-card maintained for every vaccine recipient is not handed to their guardians until the two doses are completed. In fact, there is no written documentation for the guardians to know about the vaccine administered to their daughters at school. This puts guardians in a blind situation, making them solely dependent on the schoolteachers' judgment about the well-being of their daughters and depriving them of being able to make their own decisions.

The HPV vaccine, like all other EPI vaccines used in Bangladesh, is administered with WHO approval but without any country-specific trial or licensure by any local drug administration authority. Hence, post-marketing vaccine surveillance is poor. This is a concern because there is lack of data on long-term adverse effects associated with HPV vaccinations in Bangladesh. Long-term follow up of HPV vaccine recipients is essential (De Vincenzo et al. 2014). Depriving the vaccinated girls of more organized follow-up, and hence not ensuring immediate identification and treatment of any vaccine-related adverse effects, poses a major ethical concern.

Another critical ethical dilemma about the vaccination program is the female-only strategy that the HPV vaccination program seems to adhere to. In Bangladesh, women represent almost half of the population. Despite the growing involvement of women in the workforce over the recent years, significant economic and cultural barriers still exist in the society for the women to overcome. Further, increased representation in the government and non-government sectors does not guarantee women's increased participation in the decision-making process (Panday 2008) or has not lessened the violence against women (Abusaleh and Mitra 2016). Women have to go along any decision regarding sex in familial life. In this circumstance, vaccinating only females may lead people to dismiss the disease as a women-related concern, which might increase sexual irresponsibility in the male partner. Further, seeing the female classmates to participate in special health education session and to be vaccinated for HPV might have the chance to create a false sense of security among male classmates. Thus, these boys may perceive HPV infection as a mere women-related issue ignoring the important role of men in HPV transmission. The ultimate societal impact of these phenomena should be identified at the outset to preserve ethical values revolving HPV vaccination. As a way to this, proper health education regarding HPV infection should be given to adolescent boys as well.

Vaccination is known to be important for ages to boost up immune system and prevent diseases. In countries like Bangladesh, government vaccination programs are the most successful public health initiatives. It is the high time to discuss about the ethical concerns to preserve public trust on immunization programs in Bangladesh. Given the fact that about 84 percent new cases of cervical cancer patient were from less developed region in 2018 (WHO 2019), primary prevention through HPV vaccination becomes more emphasized. As HPV vaccine is a new addition to existing immunization programs, proper measures should be taken at both government and civil society level to maintain the highest standard of ethics in every sphere of the implementation system.

References

Abusaleh K, Mitra A (2016) Trends and patterns of violence against women in Bangladesh. Glob J Hum Soc Sci 16(6):28–34

Basu P, Nessa A, Majid M, Rahman JN, Ahmed T (2010) Evaluation of the national cervical cancer screening programme of Bangladesh and the formulation of quality assurance guidelines. J Fam Plann Reprod Health Care 36(3):131–134. https://doi.org/10.1783/147118910791749218

Bruni L, Barrionuevo-Rosas L, Albero G, Aldea M, Serrano B, Valencia S, Brotons M, Mena M, Cosano R, Muñoz J, Bosch F, de Sanjosé S, Castellsagué X (2016) Human Papillomavirus and Related Diseases in the World. Summary Report. ICO Information Centre on HPV and Cancer (HPV Information Centre)

Clifford G, Gallus S, Herrero R, Munoz N, Snijders P, Vaccarella S et al (2005) Worldwide distribution of human papillomavirus types in cytologically normal women in the International Agency for Research on Cancer HPV prevalence surveys: a pooled analysis. Lancet 366 (9490):991–998. https://doi.org/10.1016/S0140-6736(05)67069-9

Copenhagen Consensus Center. Controlling the Burden of Non-Communicable Diseases in Bangladesh: Benefit-cost Analysis of Prevention Policies and Interventions Bangladesh priorities (2016) https://www.copenhagenconsensus.com/bangladesh-priorities/non-communicable-diseases. Accessed 13 Mar 2020

De Vincenzo R et al (2014) Long-term efficacy and safety of human papillomavirus vaccination. Int J Women's Health 6:999–1010. https://doi.org/10.2147/IJWH.S50365

Gallagher KE, LaMontagne DS, Watson-Jones D (2018) Status of HPV vaccine introduction and barriers to country uptake. Vaccine. The Authors 36(32):4761–4767. https://doi.org/10.1016/j.vaccine.2018.02.003

Harper DM, Nieminen P, Paavonen J, Lehtinen M (2010) Cervical cancer incidence can increase despite HPV vaccination. Lancet Infect Dis 10(9):594–595. https://doi.org/10.1016/S1473-3099(10)70182-1

Lippman A, Melnychuk R, Shimmin C, Boscoe M (2007) Human papillomavirus, vaccines and women's health: questions and cautions. Can Med Assoc J 177(5):484–487. https://doi.org/10.1503/cmaj.070944

Nack A (2002) Bad girls and fallen women: chronic STD diagnoses as gateways to tribal stigma. Symb Interact 25(4):463–485. https://doi.org/10.1525/si.2002.25.4.463

Navarro-Illana P, Aznar J, Díez-Domingo J (2014) Ethical considerations of universal vaccination against human papilloma virus. BMC Med Ethics 15(1):29 https://doi.org/10.1186/1472-6939-15-29

Panday PK (2008) Representation without participation: quotas for women in Bangladesh. IntPolitSci Rev 29(4):489–512. https://doi.org/10.1177%2F0192512108095724

Paxman JM, Zuckerman RJ, World Health Organization (1987) Laws and policies affecting adolescent health / by John M. Paxman and Ruth Jane Zuckerman. World Health Organization. https://apps.who.int/iris/handle/10665/38497 Accessed 13 Mar 2020

Raffle AE (2007) Challenges of implementing human papillomavirus (HPV) vaccination policy. BMJ 335(7616):375. https://doi.org/10.1136/bmj.39273.458322.BE

Sherris J, Wittet S, Kleine A, Sellors J, Luciani S, Sankaranarayanan R et al (2009) Evidence-based, alternative cervical cancer screening approaches in lowresource settings. Int Perspect Sex Reprod Health 35(3):147–152

Sussman AL, Helitzer D, Sanders M, Urquieta B, Salvador M, Ndiaye K (2007) HPV and cervical cancer prevention counseling with younger adolescents: implications for primary care. Ann Fam Med 5(4):298–304. https://doi.org/10.1370/afm.723

Uddin MJ, Adhikary G, Ali MW, Ahmed S, Shamsuzzaman M, Odell C et al (2016) Evaluation of impact of measles rubella campaign on vaccination coverage and routine immunization services in Bangladesh. BMC Infect Dis 16(1):411. https://doi.org/10.1186/s12879-016-1758-x

Waller J, Marlow LA, Wardle J (2007) The association between knowledge of HPV and feelings of stigma, shame and anxiety. Sex Transm Infect 83(2):155–159. https://doi.org/10.1136/sti.2006.023333

World Health Organization (WHO) (2019) Human papilloma virus (HPV) and cervical cancer. https://www.who.int/news-room/fact-sheets/detail/human-papillomavirus-(hpv)-and-cervical-cancer Accessed 13 Mar 2020

World Health Organization (2014) Considerations regarding consent in vaccinating children and adolescents between 6 and 17 years old. https://apps.who.int/iris/bitstream/handle/10665/259418/WHO-IVB-14.04-eng.pdf Accessed 13 Mar 2020

Zimmerman RK (2006) Ethical analysis of HPV vaccine policy options. Vaccine. 24(22):4812–4820. https://doi.org/10.1016/j.vaccine.2006.03.019

Ethical Challenges Using Human Tumor Cell Lines in Cancer Research

Wilhelm G. Dirks

4.1 Poor, Black, and Uneducated: Henrietta Lacks Wrote Medical History—Involuntarily

In the spring of 1951, 30-year-old Henrietta Lacks visited the Johns Hopkins Hospital in Baltimore to have severe abdominal pain treated. At the time, neither Mrs. Lacks nor the attending physician Howard Jones suspected that she would die of cervical cancer less than six months later. Treatment on the ward for black women was free of charge, and in the 1950, it was justified that the tissue removed should benefit research. Mrs. Lacks was neither informed about the removal of a biopsy nor asked for her permission to conduct research with the tissue sample (Skloot 2010). Her family doctor sent the samples taken on 8 February to the laboratory of the scientist George Otto Gey who put them into a mixture of chicken plasma, an extract of calf embryos and human umbilical cord blood and supplied them in an incubator (Masters 2002). HeLa cells—initial letters of the patient's name—doubled overnight, and a few weeks later, scientist Dr. Gey had millions of human cells at his disposal which were available to research worldwide for the first time in medical history (Scherer et al. 1953) (Fig. 4.1).

W. G. Dirks (✉)
Leibniz Institute DSMZ, German Collection of Microorganisms and Cell Cultures GmbH, Inhoffenstraße 7 B, 38124 Braunschweig, Germany
e-mail: wdi@dsmz.de

© Springer Nature Switzerland AG 2021
A. W. Bauer et al. (eds.), *Ethical Challenges in Cancer Diagnosis and Therapy*,
Recent Results in Cancer Research 218,
https://doi.org/10.1007/978-3-030-63749-1_4

4.2   Cancer Research Using Immortal Tumor Cell Lines

The establishment of HeLa as the first human continuous cell line provided a coveted standard model for the investigation of cancer pathophysiology to avoid differences between donors and to allow the reproducibility of experimental data, but above all to allow the renewal of the original biological material (Lucey et al. 2009). A few years later at Ibadan University in Nigeria in 1963, Robert Pulvertaft established the Raji cell line, the first human continuous hematopoietic cell line from a Nigerian patient affected by Burkitt's lymphoma (Pulvertaft 1964). Although the Raji cell line has successively proven to be a model system resulting from infection with the Epstein–Barr virus, the definition of the culture conditions necessary for growth in vitro paved the way for the stabilization of new cell lines growing in suspension. In addition, the availability of recombinant growth factors and conditioned media, particularly in the 1980 and 1990, enabled the stabilization of a number of hematopoietic cell lines covering almost all steps of the classification of myeloid and lymphatic leukemia (Drexler et al. 1999). The total volume of publications of both historical cell lines with regard to cancer research and healthcare amounts for HeLa to over 16,900 publications (milestone is the development of the anti-polio vaccine) and over 1600 papers for Raji (milestone is the mechanisms of infection by Epstein–Barr virus) (Mirabelli et al 2019).

4.3   Early Crisis: The Use of False Cell Lines as Cancer Models

In 1966, scientist Stanley Gartler discovered that HeLa cells that had apparently cross-contaminated numerous cell culture approaches worldwide (Gartler 1968). Due to the high proliferation rate of HeLa and with low demands on the cell culture media, a single HeLa cell introduced into an existing cell culture as an impurity due to missing cell culture guide lines can overgrow the existing culture. In the 1960s, scientists had only very limited possibilities to detect the contamination of a cell culture approach with cells of the same species, as there were no genetic analysis methods yet. An electrophoretic technique for determining a specific isoenzyme pattern of cell lines enabled Stanley Gartler and coworkers to prove that this pattern was identical in many of the cell lines he investigated and could at the same time be unambiguously assigned to that of a black donor, although many of the cell lines investigated were allegedly derived from white donors.

This result was subsequently often referred to as the HeLa bomb because it called into question much of the scientific knowledge gained from cell culture lines to that date (Del Carpio 2014). This example shows that cross-contamination is a neglected and chronic problem of cell culture that has existed since its inception in the 1950 and has hardly changed in importance to this day. Cross-contamination or viral or microbial infections occur regardless of the size or economic status of an academic or industrial institute and can significantly undermine the reliability of scientific data. With a depressing regularity, datasets cannot be reproduced or even publications must be withdrawn if the data were generated with wrong cell lines (Baker 2016).

4.4   STR Genotyping: The Beginning of the End in Cell Line Misidentification?

The example of the alleged endothelial cell line ECV-304 shows the damage and misleading effects that any use of wrong cell lines can cause. The isolation and culture of human vascular endothelial cells is associated with a number of specific problems, including a demanding requirement for exogenous growth factors, mixed cell populations from pooled vascular preparations, and a relatively low proliferation capacity. Thus, the description of ECV304 as a spontaneously transformed cell line from human umbilical vein endothelial cells (HUVEC) was highly regarded by science and industry since it represented a potentially significant advance in this field of research (Takahashi et al. 1990). ECV-304 was already distributed by the major cell banks in America and Asia until 1999, when the cell line was included in the German Biological Resource Bank DSMZ, where a match was found between short tandem repeat (STR) profiles of ECV-304 and the human bladder carcinoma cell line T-24 (Dirks et al. 1999a). A comprehensive review finally revealed that the ECV-304 cell line was cross-contaminated at source and that ECV-304 was a virtual cell line that never existed (Dirks et al. 1999b). For the cell line ECV-304 alone, more than 2500 publications exist to date, which represent a financial loss in the hundreds of millions of dollars with regard to publication efforts. To determine the extent of the problem of virtual cell lines, a further study was performed at the DSMZ, where new published cell lines were obtained directly from the establishing laboratories and a widespread intra-species cross-contamination of human tumor cell lines was found at a percentage of 18%. The misidentified cell lines found were unwittingly used as inappropriate tumor models in several thousand potentially misleading publications (MacLeod et al. 1999). Since 2010, the globally recognized STR9 typing, which was developed and published by a working group of the standard developing organization (SDO) of ATCC, is considered a milestone in quality control with regard to authentication of human cell lines (Alston-Roberts et al. 2010).

4.5   Fetal Bovine Serum (FBS), Fetal Calf Serum (FCS) or Newborn Calf Serum (NCS)

Fetal bovine serum (FBS) is derived from the blood of cow fetuses and is a major component of most culture media required for mammalian cell culture. However, the term FCS or NCS is hardly used, and FBS is more common. The use of FBS in routine cell culture is an embedded practice which is taught in almost any available cell culture training. In the spirit of "never change a winning team," there appears, from a technical point of view, no need to change this methodology. Today's leading global cell banks offer almost exclusively FBS dependent cell cultures. Although the EU adopted a directive on the protection of animals used for scientific purposes (Directive 2010/63/EU), it does not affect the production of FBS since it takes into account only unborn animals from the third trimenon of development. To obtain FBS, the uterus of freshly slaughtered pregnant cows are removed and blood is taken from the non-anesthetized fetus by heart puncture.

Animal rights organizations have been calling for replacement of FBS in cell culture for years. To reduce the use of FBS in the 3R context and possibly even replace it in the long term, chemically defined media (CDMs) should be the ultimate goal for cell culture systems. In particular, when CDMs are inapplicable, human platelet lysate (hPL) represents a promising non-animal serum alternative, which could increase the reliability of biomedical research and enable good manufacturing practice (GMP) compliant applications (Bieback 2013). Acceptance and use of FBS-free media in cell culture laboratories is not widespread worldwide, in part of the unavoidable time-consuming and cost-intensive adaptation of the cells. New FBS-free alternatives should therefore be systematically established for culture and cryopreservation for the most common human cell lines as well as frequently used human primary cells. In order to scientifically substantiate their suitability, growth parameters, physiology, and the genomic stability of the cells should be recorded. Since cell banks are significantly involved in the establishment of new standards in the sense of a Good Cell Culture Practice (GCCP), the efforts to establish chemical defined media could sustainably and globally lead to a significant reduction of FBS use in cell culture laboratories and thus contribute to the avoidance of animal suffering and to better reproducibility of scientific data (Bieback et al. 2010).

Cell culture methods are intended to be highly standardized procedures to investigate changes in viability, growth, and cell communication by varying single parameters such as adding chemicals of interest. However, FBS is a variable and undefined medium component with a complex composition that is still not fully understood. It may contain generally unpredictable factors, which might change between batches, for maintenance of the cell culture and impact upon responses. One example for such problems caused by FBS comes from translational research on cancer, where tumor cell lines are often used to model carcinogenesis. An indispensable condition for fast implementation of new clinical approaches is that researchers worldwide use identical models to generate results that can validate each other's findings. Global Biological Resource Centers (BRCs) are equipped with authentication standards to ensure an optimal use of these models (Capes-Davis and Neve 2016; Barallon et al. 2010). A recent survey revealed a reproducibility crisis in biomedical science, since more than 70% of researchers have failed to reproduce published experiments (Baker 2016), which in cancer research can be partly attributed to the use of different batches of FBS, as will be discussed below.

Furthermore, the fast growing knowledge from intra-tumor across inter-patient to intra-cell line heterogeneities demands a comprehensive maintenance and safe-guarding of a sufficient number of models to represent the genomic diversity observed across human cancers. The qualitative and quantitative variations of FBS batches can cause selection and sub-clonal outgrowth of tumor cell lines leading to a bottlenecking selection procedure of sidelines within a cell culture population. Heterogeneity of primary tumor cells represents one of the major disadvantages compared to continuous cell lines, since it is proposed that cell lines originate from a single neoplastic cell. Recently, the presence of two clones in one continuous cell line has been described, indicating clonal evolution within a cell culture population (Quentmeier et al. 2013). Different FBS qualities could thus play a decisive role in a dynamic cell culture in this regard.

4.6 Is Chemically Undefined FBS Part of the Problem of Non-reproducibility of Data?

BRCs generally use high quality FBS, sufficient for proliferation of the majority of the continuous cell lines. FBS lot charge exchanges at cell banks require extensive testing on a panel of cell lines representing different tissues and applications for a time period of at least two weeks, since one may not see the differentiating or apoptotic effects of the new FBS lot immediately after usage. Intra-cellular stores could initiate proliferation and falsify the results in short term testing, and nutritional deficiencies could cause cell lines to lose or gain genetic and phenotypic functions. The worst-case scenario is that bottlenecking selection procedures for the effects of newly purchased FBS batches on the different cell types are visible or measurable only in the rarest cases. Elimination of ancestral clones by sequential selection, possibly by unsuitable FBS charges on sophisticated cell culture, could result in replacement of novel clones which are genetically still identical with regard to STR profiles, but equipped with modified features (Kasai et al. 2016). A recent comparison of experimental methods for reproducible pharmacogenomic profiling of cancer cell line panels highlighted evidence that even the amount of FBS in growth media could have an impact (Haverty et al. 2016).

An additional potential issue is associated with the use of charcoal to strip out endogenous hormones, growth factors, and cytokines from serum. Charcoal stripped FBS is commonly used to study the effects of steroid hormones in vitro, but is prone to a high lot-to-lot variability (Sikora et al. 2016). A 2005 study found that charcoal stripping of FBS unexpectedly affected the commitment of bone progenitor KS483 cells, highly stimulating adipogenesis compared to normal FBS containing medium, which drives KS483 cells to differentiate into only osteoblasts (Dang and Lowik 2005). As a conclusion, there is an unmistakable demand for chemically defined media for achieving data reliability and for overcoming the reproducibility crisis caused by FBS charges of non-definable qualities (van der Valk et al. 2010, 2018).

4.7 Privacy and Ethical Challenges of Next-Generation Sequencing (NGS) Data

Recent advancements in genomics and bioinformatics have led to vast amounts of genomic data being generated in clinical and research settings. In order to obtain a better understanding of these data and identify potential correlations between diseases and underlying genetic factors, sharing genomic data in research and clinical settings is deemed necessary. Next-generation sequencing (NGS) enables the sequencing of the entire genome and transcriptome more cost-effectively and faster than previous techniques. NGS offers possibilities to advance medical diagnostics and treatment, but also raises complicated ethical questions that need to be clarified. The use of NGS in clinical research has features that require traditional ethical frameworks to protect research participants and patients by (i) data protection, (ii) informed consent, (iii) return of results, and (iv) profit participation. Especially, NGS data contain sensitive health and non-health information about individuals and could be used for tracing family members. Therefore, the application of adequate data protection safeguards when processing genetic data for research or clinical purposes is of paramount importance.

One of the most important legal instruments for the protection of personal data in the EU is the new General Data Protection Regulation (GDPR), which entered into force in May 2016 and repealed Directive 95/46/EC with the aim of improving the effectiveness and harmonization of the protection of personal data in the EU. GDPR lays down a number of new rules: Continued use of genetic data for scientific research purposes is allowed without additional consent if the specific conditions are met. The new regulation has already raised concerns among different stakeholders about the challenges that may arise in the implementation in different countries. In particular, the proposed definition of pseudonymized data has been

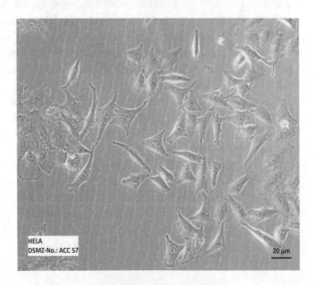

Fig. 4.1 Bright field light microscopic image of HeLa cells in culture (DSMZ ACC 057) on the right (W. G. Dirks, DSMZ).

HELA
DSMZ-No.: ACC 57   20 µm

criticized because it leaves too much room for interpretation and could affect the harmonization of data protection between countries.

To close the circle back to the HeLa story: The interest in Henrietta Lacks' cells soon became more than just a noble quest for knowledge. For example, the company *Microbiological Associates*—which became later a part of biotech giant *Life Technologies*—started out selling HeLa cells. Today, more than 17,000 US patents involve HeLa cells one way or another, and HeLa is still one of the most popular cell lines in the world. Several family members of Henrietta Lacks, the unwitting donor of the widely used HeLa cell line, say that they were never compensated for the cell line. The story of Henrietta Lacks was documented in a book *The Immortal Life of Henrietta Lacks* (Skloot 2010) and highlighted how the paucity of informed consent affected her family. In 2013, family members worked out a deal with the National Institutes of Health for the appropriate sharing of the HeLa genome with researchers. At the time, commercialization was discussed during negotiations between family Lacks and the NIH, but that science was the focus. "I was with the Lacks family as they did an interview the other day, and what they said basically was, 'Money is not our big concern in this right now.'".

References

Alston-Roberts C, Barallon R, Bauer SR, Butler J, Capes-Davis A, Dirks WG, Elmore E, Furtado M, Kerrigan L, Kline MC, Kohara A, Los GV, MacLeod RA, Masters JR, Nardone M, Nardone RM, Nims RW, Price PJ, Reid YA, Shewale J, Steuer AF, Storts DR, Sykes G, Taraporewala Z, Thomson J (2010) Cell line misidentification: the beginning of the end. Nat Rev Cancer 10(6):441–448. https://doi.org/10.1038/nrc2852

Baker M (2016) Is there a reproducibility crisis? Nature 533(7604):452–454

Barallon R, Bauer SR, Butler J et al (2010) Recommendation of short tandem repeat profiling for authenticating human cell lines, stem cells, and tissues. Vitro Cell Dev Biol Anim 46:727–732. https://doi.org/10.1007/s11626-010-9333-z

Bieback K (2013) Platelet lysate as replacement for fetal bovine serum in mesenchymal stromal cell cultures. Transfus Med Hemoth 40:326–335. https://doi.org/10.1159/000354061

Bieback K, Ha VA, Hecker A et al (2010) Altered gene expression in human adipose stem cells cultured with fetal bovine serum compared to human supplements. Tissue Eng Part A 16:3467–3484. https://doi.org/10.1089/ten.tea.2009.0727

Capes-Davis A, Neve RM (2016) Authentication: a standard problem or a problem of standards? PLoS Biol 14:e1002477. https://doi.org/10.1371/journal.pbio.1002477

Del Carpio A (2014) The good, the bad, and the HeLa - Perspectives on the world's oldest cell line. Berkley Science Review

Dang Z, Lowik C (2005) Removal of serum factors by charcoal treatment promotes adipogenesis via a MAPK-dependent pathway. Mol Cell Biochem 268:159–167. https://doi.org/10.1007/s11010-005-3857-7

Directive 2010/63/EU of the European Parliament and of the Council. Official Journal EU. https://eur-lex.europa.eu/legal-content/DE/ALL/?uri=CELEX%3A32010L0063

Dirks WG, MacLeod RA, Jäger K, Milch H, Drexler HG (1999a) First searchable database for DNA profiles of human cell lines: sequential use of fingerprint techniques for authentication. Cell Mol Biol (Noisy-le-grand) 45(6):841–53

Dirks WG, MacLeod RA, Drexler HG (1999b) ECV304 (endothelial) is really T24 (bladder carcinoma): cell line cross- contamination at source. Vitro Cell Dev Biol Anim 35(10):558–560

Drexler HG, MacLeod RAF, Uphoff CC (1999) Leukemia cell lines: In vitro models for the study of Philadelphia chromosome-positive leukemia. Leuk Res 23:207–215

Gartler SM (1968) Apparent HeLa cell contamination of human heteroploid cell lines. Nature 5130:750–751

Haverty PM, Lin E, Tan J et al (2016) Reproducible pharmacogenomic profiling of cancer cell line panels. Nature 533:333–337. https://doi.org/10.1038/nature17987

Kasai F, Hirayama N, Ozawa M et al (2016) Changes of heterogeneous cell populations in the Ishikawa cell line during long-term culture: Proposal for an in vitro clonal evolution model of tumour cells. Genomics 107:259–266. https://doi.org/10.1016/j.ygeno.2016.04.003

Lucey B, Nelson-Rees WA, Hutchins GM (2009) Henrietta Lacks, HeLa Cells, and Cell Culture Contamination. Arch Pathol Lab Med 133:1463–1467

MacLeod RA, Dirks WG, Matsuo Y, Kaufmann M, Milch H, Drexler HG (1999) Widespread intraspecies cross-contamination of human tumour cell lines arising at source. Int J Cancer 83 (4):555–563

Masters JR (2002) HeLa cells 50 years on: The good, the bad and the ugly. Nat Rev Cancer 2:315–319

Mirabelli P, Coppola L, Salvatore M (2019) Cancer Cell Lines Are Useful Model Systems for Medical Research. Cancers (Basel) 11 (8)

Pulvertaft RJV (1964) Cytology of Burkitt's Tumour (African Lymphoma). Lancet 1:238–240

Quentmeier H, Amini RM, Berglund M et al (2013) U-2932: Two clones in one cell line, a tool for the study of clonal evolution. Leukemia 27:1155–1164. https://doi.org/10.1038/leu.2012.358

Scherer WF, Syverton JT, Gey GO (1953) Studies on the propagation in vitro of poliomyelitis viruses. IV. Viral multiplication in a stable strain of human malignant epithelial cells (strain HeLa) derived from an epidermoid carcinoma of the cervix. J Exp Med 97:695–710

Sikora MJ, Johnson MD, Lee AV, Oesterreich S (2016) Endocrine response phenotypes are altered by charcoal-stripped serum variability. Endocrinology 157:3760–3766. https://doi.org/10.1210/en.2016-1297

Skloot R (2010) The immortal life of henrietta lacks. (MacMillan, ISBN 978–4000.5217–2)

Takahashi K, Sawasaki Y, Hata J-I, Mukai K, Goto T (1990) Spontaneous transformation and immortalization of human endothelial cells. Vitro Cell Dev Biol 25:263–274

Van der Valk J, Brunner D, De Smet K et al (2010) Optimization of chemically defined cell culture media—replacing fetal bovine serum in mammalian in vitro methods. Toxicol In Vitro 24, 1053–1063. https://doi.org/10.1016/j.tiv.2010.03.016

Van der Valk J, Bieback K, Buta C, Cochrane B, Dirks W, Fu J, Hickman J, Hohensee C, Kolar R, Liebsch M, Pistollato F, Schulz M, Thieme D, Weber T, Wiest J, Winkler S, Gstraunthaler G (2018) Fetal bovine serum (FBS): past—present—future. Altex 35(1):99–118

Risk-Adjusted Prevention. Perspectives on the Governance of Entitlements to Benefits in the Case of Genetic (Breast Cancer) Risks

5

Friedhelm Meier, Anke Harney, Kerstin Rhiem, Silke Neusser, Anja Neumann, Matthias Braun, Jürgen Wasem, Stefan Huster, Peter Dabrock, and Rita Katharina Schmutzler

5.1 Should People at High and Moderate Cancer Risks Be Entitled to Benefits from the Statutory Health Insurance System?

5.1.1 The Medical Perspective

5.1.1.1 Disease as a Multidimensional Concept

Phenomena of a very heterogeneous nature can be summarized under the term disease. A distinction is made between infectious diseases, degenerative diseases, systemic diseases and so on. In contrast to the pathological classification of

F. Meier (✉)
Systematic Theology II (Ethics), University of Tübingen, Liebermeisterstraße 12, 72076 Tübingen, Germany
e-mail: friedhelm.meier@uni-tuebingen.de

A. Harney · S. Huster
Medical Faculty, Institute for Social and Health Law, University of Bochum, Bochum, Germany

K. Rhiem · R. K. Schmutzler
Center for Hereditary Breast and Ovarian Cancer and Center for Integrated Oncology (CIO), University Hospital Cologne, Cologne, Germany

S. Neusser · A. Neumann · J. Wasem
Institute for Healthcare Management and Research, University of Duisburg-Essen, Essen, Germany

M. Braun · P. Dabrock
Systematic Theology II (Ethics), University of Erlangen-Nuremberg, Erlangen-Nuremberg, Germany

© Springer Nature Switzerland AG 2021
A. W. Bauer et al. (eds.), *Ethical Challenges in Cancer Diagnosis and Therapy*,
Recent Results in Cancer Research 218,
https://doi.org/10.1007/978-3-030-63749-1_5

47

diseases, there are different descriptive dimensions of disease. These can be precisely differentiated as follows:

1. *Disease*: Disease as biomedical attribution.
2. *Illness*: Illness as the experience of being ill, self-attributed.
3. *Sickness*: Sickness as a legal attribution of disease, implying an entitlement to benefit.

These dimensions are by no means always congruent with each other. For example, a patient may feel healthy despite a tumour diagnosis (*disease*) or a person may experience themselves as *ill* without having been diagnosed with a *disease*. In the first case, the person receives treatment in the form of adequate tumour therapy (*sickness*). In contrast, a person who only feels ill is not considered *sick* under social law, which is why there is no entitlement to medical treatment and reimbursement of costs by the healthcare system. A requirement for the provision of services by the statutory health insurance system is therefore the presence of a disease. Legally, a certain understanding of *disease* is assumed here. In Germany, while *disease* is not itself defined in law, the definition has been developed by jurisdiction. According to this definition, a *disease* exists if (1) an irregular physical or mental condition exists which (2) has a negative effect on the body or mental function and (3) causes a need for treatment or inability to work (BSG 35: 10–15).

5.1.1.2 The Development of Systems Medicine

The concept of *disease* as controlling benefit claims is international. However, this coupling of *sickness* and *disease* cannot adequately address the *risks of disease*. Since the decoding of the human genome in 2001, medical research has shown that, on the one hand, in the case of certain biomedical attributions, the risk of disease can be determined with increasing precision using genetic diagnostic procedures. On the other hand, preventive measures are available which can minimize risks, for example in the case of hereditary cancers.

A paradigm shift is taking place on the research side, with a strongly preventive orientation beginning to apply to classical curative medicine. This is particularly obvious in the contemporary development of systems medicine (Dabrock 2016). This type of medicine uses bioinformatic and biostatistical methods to examine anamnesis, environmental and lifestyle data in order to construct algorithmically determined *risks of disease*. With big data, risk profiling becomes more precise. Now small patient strata can be identified, enabling a *disease* to be treated as precisely as possible (Hood 2013).

Genetic diagnostics can identify carriers of pathogenic germ line mutations even before the manifestation of the disease. This opens up promising opportunities to offer risk-reduction measures to individuals at high and moderate risk of disease in order to delay or even prevent its manifestation. However, according to the guidelines defining the term *disease* in health law, pathogenic germ line mutations do not automatically classify as *disease*. The classical concept of disease cannot adequately address *risks of disease*. Consequently, persons at risks are not entitled to benefits (they are not recognized as *sick* under health law).

Against this background, the following questions arise:

1. Whether persons at high and moderate risk should be entitled to benefits for risk-reduction measures;
2. If so, how such entitlements to benefits can be adequately regulated.

This involves further questions:

3. Which groups of risk this new framework of entitlements to benefits applies to; and.
4. Which risk-reduction measures should be allocated to which risks.

5.1.1.3 The Case of Hereditary Breast Cancer

The case of hereditary breast cancer provides a concrete example for discussion of these questions. In this case, a large number of low-penetrant, moderately penetrant and highly penetrant pathogenic mutations have been researched, risk communication is profiled on the basis of many years of experience and various risk-reduction measures are available.

Pathogenic Germ Line Mutations

In Germany, there are about 70,000 new cases of breast cancer every year (Robert Koch Institut 2015). A familial clustering is found in about 30%, or about 19,000 cases (Rhiem et al. 2019). Pathogenic germ line mutations in various breast cancer risk genes can be considered for these cases. Depending on the specific risk gene, there is a different lifetime risk of developing breast cancer in women. In research and practice, three groups of risk genes are therefore known to exist. With a lifetime risk of more than 40% (odds ratio/OR > 5.0) highly penetrating pathogenic mutations in high-risk genes, such as *BRCA1/2* or *TP53*, are underlying. Lifetime risks of 21–40% (OR 1.5–5.0) are associated with the group of moderately penetrating risk genes such as *CHEK2* or *ATM*. Finally, risk genes with a lifetime risk of 11–20% (OR < 1.5), such as *TOX3* or *FGFR2*, are classified as low-penetrating risk genes. The high-risk genes *BRCA1* and *BRCA2*, which became particularly well known through the 'Jolie effect' (Evans 2014), have been identified in approximately 24% of all familial breast cancers (Kast et al. 2016). It is expected that further risk genes will be identified by research and that the interaction between individual risk genes will be more clearly defined in terms of familial cancer incidence than has been the case so far (Meindl et al. 2010; Hemminki et al. 2010; Antoniou et al. 2008; Easton et al. 2007). The categorization of risk genes as highly penetrant, moderately penetrant and low-penetrant is helpful, but imprecise against the background of the current state of medical research. This is because risk calculation takes into account as many correlating factors as possible (Kuchenbaecker et al. 2017). This becomes clear in cases where a high number of familial breast cancer cases correlates with a moderate risk gene, indicating that the risk does not depend solely on pathogenic mutation. In order to do justice to this fact, the question of benefit entitlements must not be restricted to the group of female carriers of mutations in high-risk genes. For this reason, the cumbersome but factually correct term *persons at high and moderate (breast cancer) risk* will be used in this chapter. We know that men can also be carriers of risk mutations. However, since this group is small, compared to the affected women, the following focuses solely on women.

Risk of Disease—A Multifactorial Construct
Pathogenic mutation can be understood as the basal parameter of risk assessment. However, the concept of risk would be too narrow if it were reduced to genetic factors alone. Rather, risk must be described as a multifactorial construct made up of heterogeneous factors. For example, reproductive/hormonal factors, physical activity, body weight or alcohol consumption influence the level of breast cancer risk (Nationaler Krebsplan 2012). Three areas of risk factors can be distinguished:

1. Medical data such as personal or family cancer history, age, BMI (body mass index), genetic predisposition, etc.
2. Behavioural and social factors such as physical activity, eating habits, alcohol consumption, smoking, stress, social networks, low pregnancy and birth rates, etc.
3. Environmental factors such as exposure to harmful substances, e.g., in traffic or at work.

The interaction of individual factors is statistically identified by correlations (Jones et al. 2017). It is therefore not possible to identify the proportion of risk factors in individual cases.

Identification of Persons at High and Moderate Risks: Family History and Genetic Testing
In order to identify persons at high or moderate breast cancer risk, the following criteria are used to analyze familial cancer burden (Kast et al. 2016):

- three women with breast cancer regardless of age at the onset of the disease
- two women with breast cancer, one of whom was diagnosed before the age of 51
- a woman with breast cancer and a woman with ovarian cancer
- two women with ovarian cancer
- one woman with breast cancer or ovarian cancer and one man with breast cancer
- a woman with breast cancer before the age of 36
- a woman with bilateral breast cancer whose first disease was diagnosed before the age of 51
- a woman with breast and ovarian cancer
- a woman with triple-negative breast cancer before the age of 50 (Engel et al. 2018)
- a woman with ovarian cancer before the age of 80 (Harter et al. 2017).

In the largest study of its kind in the world, the German Consortium for Hereditary Breast and Ovarian Cancer showed that if one of these criteria is met, at least 10% of mutations are detected; in the case of *BRCA1/2* mutations, the proof is as high as 24% (Kast et al. 2016; Meindl et al. 2011). Therefore, these criteria have been included in the German national recommendations as well as in the data collection forms for the certification of breast cancer and gynaecological cancer centres (S3-*Leitlinie Früherkennung* (Guidelines for Early Detection)). Provided that the familial criteria are met, genetic testing is offered (§ 3 VIII GenDG).

Consulting Situation: Divergences in Risk Assessment Between Doctors and Patients

It follows from the different dimensions of disease that there may be a significant divergence between risk assessments by patients and physicians. Studies on risk communication and risk perception initiated by the German Consortium of Hereditary Breast and Ovarian Cancer have shown that the majority of *BRCA1/2* mutation carriers who

1. overestimate their individual risk of disease (80% of those affected),
2. show pathological anxiety values, and
3. have a higher degree of irritability, stress, physical complaints and emotional behaviour, and are younger, decide on a prophylactic mastectomy (Wassermann et al. 2017).

If the overestimation of risk correlates with an invasive and irreversible measure, risk communication is especially challenging for doctors. In this respect, the close linking of medical research with the translation of current data into clinical consultations is consistent, as is the case at the German Consortium for Hereditary Breast and Ovarian Cancer's 21 university centres. In this way, genetic/risk literacy and risk communication by doctors is systematized and oriented to the current state of research.

Preventive Measures

Different options are available for persons at moderate to high breast cancer risk:

1. Carriers of high-risk or moderate-risk genes can take advantage of a risk-adjusted screening programme for breast cancer in the German Consortium's specialist centres.
2. Women with a family history, in whom no mutation has yet been detected, because the risk gene that is probably present is not yet known, are also offered this risk-adjusted screening programme (the *Boadicea* risk calculation programme). At present, five different examination algorithms have been established in the German Consortium's centres. These algorithms are adapted to the risk of breast cancer with regard to age at the start of the programme, examination intervals and diagnostic methods. As an example, for healthy *BRCA1/2* mutation carriers aged over 25, the programme includes breast ultrasound every

six months, a breast MRI scan every year and a mammography every two years between the ages of 40 and 70. Female carriers of mutations in moderate-risk genes (e.g. *CHEK2*) start with intensified surveillance at the age of 30. They receive annual examinations including mammography (starting at age 40, every two years), MRI and ultrasound of the breast up to the age of 70. Women with a statistically increased breast cancer risk but without a detected mutation can participate in the intensified surveillance programme between 30 and 50 years of age.

In addition to intensified surveillance, there are also surgical risk-reduction measures. Here, women with *BRCA1* and *BRCA2* mutations have basically two options:

3. Risk-reduction mastectomy is the most effective measure to reduce the risk of hereditary breast cancer. In the case of bilateral prophylactic mastectomy in healthy *BRCA1/2* germ line mutation carriers, the breast cancer risk is reduced to approximately 2%, depending on the surgical procedure (Lostumbo et al. 2010). According to retrospective analyses, *BRCA* mutation carriers who have undergone risk-reduction mastectomy show a high level of satisfaction with their decision (approx. 85%) due to the risk reduction (Frost et al. 2000; Lodder et al. 2001). However, 16–37% of women report having suffered surgical complications (Gahm et al. 2010) requiring additional surgical interventions (Frost et al. 2000; Zion et al. 2003). In addition to the follow-up interventions, negative effects on their own body image and sex life are felt by 23% of those affected, with 11% expressing regret regarding their decision (Zion et al. 2003). These 11% of women dissatisfied after a risk-reduction mastectomy indicate that the counselling process requires further research and development. However, it would hardly be possible to completely prevent dissatisfaction.

4. Women carrying a pathogenic mutation in an ovarian cancer risk gene (e.g. *BRCA1/2, RAD51C/D, BRIP1*) can also opt for a risk-reduction bilateral salpingo-oophorectomy (RRSO). Ovarian cancer risk will be reduced by 96%, while ovarian cancer screening is not efficient (Domcheck et al. 2010). While a previous meta-analysis (Xiao et al. 2019) demonstrated a significant reduction in breast cancer incidence after RRSO, most recent studies have failed to find a significant reduction in breast cancer risk associated with RRSO (Heemskerk-Gerritsen et al. 2015; Mavaddat et al. 2020).

5. Chemoprevention is another risk-reduction option. Treatment with an oestrogen receptor modulator such as tamoxifen or raloxifen is also considered an appropriate preventive measure. However, this option is associated with menopausal symptoms in pre-menopausal women. Other side effects of tamoxifen treatment are thrombosis, pulmonary embolism and endometrial cancer; postmenopausal women may also develop osteoporosis. In addition, anti-hormonal treatment has mainly been carried out in patients are already suffering from breast cancer. The only long-term study shows higher mortality in the group that took tamoxifen prophylactically (Cuzick et al. 2015). In

Germany, tamoxifen for breast cancer prevention is therefore only recommended in studies (King et al. 2001). However, the US Food and Drug Administration (FDA 1998) as well as the National Institute for Health and Clinical Excellence (NICE) in the UK have recommended an indication at least of tamoxifen for breast cancer risk reduction (Bevers et al. 2010; Wise 2013; Smith et al. 2016). Since the side effects of oestrogen receptor modulators in particular lead to low compliance when taken, other chemopreventive approaches are being pursued. Denusomab, an anti-RANKL antibody that inhibits RANKL might constitute such a novel preventative therapy as it can be demonstrated that RANKL inhibition suppresses tumour onset in BRCA-deficient mouse models. Therefore, an international prevention study with Denosumab in *BRCA1* mutation carriers between 25 and 55 years of age has recently been initiated (Clinical Trials for BRCA-P; Nolan et al. 2016).

5.1.1.4 Interim Conclusion

Based on the paradigmatic case of hereditary breast cancer, it is obvious that the line between the biomedical definition of disease and biomedical risks is blurred. One reason for this is that the *risk of disease* is increasingly precisely determined based on breast cancer risk genes already being researched. Therefore, further stratifications can already be made within the risk collective. In this respect, clinical measures, i.e., risk-adjusted surveillance, risk-reduction surgery and chemoprevention, that are already available require a novel concept if they are to be included within the healthcare system.

5.1.2 The Legal Perspective

In Germany, the entitlement of insured persons to benefits from the Statutory Health Insurance Fund is regulated by social law. This raises the question of how the health insurance system currently takes account of persons with a genetic breast cancer risk. It is difficult to control *risks of disease* with the concept of medical treatment (*Krankenbehandlung*), which is essentially used to define entitlement to benefits. Persons with a high and moderate risk of breast cancer tend to be considered *healthy* under social law. Risk-reduction mastectomy, for example, is consequently not a standard benefit (*sickness* status). However, since health insurers are also aware of the seriousness of the diagnosis of a pathogenic *BRCA1/2* mutation, the Medical Review Board of the Statutory Health Insurance Fund usually routinely recommends risk-reduction mastectomy based on individual case applications. This shows that the case group of female carriers of high-risk genes is being specifically addressed. Carriers of moderate-risk genes, however, are not routinely included.

If the Medical Review Board does not recommend the reimbursement of a medical service from the Health Insurance Fund in an individual case, the only option open to affected persons is legal action. However, the medical care of persons at high and moderate (breast cancer) risks cannot be adequately resolved through individual court decisions. From a medical point of view, there is not *one single* risk of disease. The *risk of disease* is a multifactorial construct (see above) comprising highly heterogeneous and therefore distinguishable entities and types of disease risks. These differences should be reflected in the legal system. If benefits are granted, the *risk of disease* must be represented in social law as a separate category from benefits for the treatment of the sick.

Court decisions in individual cases do not create a general obligation and are therefore not a suitable instrument to reflect existing differences and to create legal certainty for risk groups. However, such medical questions can hardly be clarified individually in court. People at high and moderate (breast cancer) risks represent a completely new group for the legal system. Political and parliamentary decision-making processes are involved. Should such decisions, from an institutional point of view, be left to the judicial system, public visibility and legal certainty will inevitably be lost in the focus on the individual case. The criteria according to which '*risks of disease*' are medically safeguarded necessarily remain diffuse. In the long run, therefore, separate legal regulations are needed (Huster and Harney 2016; Meier et al. 2018).

5.1.3 The Health Economics Perspective

From a health economics perspective, the question of the effect of entitlement to benefits of persons at high risk of (breast) cancer on the economic indicators of the relevant healthcare system needs to be addressed. In the case of hereditary breast cancer, on the one hand, there is the budgetary burden on health insurance entities caused by increasing demand for genetic testing, surgical interventions or intensified surveillance. On the other hand, early diagnosis or even prevention of breast and ovarian cancer may result in cost saving. A number of models have been developed internationally to analyze the cost-effectiveness of different intervention strategies in hereditary breast and ovarian cancer (Anderson et al. 2006; Balmana et al. 2004; Cott Chubiz et al. 2013; de Bock et al. 2013; Grann et al. 2011; Griffith et al. 2004; Kwon et al. 2013). However, these studies differ considerably in terms of design, target population and the intervention strategies investigated. The same applies to the German context (Schrauder et al. 2017).

In the absence of reliable results for the German context, we have investigated the budgetary impact on the German healthcare system of genetic testing and subsequent therapy in *BRCA1/2* mutation carriers (Neusser et al. 2019). Based on data from the German Consortium for Hereditary Breast and Ovarian Cancer, we developed a Markov model in the form of a cohort simulation. It analyzes a population of female relatives of hereditary breast cancer patients. Mutation carriers are offered intensified surveillance, and women with a *BRCA1* or *BRCA2* mutation can decide on risk-reduction mastectomy and/or ovariectomy. We compared two scenarios: steady demand for predictive genetic testing; and rising demand. The model contains 49 health states, starts in 2015 and runs for 10 years. Costs were evaluated based on statutory health insurance. The model demonstrated that steady demand leads to an expenditure of €49.8 million over a 10-year period. Rising demand leads to additional expenditure of €125.5 million.

The main cost driver is genetic analysis, while there are cost savings in the treatment of breast and ovarian cancer. The outcomes of rising demand for intensified surveillance are remarkable. In the rising demand scenario, a total of 104 deaths caused by breast and ovarian cancer can be avoided compared to the steady demand scenario. In addition, 181 breast and 91 ovarian carcinomas are avoided as a result of risk-reduction surgery. From the health economics perspective, therefore, it is clear that an improvement in health outcomes brings with it additional costs for the healthcare system. Societal debate should show whether these benefits justify the costs.

5.1.4   The Ethical Perspective

Based on the medical, socio-legal and health economics explanations, the social-ethical perspective asks to what extent legal integration of persons at high and moderate risk is required in order to establish fair conditions for participating in medical services. In the German healthcare system, there is currently unequal treatment. Factor V Leiden mutation carriers are entitled to benefits for their increased risk of thrombosis (Kassenärztliche Bundesvereinigung 2020). However, factor V Leiden mutation carriers, like carriers of mutations in breast cancer risk genes, do not have a manifest '*disease*', only a *risk of disease*. They are entitled to benefits on the basis of an existing *risk of disease* and are treated with heparin or phenprocoumon. Female carriers of mutations in breast cancer risk genes, especially *BRCA1/2* germ line mutation carriers, are not entitled to benefits. In this respect, comparable cases are treated unequally. Moreover, the health economics explanations have shown that alongside the additional budgetary burden, diseases and deaths can be avoided. From a social-ethical perspective, the aim is to develop criteria and standards that can guarantee active social participation, especially of vulnerable and disadvantaged persons (Dabrock 2012). In other words, not only should equal claims be treated equally, but depending on the preconditions, individuals may also need varying degrees of support to achieve recognition of their claims (Schnell 2017). Finally, the legal integration of persons at high and moderate (breast cancer) risks can make those affected truly capable of taking responsibility for their own health (Hruschka 2014).

5.1.5   Interim Conclusion

The arguments for an explicit entitlement to benefits for persons at high and moderate breast cancer risks outweigh the counter-arguments. This is because the existing unequal treatment in law, the ability to participate equally in medical treatment and a proven number of avoidable deaths outweigh the additional budgetary burden on health insurance funds in this specific case. In this respect, we believe that persons at high and moderate breast cancer risks should be legally integrated. In other cases of hereditary diseases, the extent to which analogous conditions can be found must be specifically proved, so that a corresponding conclusion can be reached. The fact that this applies not only to German social law and the German healthcare system, but also in principle to all countries with universal healthcare is a desideratum, which can only be indicated here, but not specifically proven. In our opinion, the German context stands here as *pars pro toto*. In the following we will therefore look at how entitlement to benefits for persons at high and moderate (breast cancer) risk could be adequately implemented in healthcare.

5.2 How Can the Entitlements to Benefits of Persons at High and Moderate Risk Be Regulated?

5.2.1 Medical Need

The first and fundamental question is how to justify the medical treatment needs of persons at high and moderate (breast cancer) risk. Two options are conceivable here. First, it is clear that a *risk of disease* cannot easily be assigned to the concept of illness under social law, as the criterion of *physical functional impairment* does not apply. However, this difficulty could still be overcome with the following argument. In the presence of a pathogenic mutation there is a functional disturbance in the metabolism. Although this is not noticeable externally, an abnormal function of the metabolism can be understood as a *disease* (Boorse 2012). This argument, however, results in '*disease*' being equated with '*risk of disease*'. In terms of law, the loss of the clarity of the term *disease* may be acceptable. Socially, however, this implies a comprehensive pathologization, according to which every person with a pathogenic mutation is considered *diseased*. This may, at micro level, affect the doctor–patient relationship or, at macro level, encourage additional influence from commercial stakeholders (Contino 2016).

A second possibility would be to understand the *risk of disease* not as a curative but as a need for preventive treatment. A treatment would therefore have to be borne by the healthcare system if the *risk of disease*, taking into account all modulating factors, requires intervention according to the current state of medical knowledge. This position implies that, in addition to acute care, there is also a domain of preventive medicine, controlled not by the term *disease*, but by its own coding. This coding could include entitlements to benefits for persons at high and moderate (breast cancer) risk, if the persons concerned have a detectable risk of disease requiring intervention for their specific risk collective that differs significantly from the average risk of disease of the entire population. Since in the case of a high and moderate (breast cancer) risk the assumption of a need for preventive treatment implies less problematic consequences for society than are to be feared from the assumption of a need for curative treatment (comprehensive pathologization), we use the concept of the need for preventive treatment in the following.

5.2.2 The 'Healthy Sick' Model

In order to properly develop the multidimensional question of entitlement to benefits based on an existing (breast cancer) risk, a look at the five criteria of the 'healthy sick' model is helpful (Meier et al. 2017):

1. In view of the fact that genetic risk can diverge enormously within a lifetime and that there are several preventive measures available for certain diseases that differ in their depth of intervention (e.g., from intensified surveillance to risk-reduction mastectomy), the preventive measures must be classified as *risk-sensitive and proportionate.* On the one hand, a distinction must be made between a *risk of disease* that requires intervention and one that does not. Accordingly, the *risk of disease* would require intervention if the genetic risk was of such a nature that the absence of a medical intervention would be negligent. Negligence would apply if, for example, a serious cancer or death is imminent. Here, there would be a medical necessity (Schöne-Seifert et al. 2018). Consequently, on the one hand, not everyone who belongs to the breast cancer risk group is entitled to a risk-reduction mastectomy. On the other hand, various preventive measures are available within the area of the interventional risk of a disease that requires intervention, and since the depth of these measures varies greatly, this area must be specifically differentiated. The preventive measure selected should correspond to the requirements of the respective *risk of disease.*
2. Because risk is a multifactorial construct, risk assessment is only comprehensive when other factors (including psychological and lifestyle factors) are taken into account in addition to genetic factors. Consequently, the risk assessment must be carried out in a *risk-sensitive, life-oriented* manner.
3. The quantitative recording of persons affected on the basis of collected data should correspond to a *qualitative-narrative* criterion, according to which persons affected should be given an appropriate place in the risk assessment. In this way, in the dialogue between doctor and patient space can be created for biographical-family experiences and individual patterns of interpretation in order to identify possible *obstacles to understanding* and to promote a decision process that is as reflective as possible.
4. The first three criteria outline a highly complex situation, which can only succeed if the complexity is applied in a legally *pragmatic* manner. In other words, a procedure must be found that relates the individual risk profile to general entitlement to benefits in such a way that access to preventive measures is transparent.
5. Finally, the legal integration of people at high and moderate risk must be considered in the macro context of budgetary resources. Whether the health system can bear additional costs in the event of risk of disease groups, which is

not a relief for health insurers, as in the case of inherited breast cancer, has to be negotiated for the respective group within the highly sensitive budget assessment. Without doubt, however, it is clear that these groups of people can only be considered in a *financially proportionate* manner that takes into account both the priority of curative medical therapies and the paradigm shift in medicine described above (ZEKO 2007).

5.2.3 The Problem of Existing Categories in Health Legislation

Using the five *healthy sick* model criteria and the need for preventive treatment for persons at high and moderate risk, does existing law provide entitlement to benefits for persons at high and moderate (breast cancer) risk or should new legal concepts be established?

First, we consider the categories of German social law which could prima facie regulate entitlements for persons at high and moderate (breast cancer) risk. Second, we focus on the function of the term *disease*, which, as we have seen, is essentially used to regulate access to healthcare services under German law. These considerations should also be useful for the healthcare systems of other countries such as Austria, Denmark, Great Britain and the US. It is, after all, the conditions for access to health services, not the different financing systems, that are ultimately decisive for the provision of preventive measures. Access to medical services in the countries mentioned is regulated by the concept of medical necessity, which is based first of all on the diagnosis of manifest disease (Wendt 2013, 204ff; Schöne-Seifert et al. 2018). Thus, the various healthcare systems are essentially linked to the concept of *disease* and are mainly curatively oriented (Kettner 2018), with preventive medicine playing a subordinate role.

The legal concepts of German social law cannot adequately regulate entitlement to benefits for persons at high and moderate (breast cancer) risk. For example, risk-reduction mastectomy, the most effective way of minimizing the risk of damage in the case of hereditary breast cancer, represents an intervention in healthy tissue. No legal concept exists providing for prophylactic or risk-reduction surgery. The category of *prevention or health promotion* (§ 20 SGB V) promotes only the maintenance of health by influencing environmental, social and behavioural factors. The category of *early detection of diseases* (§ 25 SGB V) includes diagnostic procedures, but no prophylactic or risk-reduction surgery. Finally, while *preventive medical care* (§ 23 para. 1 no. 3 SGB V) includes provision of medicines, bandages, remedies and aids to prevent *disease*, this concept cannot be applied to prophylactic surgery. We do not recommend extending the scope of any of these categories to include risk-reduction mastectomy, which we believe would cause the intended guiding function of this legal concept to be lost.

Preventive surgery such as risk-reduction mastectomy can only be performed on an in-patient basis. In-patient operations, however, require a diagnosis of *disease*, as this is decisive for medical treatment. Medical treatment is defined as necessary "in order to recognise a disease, to cure it, to prevent its progression or to alleviate symptoms" (§ 27 I 1 SGB V). But risk of disease cannot simply be qualified as a *disease* in terms of social law. In the case of carriers of high-risk genes for breast cancer, the *risk of disease* could logically be understood—*ultima ratio*—as a *disease* in terms of German social law if (1) the *risk of disease* is unacceptable and (2) the risk can only be minimized by means of an in-patient operation, since, according to current medical knowledge, no alternative treatment offers the same promising result (Hauck 2016).

If a pathogenic mutation in the high-risk genes *BRCA1/2* qualifies as a *disease*, then risk-reduction mastectomy, together with the necessary genetic testing and subsequent autologous or heterologous breast reconstruction, can be understood as medical treatment. In this case, the costs of these measures would be borne by the health insurers (Hauck 2016). This pragmatic solution starts from the perspective of risk-reduction services. However, since risk-reduction mastectomy is an operation and can only be carried out on an in-patient basis, carriers of mutations in such genes can only be entitled to benefits based on the concept of 'medical treatment'. This implies that *BRCA1/2* germ line mutation carriers have a need for curative treatment; a *disease* is therefore assumed in the sense of the statutory health insurance.

In other words, while there is no biomedical *disease*, a sickness status is assumed in terms of social law (Hauck 2016). However, with no fundamental regulation of this growing group of patients at risk, there remains only assessment on a case-by-case basis, an approach that fails to clarify (1) which *risks of disease* require intervention and (2) which measures are appropriate for which *risk of disease*. Court rulings on individual cases do not clarify the basic problem and create legal uncertainty. In the medium term, social law (not only in Germany) must recognize that a paradigm shift in medicine is taking place, with effective preventive measures offered to persons at high and moderate (breast cancer) risk. In the long term, the 'disease' concept guidance is fundamentally inadequate for this purpose.

5.2.4 'Risk-Adjusted Prevention'

In our opinion, there is currently no legal concept in any universal healthcare system worldwide that takes the paradigm shift in medicine seriously and thus recognizes prophylactic surgery as a benefit claim for persons at high and moderate risks. We therefore recommend the establishment of a new legal concept of *risk-adjusted prevention* in all universal healthcare systems that

1. have conditions equivalent to those of the German healthcare system discussed here,
2. take the paradigm shift in medicine seriously and assign prevention-oriented medicine to the classical curative medical model, and

3. are seriously concerned about the well-being of persons at high and moderate (breast cancer) risk.

This term is based on the term *risk-adjusted cancer screening* which is commonly used in medicine. Although the term *risk-adjusted cancer screening* implies the opportunity for targeted prevention, it emphasizes the identification of risk collectives and corresponding cancer screening tests. The term 'risk-adjusted prevention' seems appropriate for what is basically a screening programme that places more emphasis on targeted cancer prevention through effective medical measures, with the aim of establishing a social law entitlement to benefits beyond individual case decisions for groups that carry a risk requiring intervention.

5.3 Regulation of Entitlements to Benefit Based on 'risk-Adjusted Prevention' for Specific Risk Collectives

In addition to the specific case of persons at high and moderate breast cancer risk, this raises the question of which case groups should legally be entitled to benefits within risk collectives, and the criteria on which this allocation should be based. In principle, the genetic risk of these case groups must create a demand for intervention in the sense of a medical necessity, as explained above. Consequently, in making a distinction within risk collectives between risks that do and do not require intervention, the following extremes must be avoided:

1. The legal terms and conditions should not be set so high that the group of cases is ultimately limited from the outset by certain high-risk variants (*unacceptable risk*—see above). In this case, risk as a multifactorial construct would not be adequately taken into account. In the specific case of hereditary breast cancer, it has become clear that carriers of mutations even in moderate risk genes may have an explicitly high risk.
2. However, the allocation of preventive measures to the respective risk should not depend solely on subjective risk perception (*illness* factors). Subjective needs alone cannot be sufficient criteria for entitlement to benefits, especially since the divergence in the perception of breast cancer risks already indicates how difficult risk assessments can be (see above).

5.4 Allocation of Prophylactic Measures to Individual Risk

Since available preventive measures vary in their depth of intervention, a clear allocation of risks and preventive measures should be made within the group of persons by forming case groups. The following principles should be observed in the allocation of preventive measures to *disease risks* when either (1) *risk-adjusted prevention* is introduced as a new legal concept that reflects the entitlement to benefits of persons at high and moderate risk, or (2) legal regulations are established that apply to an equivalent outcome under national health law.

1. In principle, risk-sensitive and proportionate criteria must be used to make a distinction between risks requiring intervention and risks not requiring intervention.
2. Within the range of any risk requiring intervention, there must be further differentiation in accordance with the risk-sensitive and proportionate criteria, since only in this way can the various preventive measures correspond to a specific risk of disease.
3. Since risk is a multifactorial construct, as many risk factors as possible should be taken into account for precise individual risk assessment. In addition to basic genetic factors, non-genetic factors, such as *illness*, environmental and lifestyle factors, should be considered.

It follows that defining allocation criteria in legal terms for particular groups of cases is likely to be difficult. However, a debate on these criteria is only meaningful for risk collectives for which there are effective medical preventive measures. The availability of intervention measures is thus an indispensable criterion for the formation of a benefit claim for specific risk collectives. Risk collectives to which this criterion does not apply—i.e., for which there are no intervention measures such as risk-reduction surgery—should be assigned to the risk-adjusted cancer screening programmes.

The allocation procedure is illustrated graphically in Fig. 5.1

The allocation of case groups being considered in this sense must take the following criteria in particular into account:

1. The potential amount of harm indicates what harm is associated with a particular risk of disease. In the case of a pathogenic *BRCA1/2* mutation, this could be breast cancer or, ultimately, death.

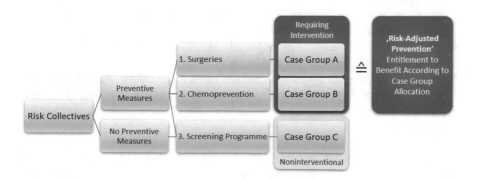

Fig. 5.1 Illustration of the concept of risk-adjusted prevention

2. The likelihood of occurrence of the harm is also generally indicated simply as *risk*. This construed value of heterogeneous factors indicates the individual probability of occurrence of the possible damage (*disease*).
3. In some groups of cases, the manifestation of a '*disease*' for which a genetic predisposition exists can be attributed to certain age groups.
4. Early diagnostic methods increase the chance of diagnosing breast cancer in an early form, for example, so that there is a good therapeutic chance of curation. However, the risks of chemotherapy may be accepted.
5. As in the case of hereditary breast cancer, preventive measures can reduce the risk of breast cancer, but at the same time involve considerable intervention risks. The benefits and risks of the measures must therefore be compared.

As a guide, the application of these five criteria is complemented by the following propositions:

1. The higher the potential harm on manifestation of the disease and the higher the probability of the occurrence of harm, the more likely it is that invasive prophylactic measures to prevent harm and the risks associated with them are required.

The reverse must apply:

2. The lower the potential harm and the probability of harm occurring, the more likely it is that (invasive) high-risk preventive measures are refused and alternative forms of prevention offered that promise a lower treatment risk.

This allocation procedure is an appropriate framework for action for the following reasons:

1. It creates legal certainty for the parties concerned by providing a clear legal framework that goes beyond individual case-law decisions.
2. It provides the flexibility to adapt the case groups based on new medical research results.
3. It is appropriate because risk profiling takes into account as many risk-modulating factors as possible.
4. Patients can independently manage their individual well-being and health irrespective of their financial circumstances.
5. It pre-empts criticism of systems medicine by categorically assigning patients to a treatment spectrum on the basis of quantitative numerical values. Qualitative components are also taken into account in the dialogue between patients and physicians.

This procedure could be implemented in the short term for well-researched *disease risks* and in the long term for less well-researched risk and disease patterns. However, these health policy recommendations cannot be more concrete, first, because the criteria for the case groups require a more comprehensive framework than is given here, and second, because more specific recommendations must be made in national health laws.

5.5 Health Policy: Two Routes for National Health Laws

Health policy recommendations for such a highly complex topic at international level are only meaningful if a concrete context is considered. In this chapter we have drawn attention to the international context at appropriate points, but it is clear that the German healthcare system as a whole cannot be transferred to other, different, national contexts. Nevertheless, medical developments and their ethical evaluation have analogous (if not equal) implications for all universal healthcare systems. This can be seen in concrete terms in the legal concept of risk-adjusted prevention and the regulations presented here.

For all universal healthcare systems that have a legal system equivalent to Germany's, we recommend the implementation of risk-adjusted prevention, as explained in this chapter. For all universal healthcare systems whose legal system is not equivalent to Germany's, we recommend taking equivalent measures to provide preventive health services, in accordance with national health legislation, to persons at high and moderate (breast cancer) risk.

Only when persons at high and moderate (breast cancer) risk are integrated into the healthcare system will the paradigm shift in medicine be adequately taken into account. The possibility of unequal treatment within legal systems will thus be eliminated and carriers of mutations in high and moderate (breast cancer) genes will be enabled to deal with their health in a responsible manner.

Acknowledgements This work was realized within the SYSKON project Re-configuration of Health and Disease. Ethical, Psychosocial, Legal and Health Economics Challenges of Systems Medicine (FKZ 01GP1407). The authors are grateful for the generous support of the German Federal Ministry of Education and Research.

References

Anderson K, Jacobson JS, Heitjan DF et al (2006) Cost-effectiveness of preventive strategies for women with a BRCA1 or a BRCA2 mutation. Ann Int Med 144:397–406. https://doi.org/10.7326/0003-4819-144-6-200603210-00006

Antoniou AC, Spurdle AB, Sinilnikova OM et al (2008) Common breast cancer predisposition alleles are associated with breast cancer risk in BRCA1 and BRCA2 mutation carriers. Am J Hum Genet 82(4):937–948. https://doi.org/10.1016/j.ajhg.2008.02.008

Balmana J, Sanz J, Bonfill X et al (2004) Genetic counseling program in familial breast cancer: analysis of its effectiveness, cost and cost-effectiveness ratio. Int J Cancer 20:112(4):647–652. https://doi.org/10.1002/ijc.20458

Bevers TB, Armstrong DK, Arun B et al (2010) Breast cancer risk reduction. J Natl Comp Canc Netw 8:1112–1146. https://doi.org/10.6004/jnccn.2015.0105

Boorse C (2012) Gesundheit als theoretischer Begriff. In: Schramme T (ed) Krankheitstheorien. Suhrkamp, Berlin, pp 63–110

BSG 35:10–15

Clinical Trials for BRCA-P. https://www.clinicaltrialsregister.eu/ctr-search/search?query=brca-p. Accessed 8 May 2020

Contino G (2016) The medicalization of health and shared responsibility. New Bioeth 22(1):45–55. https://doi.org/10.1080/20502877.2016.1151253

Cott Chubiz JE, Lee JM, Gilmore ME et al (2013) Cost-effectiveness of alternating magnetic resonance imaging and digital mammography screening in BRCA1 and BRCA2 gene mutation carriers. Cancer 119(6):1266–1276. https://doi.org/10.1002/cncr.27864

Cuzick J, Sestak I, Cawthorn S et al (2015) Tamoxifen for prevention of breast cancer: extended long-term follow-up of the IBIS-I breast cancer prevention trial. Lancet Oncol 16(1):67–75. https://doi.org/10.1016/S1470-2045(14)71171-4

Dabrock P (2012) Befähigungsgerechtigkeit. Ein Grundkonzept konkreter Ethik in fundamentaltheologischer Perspektive. Gütersloher Verlagshaus, Gütersloh

Dabrock P (2016) Soziale Folgen der Biomarker-basierten und Big-Data-getriebenen Medizin. In: Hurrelmann K, Richter M (eds) Soziologie von Gesundheit und Krankheit. Springer, Berlin, pp 287–300

de Bock GH, Vermeulen KM, Jansen L et al (2013) Which screening strategy should be offered to women with BRCA1 or BRCA2 mutations? A simulation of comparative cost-effectiveness. Br J Cancer 108(8):1579–86. https://doi.org/10.1038/bjc.2013.149

Domchek SM, Friebel TM, Singer CF et al (2010) Association of risk-reducing surgery in BRCA1 or BRCA2 mutation carriers with cancer risk and morality. JAMA 304(9):967–975. https://doi.org/10.1001/jama.2010.1237

Easton DF, Pooley KA, Dunning AM et al (2007) Genomewide association study identifies novel breast cancer susceptibility loci. Nature 447(7148):1087–1093. https://doi.org/10.1038/nature05887

Engel C, Rhiem K, Hahnen E et al (2018) Prevalence of pathogenic BRCA1/2 germline mutations among 802 women with unilateral triple-negative breast cancer without familial cancer history. BMC Cancer 18(1):265. https://doi.org/10.1186/s12885-018-4029-y

Evans DG, Barwell J, Eccles DM et al (2014) The Angelina Jolie effect: how high celebrity profile can have a major impact on provision of cancer related services. Breast Cancer Res 16(5):442. https://doi.org/10.1186/s13058-014-0442-6

FDA (1998). https://www.accessdata.fda.gov/drugsatfda_docs/appletter/1998/17970s39.pdf. Accessed 10 May 2020

Frost MH, Schaid DJ, Sellers TA et al (2000) Long-term satisfaction and psychological and social function following bilateral prophylactic mastectomy. JAMA 284(3):319–324. https://doi.org/10.1001/jama.284.3.319

Gahm J, Wickman M, Brandberg Y (2010) Bilateral prophylactic mastectomy in women with inherited risk of breast cancer–prevalence of pain and discomfort, impact on sexuality, quality of life and feelings of regret two years after surgery. Breast 19(6):462–469. https://doi.org/10.1016/j.breast.2010.05.003

Grann VR, Patel PR, Jacobson JS et al (2011) Comparative effectiveness of screening and prevention strategies among BRCA1/2-affected mutation carriers. Breast Cancer Res 125 (3):837–847. https://doi.org/10.1007/s10549-010-1043-4

Griffith GL, Edwards RT, Gray J (2004) Cancer genetics services: a systematic review of the economic evidence and issues. Br J Cancer. https://doi.org/10.1038/sj.bjc.6601792

Harter P, Hauke J, Heitz F et al (2017) Prevalence of deleterious germline variants in risk genes including BRCA1/2 in consecutive ovarian cancer patients (AGO-TR-1). PLoS One 12(10): e0186043. https://doi.org/10.1371/journal.pone.0186043

Hauck E (2016) Erkrankungsrisiko als Krankheit im Sinne der gesetzlichen Krankenversicherung? NJW 37:2695–2700s

Heemskerk-Gerritsen BAM, Seynaeve C, van Asperen CJ, et al (2015) Breast Cancer Risk After Salpingo-Oophorectomy in Healthy BRCA1/2 Mutation Carriers: Revisiting the Evidence for Risk Reduction. JNCI J Natl Cancer Inst 107(5):djv033. https://doi.org/10.1093/jnci/djv033

Hemminki K, Müller-Myshok B, Lichtner P et al (2010) Low-risk variants FGFR2, TNRC9 and LSP1 in German familial breast cancer patients. Int J Cancer. https://doi.org/10.1002/ijc.24986

Hood L (2013) Systems biology and P4 medicine: Past, present and future. Rambam Maimonides Med J 30:4(2):e0012. https://doi.org/10.5041/RMMJ.10112

Hruschka J (2014) Themenschwerpunkt: Grund und Grenzen der Solidarität in Recht und Ethik. In: Jahrbuch für Recht und Ethik 22. Duncker & Humblot, Berlin

Huster S, Harney A (2016) Anmerkung zu VG Darmstadt, Urt. v. 14.5.2015, Az.: 4 1 K 491/13. DA, MedR 367, 369

Jones ME, Schoemaker MJ, Wright LB et al (2017) Smoking and risk of breast cancer in the generations study cohort. Breast Cancer Res. https://doi.org/10.1186/s13058-017-0908-4

Kassenärztlichen Bundesvereinigung (2020) Einheitlicher Bewertungsmaßstab (EBM). https://www.kbv.de/media/sp/EBM_Gesamt___Stand_1._Quartal_2020.pdf; Accessed 10 May 2020

Kast K, Rhiem K, Wappenschmidt B et al (2016) Prevalence of BRCA1/2 germline mutations in 21 401 families with breast and ovarian cancer. J Med Genet. https://doi.org/10.1136/jmedgenet-2015-103672

Kettner M (2018) Einheit und Differenz von kurativer und wunscherfüllender Medizin. In: Ringkamp/Wittwer (ed) Was ist Medizin? Verlag Karl Alber, Freiburg/München, pp 19–41

King MC, Wieand S, Hale K et al (2001) Tamoxifen and breast cancer incidence among women with inherited mutations in BRCA1 and BRCA2: national surgical adjuvant breast and bowel project (NSABP-P1) breast cancer prevention trial. JAMA 286(18):2251–2256. https://jamanetwork.com/journals/jama/fullarticle/1108388

Krebs in Deutschland (2015) Eine gemeinsame Veröffentlichung des Robert Koch-Institut (ed) und der Gesellschaft der epidemiologischen Krebsregister in Deutschland e. V. 10. Ausgabe, 2015. https://www.krebsdaten.de/Krebs/DE/Content/Publikationen/Krebs_in_Deutschland/kid_2015/krebs_in_deutschland_2015.pdf;jsessionid=AAFA4585AE4BD2B35F2FC3351EE49072.1_cid381?__blob=publicationFile. Accessed 10 May 2020

Kuchenbaecker KB, Hopper JL, Barnes et al (2017) Genomewide association study identifies novel breast cancer susceptibility loci. Nature. risks of breast, ovarian, and contrallateral breast cancer for BRCA1 and BRCA2 mutation carriers. JAMA. https://doi.org/10.1001/jama.2017.7112

Kwon JS, Tinker A, Pansegrau G et al (2013) Prophylactic salpingectomy and delayed oophorectomy as an alternative for BRCA mutation carriers. Obstet Gynecol. https://doi.org/10.1097/AOG.0b013e3182783c2f

Leitlinienprogramm Onkologie (Deutsche Krebsgesellschaft, Deutsche Krebshilfe, AWMF): S3-Leitlinie Früherkennung, Diagnose, Therapie und Nachsorge des Mammakarzinoms, Version 4.1, 2018 AWMF Registernummer: 032-045OL, https://www.leitlinienprogramm-onkologie.de/leitlinien/mammakarzinom/. Accessed 11 May 2020

Lodder L, Frets PG, Trijsburg RW et al (2001) Psychological impact of receiving a BRCA1/BRCA2 test result. Am J Med Genet 98(1):15–24

Lostumbo L, Carbine NE, Wallace J (2010 Prophylactic mastectomy for the prevention of breast cancer. Cochrane Database. Syst Rev. https://doi.org/10.1002/14651858

Mavaddat N, Antoniou AC, Mooij TM et al (2020) Risk-reducing salpingo-oophorectomy, natural menopause, and breast cancer risk: an international prospective cohort of BRCA1 and BRCA2 mutation carriers. Breast Cancer Res 22(1):8. https://doi.org/10.1186/s13058-020-1247-4

Meier F, Ried J, Braun M et al (2017) 'Healthy sick' oder: Wie genetisches Risiko den Krankheitsbegriff des GKV-Systems aushebelt. Gesundheitswesen. https://doi.org/10.1055/s-0043-10986

Meier F Harney A, Rhiem et al (2018) 'Risikoadaptierte Prävention' . Governance Perspective für Leistungsansprüche bei genetischen (Brustkrebs-)Risiken. Springer, Wiesbaden. https://www.springer.com/de/book/9783658208004

Meindl A, Hellebrand H, Wiek C et al (2010) Germline mutations in breast and ovarian cancer pedigrees establish RAD51C as a human cancer susceptibility gene. Nat Genet 42:410–414. https://doi.org/10.1038/ng.569

Meindl A, Ditsch N, Kast K et al (2011) Hereditary breast and ovarian cancer: new genes, new treatments, new concepts. Dtsch Ärztebl 108(19):323–330. https://doi.org/10.3238/arztebl.2011.0323

Nationaler Krebsplan. Handlungsfelder, Ziele und Umsetzungsempfehlungen, Broschüre des Bundesgesundheitsministeriums, Stand 2012. https://www.bundesgesundheitsministerium.de/fileadmin/Dateien/5_Publikationen/Praevention/Broschueren/Broschuere_Nationaler_Krebsplan_-_Handlungsfelder__Ziele_und_Umsetzungsempfehlungen.pdf. Accessed 11 May 2020

Neusser S, Lux B, Barth C et al (2019) The budgetary impact of genetic testing for hereditary breast cancer for the statutory health insurance. Curr Med Res Opin 35(12):2103–2110. https://doi.org/10.1080/03007995.2019.1654689

Nolan E, Vaillant F, Branstetter D et al (2016) RANK ligand as a potential target for breast cancer prevention in BRCA1-mutation carriers. Nat Med 22(8):933–939. https://doi.org/10.1038/nm.4118

Rhiem K, Bücker-Nott HJ, Hellmich M et al (2019) Benchmarking of a checklist for the identification of familial risk for breast and ovarian cancers in a prospective cohort. Breast J 25 (3):455–460. https://doi.org/10.1111/tbj.13257

Schnell M (2017) Ethik im Zeichen vulnerabler Personen. Leiblichkeit – Endlichkeit – Nichtexklusivität. Velbrück Wissenschaft, Weilerswist

Schöne-Seifert B, Friedrich DR, Harney A et al (2018) Medizinische Notwendigkeit: Herausforderungen eines unscharfen Begriffs. Ethik Med. 325–341. https://doi.org/10.1007/s00481-018-0497-5

Schrauder MG, Brunel-Geuder L, Häberle L et al (2017) Cost-effectiveness of risk-reducing surgeries in preventing hereditary breast and ovarian cancer. Breast. https://doi.org/10.1016/j.breast.2017.02.008

Smith SG, Sestak I, Forster A et al (2016) Factors affecting uptake and adherence to breast cancer chemoprevention: a systematic review and meta-analysis. Ann Oncol. https://doi.org/10.1093/annonc/mdv590

Wassermann K, Dick J, Schmutzler RK, et al (2017) Impact of distress and personality factors on preference for preventive strategies in BRCA1/2 mutation carriers: Results of a prospective cohort study. Germany acknowledgment of research support: grant no. IIA5-2512 FSB 002 (German Federal Ministry of Health). Submitted to Cancer

Wendt C (2013) Krankenversicherung oder Gesundheitsvorsorge. Gesundheitssysteme im Vergleich. Springer, Wiesbaden

Wise J (2013) NICE recommends preventive drugs for breast cancer. BMJ. https://doi.org/10.1136/bmj.f4116

Xiao YL, Wang K, Liu Q et al (2019) Risk reduction and survival benefit of risk-reducing salpingo-oophorectomy in hereditary breast cancer: meta-analysis and systematic review. Clin Breast Cancer 19(1):e48–e65. https://doi.org/10.1016/j.clbc.2018.09.011

ZEKO Priorisierung medizinischer Leistungen im System der Gesetzlichen Krankenversicherung (GKV) Langfassung 2007. https://www.zentrale-ethikkommission.de/downloads/langfassungpriorisierung.pdf. Accessed 11 May 2020

Zion SM, Slezak JM, Sellers TA et al (2003) Reoperations after prophylactic mastectomy with or without implant reconstruction. Cancer 98(10):2152–2160. https://doi.org/10.1002/cncr.11757

The Right to Know and not to Know: Predictive Genetic Diagnosis and Non-diagnosis

6

Gunnar Duttge

6.1 Prevention Rather Than Cure

Cancer, one of the most frequent causes of death, is understandably particularly feared by the general population. At some point in their lives, 50% of people will suffer from uncontrolled, destructive growth of the body's own cells, mainly breast cancer for women and prostate cancer for men (RKI 2020). Respectable estimates suggest that the number of new cancer cases worldwide could double in the next 20 years. Medical research to develop effective therapies has long recognized the epidemiologically paramount importance of cancer. In 2019, the German Federal Ministry of Education and Research (BMBF) and the Federal Ministry of Health (BMG), together with the German Cancer Research Centre (DKFZ) and other institutions, initiated the National Decade against Cancer, which aims to further expand cancer research, but also to "further develop measures for health maintenance and prevention as well as risk-adapted early cancer detection", in particular with the help of "screening programmes and preventive examinations" (BMBF 2019). This arose from two insights. First, the survival of cancer patients has increased significantly in recent decades due to optimized chemotherapies, targeted drugs and more supportive therapies, although we remain far from the—frequently predicted—'vision zero' goal of defeating cancer as soon as possible. In some cases, the benefit of (statistically) prolonging life due to new drugs contrasts with serious side effects of drug administration. Second, the idea that the 'best medicine' is early detection and treatment of tumours long before the first symptoms appear has probably been neglected for many years in Germany. Early detection is not only

G. Duttge (✉)
Center for Medical Law, Georg-August-University Göttingen,
Platz der Göttinger Sieben 6, 37073 Göttingen, Germany
e-mail: lduttge@gwdg.de

© Springer Nature Switzerland AG 2021
A. W. Bauer et al. (eds.), *Ethical Challenges in Cancer Diagnosis and Therapy*,
Recent Results in Cancer Research 218,
https://doi.org/10.1007/978-3-030-63749-1_6

essential for successful healing but also protects the 'not yet sick' in the sense of the care required (Beauchamp and Childress 2009: 165–224).

Cancer is primarily caused by increased age, and also by exogenous factors such as lifestyle and environmental influences. However, for some of them, a genetic predisposition (so-called driver mutations) or at least genetic co-relevance significantly increases the statistical risk of cancer (Griesinger 2020; Rahner and Steinke 2008). While the determination of a person's genotype or specific genetic characteristics after a cancer diagnosis controls which 'precision' therapies are tailored to the individual patient, for certain cancers predictive diagnostics also promises the chance of the early detection of predispositions in "healthy patients" (Brand et al. 2004, 15; Zerres 2006). The response of society as a whole can be measured by the debate about the possible consequences of identifying a mutation in the *BRCA1/2* genes associated with an increased risk of breast or ovarian cancer. The desire for certainty in the sense of a negative result, which impels the decision for a genetic diagnostic analysis in the long term, is usually impossible to fulfil because reliable predictions can only rarely be made—as in the case of the dominant inherited Huntington's chorea. Several hundred mutations of these two breast cancer genes are known, but it is not known how many of these mutations are harmful or indeed how they relate to disease (Bobbert 2012, 182; Hodgson et al. 2004). In the past, the probability of disease was undoubtedly overestimated, resulting in unnecessary preventive measures with far-reaching consequences (ovariectomy or even mastectomy). The transfer of genetic knowledge, therefore, has a dominant effect here —but by no means only here—like a "dictatorship of genes" (Mieth 2001; Lemke and Liebsch 2015), and not only for the benefit of those affected.

6.2 Ambivalence of Risk Knowledge

Predictive genetic testing inherently promises to eliminate the uncertainty of the highly personal bio-existential fate by subjecting it to one's own 'precautionary' control in order to create "in times of confusion … a piece of future certainty" (Feuerstein and Kollek 2001: 26–27). This claim is utopian, if only because the informative value of predictive genetic tests is usually limited to probabilistic information. A negative result provides no absolute certainty, and even in the case of a positive result, there is only a general probability that the genetic risk position will actually manifest itself (Eißing 2015: 63). For the majority of genetically conspicuous findings, there is also a rather low correlation between genotype and phenotype (Bobbert 2012: 179–180). For example, in breast cancer diagnosis neither a positive nor a negative 'finding' can even approximately predict the future health development of the patient (Schroeder 2015: 50). However, this leaves the central question of one's own personal fate—or more precisely, the clear identification of the individual genetically determined risk of disease—unanswered; consequently "there is always the possibility that a stressful medical intervention is unnecessary" (Feuerstein and Kollek 2001: 28).

Added to this is the limited unambiguity and safety of the genetic diagnostic test procedure, the technical quality of which is never 100% specific and sensitive. In most cases, diagnosis cannot be guaranteed to capture every single characteristic carrier; as sensitivity reduces, false-negative test results are inevitable—with a consequent erroneous, fragile feeling of security. Equally serious are false-positive test results caused by reduced specificity—with potential considerable psychological and/or physical consequences for those affected. Using the example of *BRCA* mutations, the German Ethics Council has illustrated these risks of error in concrete terms as follows (Deutscher Ethikrat 2013: 54ff.). If carriers of the mutations have a statistical risk of disease of 67%, but the probability for carriers of the non-mutated alleles is only—but still—10%, then in the case of the former the expectation 'will probably fall sick' would be wrong for as much as a third of those tested, and for the latter, the opposite relieving statement ('will probably not fall sick') would be wrong in a proportion that comes close to the overall statistical risk of the female population (13%). This calls the concept of such test procedures, which in any case can never provide a reliable attestation without residual risks for the individual, fundamentally into question.

Even if, exceptionally, a high level of deterministic-causal relationship between genetic predisposition and disease (independent of environmental influences) were established, the timing and severity of the disease pattern could not regularly be predicted based on genetic diagnostic findings. It is the concrete phenotypic effect, the expressivity of the genetic abnormality, which is usually of vital importance from the perspective of the person who has to weigh up and decide for or against acquiring this knowledge or, as a doctor, make an appropriate recommendation. As a rule, for example, it is not possible to assess whether neurofibromatosis type 1 (also known as Recklinghausen's disease) is associated with barely noticeable skin changes or with severe functional impairments due to a large number of tumours (Henn 2009: 22). The risk genes identified for breast carcinoma can also trigger very different subtypes (Zylka-Menhorn 2017). Above all, however, the possibilities of genetic diagnostics are in massive imbalance with therapeutic and preventive possibilities. A rare exception is hereditary colon cancer (familial adenomatous polyposis, FAP), in which early surgical removal is usually lifesaving and allows patients to lead a relatively unaffected social life (Bobbert 2012: 183–184). In the case of many other genetic predispositions to disease, however, the practical options for action are limited once knowledge has been acquired, either by radical measures of "preventive removal" or the "intervention logic" (Barbehön and Folberth 2019: 103) inherent in diagnostics runs completely into the void (Hildt 2009: 16). Setting aside expanding one's horizons purely out of curiosity, knowledge valued primarily for its usefulness in making concrete decisions for the individual patient is inevitably lost as soon as the practical consequences of a determined predisposition appear inevitable and fateful. At the same time, the fundamental reason for these investigations becomes questionable since medical diagnostics aim to clarify the medical status quo in order to pursue traditional medical goals such as healing or alleviation (Bobbert 2012:184–185).

6.3   Psychology and Sociology of Genetic Knowledge

This is the real-world context in which the general question arises, not least concerning cancer, as to whether a predictive genetic diagnosis is always a blessing or can sometimes also be a curse (Propping 2009). Relatively extensive empirical data are available on the psychological consequences of the reporting of findings in cases of Huntington's chorea. Although the extent of catastrophic events (suicide and attempted suicide, admission to a psychiatric clinic) remain "relatively rare" (Heinrichs 2006: 131), the increased suicide risk is significant (fourfold) and it can be assumed that in at least one-third of those affected the depression that develops will require drug treatment (Renz 2011: 99–100). Surveys indicate that far fewer risk carrier candidates can be tested than previously declare their intention to do so (Renz 2011: 95; see also Rose and Novas 2000). In any case, many people seem to know or to suspect that a positive result could have a significant impact on their lifestyle. Consent to a pre-symptomatic genetic test is primarily motivated by a desire to have children ('for the sake of the child'), but may also be prompted by biographical interest regarding further life planning. The anthropologist and theologian Günter Renz states in summary that a lack of clear motivation ("getting rid of uncertainty") increases the risk of depression after testing and that basic psychological constitution and socially constructive coping ability (overcoming psychological problems) have a considerable influence on the concrete consequences of predictive genetic diagnostics (Renz 2011: 100).

Against these generalizations, however, one might object that Huntington's disease is a very specific 'sword of Damocles' scenario (Heinrichs 2006: 131). In the case of a genetic carrier, the disease is irreversibly fatal and only knows symptomatic accompanying therapies. It is obvious, however, that even beyond this, the "abolition of the unencumbered human being" (Henn 2008: 283; Maio 2012a: 258–259) from a gene-deterministic imaginary world *cum grano salis* is not without psychological consequences, even if the data are generally still deficient (Schroeder 2015: 104ff.). For the "mortgage that weighs on the life of the healthy" is now no longer merely the abstract knowledge of the general possibility of future illness; it gains "a different relationship to reality through a scientifically objectifiable diagnosis" (Feuerstein and Kollek 2001: 29). This assumption that the simple equation "knowledge equals benefit" often does not work out for those affected, is all the more plausible as the toxic effect of incriminating information is now sufficiently known from recent nocebo research (Poser 2019: 197ff.; Wojtukiewicz et al. 2019). The phenomenon of the potentially self-destructive self-fulfilling prophecy is likely to represent a serious dimension of damage, especially when it comes to the knowledge of risks of a disease that can put an abrupt end to a familiar healthy life at any time. No knowledge is reversible, no unencumbered state can be restored afterwards (Rehmann-Sutter 2019: 197ff.; Wojtukiewicz et al. 2019: 143), so that with positive findings, the disease—although only of virtual *status futurus*—is already "burned into" the real life and identity-creating self-image of the patient in the here and now (Eißing 2015: 64). But if this kind of coercive effect is an inherent element of the satisfaction of informational curiosity, in that it obscures the possibility of life-affirming self-development and shadows the future life biography in the form of "enlightened powerlessness" (Arntz 2019: 124), then clever foresight and rational "uncertainty management" can certainly lead to conscious renunciation of such 'poisoned' knowledge (Feuerstein and Kollek 2001: 33).

According to decision theory, a potentially genetically dispositional everyone has three basic options. First, they can try to eliminate the possibly agonizing uncertainty and arrange for a genetic diagnostic analysis, but must then live with the result—with or without professional support. In most cases, no complete certainty can be established and the findings (according to § 12 (1) sentence 1. 2 German Gendiagnostikgesetz (GenDG) at least for 10 years) are not absolutely protected, even in relation to third-party interests (e.g., highly capitalized life insurers, cf. § 18 (1) sentence 1 No. 2, sentence 2 GenDG). Second, the person tested can refuse to take note of the findings until further notice, but at the same time instruct that others —e.g., doctors, family members—should be informed of the findings under certain conditions. In such a case, the possibility of a prompt and immediate pathologization is averted, but not an indirect, later confrontation, since the purpose of such a procedure would be for the findings to be very much used at a later time and thus become known (presumably also to the tested person). Although current law does not explicitly identify such power of disposition, it does recognize a right of revocation after a genetic diagnosis has been carried out and—as a consequence—a right of refusal regarding the test result (§§ 8 (2), 11 (4) GenDG), as long as the notification has not yet been made. By way of an *argumentum a maiore ad minus*, the person concerned must then also be allowed to only limit the acquisition of knowledge (factually or temporally), by simultaneously granting consent in favour of accessibility for (certain) third parties in accordance with § 11 (3) GenDG (as well as Fenger 2018, § 11 marginal no. 2 and Kern 2012, § 11 GenDG marginal no. 10: limitation to "certain objectives"). But in the end, albeit with a time lag, the problem remains of how to deal with the possibly seriously burdensome findings. The third option is that genetic diagnostic analysis is decided against from the outset, so that the decision maker can keep themselves free from the possible consequences of a positive finding by maintaining the informational *status quo*.

Nonetheless, this attitude of "blissful ignorance" (Solhdju 2017: 160), which does not try to counteract natural fate, appears *prima vista* an irrational expression of "mental inertia" or even irresponsibility, because only the best possible self-knowledge and exercise of control makes it feasible for responsible people to act on their responsibility (Harris and Keywood 2001: 421; Sass 1994: 344–345). The moral appeal to the perpetual search for the "exit from self-inflicted immaturity" (Kant 1784: 481) is in modern man's self-understanding inextricably linked to acquisition of the greatest possible quantity of knowledge, which in relation to the doctor–patient relationship emphatically clarifies the central medical-ethical and legal category of informed consent as the (supposed) core of the principle of autonomy (Beauchamp and Childress 2009: 77ff., among others). The anthropological constant (Aristotle 1994, *Metaphysics* I 1: 980 a 21) undoubtedly has its fundamental justification, according to which the *conditio humana* is shaped by the pursuit of knowledge for the purpose of being able to make necessary decisions according to reasons, so that their reasonableness does not come across as chance (Kiesel 2012: 265). But the recourse to the principle of autonomy becomes fragile when the pursuit of information increasingly becomes the manifestation of an irresistible temptation (Solhdju 2018) beyond rational decision making. Given the frequently limited informative value of the test results (see above) and deficient grasp of the complex interrelationships on the part of those affected, it is no longer possible to speak of enlightened consent, even according to the general principles. In addition, there is a behaviour-controlling effect of normalization, based on the growing relevance and accessibility of the options provided by the analysis, which suggest to the individual a social, family or moral expectation to make use of them: "The more one will be able to know, the more one will be obliged to know" (Maio 2012b: 18). The 'will to know' could, therefore, thanks to the modern guiding formula of 'self-responsibility' and 'health literacy', gradually shift from the individual to the (solidarity) community (Feuerstein 2011), to which economic interests are also relevant. In a one-sided overemphasis on the opportunities of prediction and prevention (Schroeder 2015: 115; Stockter 2011: 31), with the increasing establishment of indication-independent (pre-conceptual) carrier screening ("expanded carrier screening", ECS), not much of the much prized freedom would be left. If recent technological developments and their implementation in the social world are shaped in terms of the sociology of knowledge by the logic of "more is better" (Wehling 2019: 242), then there is less and less reason to expect that those affected will still regard and advocate their non-use as a serious option.

6.4   From 'therapeutic Privilege' to the Right not to Know

The novelty of recent developments in medicine and society lies in the promotion of an independent individual's right not to know—or more precisely, to "not want to be informed" (Duttge 2010, 35), or "informational seclusion" (Taupitz 1998: 585). If the hunger for knowledge in modern scientific medicine and health care under the sign of 'big data' has increasingly assumed the significance of an absolute paradigm in society as a whole (Duttge 2016: 664–665), while at the same time the individual has to bear the structural risk of collateral damage that is not merely marginal, then the individual should themselves make decisions in the area of conflict between 'truth' and 'well-being' according to their own personal preferences. This applies all the more as the power of self-determination, particularly concerning the knowledge of genetic data, is in principle broadly and emphatically shared (Duttge 2016: 668), as shown by a representative survey by the Göttingen BMBF *Recht auf Nichtwissen* research project (www.recht-auf-nichtwissen.uni-goettingen.de; for more details on the design and methodology see Flatau and Schulze 2019: 148).

This study also found that, on an abstract level, a large majority of people were in favour of gaining knowledge about their own genetic predispositions, and surprisingly, this was independent of whether it related to curable or incurable diseases. However, differentiation shows clearly that people with higher education and/or professional experience (doctors and nurses, medical students and laypeople) reveal a much more critical evaluation and lower acceptance of genetic testing. Health care personnel, significantly, often did not give a clear answer to assessments regarding the relevance of genetic knowledge, although they were far better qualified to give a competent answer due to their knowledge base. The obvious interpretation of this response behaviour is that "these participants were better informed about the limits of genetic diagnostics" (Lenk 2019: 170). On the whole, the temptation offered by the accessibility of genetic diagnostics without a reliable understanding of its limited benefits and, above all, the new risks and uncertainties that threaten to arise from this are also impressively demonstrated empirically here (Feuerstein and Kollek 2001: 28–29). In this respect, it is clear that the development of modern medical technology urgently needs a "subversive sting in the self-image, certainties, and routines" to protect those affected. "Not wanting to know anything about one's own genetic make-up undermines the central premise and action-guiding fiction of modern societies, according to which growing (scientific) knowledge almost inevitably translates into social progress, greater prosperity, individual freedom and security" (Wehling 2019: 236).

A legally secured subjective 'right not to know', legally enforceable in the case of conflict, provides a claim to individual assessment and decision, faced with one's own genetic make-up, that is much more effective than was previously the case. Traditionally, insight into the possibility of a damaging medical explanation was only one reason for its limitation in medical law to external determination and care in the guise of what was called 'therapeutic privilege', but there was no individual power of decision. It has long been known not only that this terminology is misconceived regarding the intended protection of the patient (Schreiber 1984: 71ff.), but above all that the legal construction as such is an inexplicable anomaly in the light of patient autonomy. However, even on the occasion of the German Patients' Rights Act (*Gesetz zur Verbesserung der Rechte von Patientinnen und Patienten* of 20 February 2013, BGBl. I 277), the legislature misjudged that the concern about "informational harm" is far better off in the hands of those affected, which requires the recognition of an "informational veto right" (for an emphatic criticism of this relapse into medical paternalism, see Duttge 2014). In the field of genetic diagnostics, since the GenDG came into force on 1 February 2010 (BGBl. 2009 I 2529), this is no longer disputed, having explicitly found its formal legal effect in § 9 (2) no. 5 (within the framework of the required content of medical education prior to the performance of a genetic diagnostic examination). Rulings in the highest court also signify approval (Federal Court of Justice, judgment of 20 May 2014— VI ZR 381/13—NJW 2014, 2190, 2191; OLG Koblenz, judgment of 31 July 2013 —5 U 1427/12—MedR 2014, 168, 172 et seq.) A guarantee under international law of due respect for any wish not to obtain knowledge of health-specific information about oneself is contained in Article 10 (2) sentence 2 of the Council of Europe's Biomedicine Convention (Convention on Human Rights and Biomedicine of the Council of Europe of 4 April 1997) – although this is not legally binding in Germany due to lack of ratification. A parallel statement—also without legal force

—is contained in the UNESCO Declaration on the Protection of Genetic Data of 17 October 2003 (Art. 10 sentence 1, 3; in addition Taupitz and Guttmann 2006: 70; in detail Molnár-Gábor 2012: 715ff.).

6.5   Content and Normative Weight of a Right not to Know

Conceptually, such an individual right contains the desired (i.e., strategic and instrumental) defense against possible 'knowledge' in order to protect oneself from its possibly high psychological and social costs. It protects the opportunity to continue an unencumbered lifestyle and the freedom to decide for oneself, according to one's own personal preferences, which knowledge one wants to accept and which one does not. This enables the individual in particular "[to evade] thus the constraints of decision making and attribution of responsibility often resulting from medical knowledge" (Wehling 2015: 22). In this respect, therefore, ignorance forms the negation of the corresponding reference object of a possible transfer of knowledge, even if the negation thesis is sometimes disputed in the relationship between knowledge and ignorance (Kraft and Rott 2019: 21ff., 35). In the sociology of knowledge, the right of refusal, therefore, concerns "specified non-knowledge", which, in contrast to knowledge, is reversible at any time (Arntz 2019: 120: "Transitional stage of future knowledge"), in that the finding and acquisition of knowledge can be made up for at a later time if necessary; moreover, this is the "prototypical case of the known unknown" (Kraft and Rott 2019: 44), because the person who wants to make use of their right not to know is, not unlike in the classic renunciation of medical education (on the basic renounce ability, see e.g. Federal Court of Justice, judgment of 28 November 1972—VI ZR 133/71—NJW 1973, 556, 558; Harmann 2010; Spickhoff 2018, § 630e BGB marginal no. 11), perfectly aware that they are renouncing available, possibly socially relevant knowledge. They are doing this in order to achieve "that an epistemic *status quo* is not undermined", be it the preconceived positive conviction of the optimist or a conscious position of informational "abstinence" and distance (Kraft and Rott 2019: 43).

Current legal discourse does not dispute that there is a constitutional foundation for the autonomy-securing potency of this information-related decision-making power by each individual. It merely disputes whether such an informational 'right to be let alone' is to be located in the basic legal doctrine of the "general right of personality" (Article 2 (1) in conjunction with Article 1 (1) of the German Basic Law)—comparable with the "right to one's own image" or "right to one's own word" (Guttmann 2007: 118–119; Retzko 2006: 144ff.)—or in its specification under information law—the so-called "right to informational self-determination". The latter is partly disputed because this special guarantee of a fundamental right has so far only become known in the jurisprudence of the Federal Constitutional Court in relation to the collection and use of personal data by third parties (recognized for the first time by the so-called 'census ruling', see BVerfGE 65, 1 et seq.). On the other hand, however, it can hardly be overlooked that the protective purpose of the fundamental rights position at issue here ultimately also aims to preserve individual self-determination in specific informational terms. It, consequently, seems more convincing to assume that there is in fact a complementary side to the right to informational self-determination. The 'data sovereignty' guaranteed by this refers not to the outcome, but only to the receipt of personal (here: predictive genetic) information (Duttge 2010: 38; Duttge 2014: 83; Damm 2006: 731–732; Damm 2012: 709; Herdegen 2000: 635; Katzenmeier 2006: A-1054; Sternberg-Lieben 1987: 1246: "Basic right to genetic self-determination"; lastly as here also Di Fabio 2020, Art. 2 para. 1 Rn 192: "negative variant of the right to informational self-determination"). This is also supported by the fact that the two aspects of informational self-determination are by no means hermetically separated from one another (also Molnár-Gábor 2019: 83, 98ff.). A person who refuses a genetic diagnostic analysis also prevents the possibility of third parties eventually learning about the findings (and drawing socially relevant consequences from them, see Brownsword and Wale 2017: 3ff;). A person who fears the unauthorized transfer of data possibly does this in order also not to be constantly confronted anew with the same incriminating information (e.g., a previous crime) (the so-called 'right to be forgotten', cf. European Court of Justice, judgment of 13 May 2014—C-131/12—NJW 2014, 2257 et seq. and of 24 September 2019—C-136/17—NJW 2019, 3503 et seq. and Federal Constitutional Court, order of 6 November 2019—1 BvR 16/13—NJW 2020, 300 et seq. and of 6 November 2019—1 BvR 276/17—NJW 2020, 314 et seq.).

The constitutional dignity of the right not to know has no bearing on its value in relation to conflicting legal interests. The legal normative anchoring in Art. 2 (1) in conjunction with Article 1 (1) of the German Basic Law makes it clear, however, that it is not an absolutely protected legal authority, meaning one that is superior per se to all other concerns, because only the innermost, absolutely "inviolable core area of private life" is considered to be such (constant case law, e.g. Federal Constitutional Court, judgment of 3 March 2004—1 BvR 2378/98 and others—BVerfGE 109, 279, 313 et seq. and of 7 December 2011—2 BvR 2500/09 and others—BVerfGE 130, 1, 22). Thus, not every unintentional acquisition of information relevant to personality immediately makes the person concerned a data object in the instrumentalizing clutches of others (Fündling 2015: 148). Nevertheless, a maximum personality of the process close to human dignity is very much in question, the evaluation of which is, therefore, assigned to the personal responsibility of the individual on the basis of a freely constituted legal community, so that within the framework of the constitutionally prescribed weighing of interests a substantial relevance can be assumed. This statement is all the more significant because the prevailing constitution of society as a whole clearly reveals a cultural bias in favour of knowledge (Wehling 2009: 105; Wehling 2015: 22; Wehling 2019: 249). The desire not to know has always been, and is increasingly being, ascribed the "status of an unnatural exception requiring justification", even though, from the perspective of freedom law, these two decision-making options are in principle equivalent (Wehling 2019: 240 and 249 with the demand for "methodological symmetry"; emphatically also Wollenschläger 2013: 170–171). The fact that this bias not only has a background premise in theoretical reasoning, but also has consequences for legal practice, is demonstrated by the case law of the Federal Constitutional Court on the rights of descendants in the case of conflicting claims within a family. Here it was even doubted whether the child in question could claim a right not to know for itself in the face of the presumed father's claim to information; in any case, "a right ... that protects a possibly incorrect assumption ... would in principle carry less weight than the right to know one's ancestry, because this alone can ultimately make a lasting contribution to the man's and the child's own search for identity" (Federal Constitutional Court, judgment of 13 February 2007—1 BvR 421/05—BVerfGE 117, 202, 230).

Such paternalism, self-empowering in the cause of a postulated 'objective reason', is effectively deterred by a subjective-legal power of defense against ignorance. This is particularly obvious in the absence of third-party involvement if the objective of any information is limited to not leaving the person concerned 'in the dark' for reasons of medical care or even for the sake of their own liability risks. Numerous (international) recommendations, however, allow an exception if unconditional respect for not wanting to know prevents easily possible therapeutic defenses against serious disease. Until recently, this was also the legal situation in Switzerland (Art. 18 Abs. 2 of *Bundesgesetz über genetische Untersuchungen beim Menschen* of 8 October 2004, https://www.admin.ch/opc/de/classified-compilation/ 20011087/index.html; also Andorno 2019: 80). Remarkably, the more recent version of this law (15 June 2018) deliberately refrained from such a reservation in order to "strengthen the right of the persons concerned not to know", because imposing findings on persons capable of judgment "no longer corresponds to the principles of patients' rights applicable today" (*Botschaft zum Bundesgesetz über genetische Untersuchungen beim Menschen* of 5 July 2017, 5667). In fact, the protection of the individual against himself on the assumption of his maturity appears to be a contradiction in terms and therefore also difficult to legitimize constitutionally (which only recently prompted the Federal Constitutional Court to declare the prohibition norm against "business-like suicide assistance" a disproportionate and therefore void law, Judgment of 26 February 2020—2 BvR 2347/15 u.a.—NJW 2020, 905ff.). The problem lies in the basic assumption of a self-evident 'maturity'. If laypeople, insufficiently informed about the closer relevance of a possible positive finding to a merely statistical risk of illness, mistrust their own decision, despite all the emphatic emphasis on the right to self-determination (according to the empirical finding of the Göttingen study, see the BMBF *Recht auf Nichtwissen* project 2016; see also Duttge 2016: 668), then—especially given the continuously expanding technical possibilities of genetic diagnostics (see the contributions on next-generation sequencing in Duttge et al. 2019)—the resilience of an informational veto cannot be taken for granted. The same applies, however, to the opposite, possibly no less hastily and thoughtlessly issued declaration of consent, so that an appropriate normative response cannot lie in a general curtailment of individual law precisely where it acquires particular relevance, but only in a procedural strengthening of the potential for reflection prior to the exercise of the right of decision and its embedding in a process of ongoing revisibility (already indicated in Duttge 2016: 668).

This also applies to the specific, much discussed problem of so-called random or additional findings in the context of medical research; here, obtaining such information would be particularly contrary to expectations, unless such a contingency is already included in the clarification discussion in advance. Contrary to many a medical-ethical 'lower case' of the individual's right of decision in favour of 'medical progress', (e.g., Schmücker 2013), the Göttingen BMBF research group has therefore made the following recommendation: The test persons must be informed in particular whether and to what extent incidental findings with regard to which disease scenarios or disease risks are possible and with what probability. In this respect, the test persons are to be informed about possible consequences of such findings as well as about the fact that their disclosure may result in severe stress. The test persons must also be informed that the research study does not include any investigations with therapeutic intent, and that no conclusions about the health status of the test person can be drawn from a lack of findings. ...If the respondent does not agree in whole or in part with the disclosure of any random findings, this must be respected if the findings were the explicit subject of the previously informed refusal. This also applies if it is a treatable disease and timely therapeutic intervention could prevent serious suffering for the test person. (BMBF *Recht auf Nichtwissen* project group 2016: 403). The problem, therefore, needs to be handled appropriately by researchers and the subject status of tested persons should not be disregarded merely for the researchers' convenience.

An essential characteristic of genetic diagnostic tests is the regular involvement of genetically related persons. This causes a specific conflict of information: one person's right to knowledge after diagnosis can easily force a confrontation for the other person, leading to loss of their "genetic innocence" (Leopoldina 2010: 49). In order to balance this tension, the German Genetic Diagnostics Act (GenDG) contains an attempt at a "Solomonic compromise": if a genetic predisposition with relevance to an avoidable or treatable disease is identified, § 10 (3) sentence 4 GenDG prohibits direct contact between the human geneticist and his relatives, but it does formulate the expectation that the person examined, "should", in the course of the subsequent human genetic counselling, recommend that their relatives themselves take advantage of human genetic counselling. However, this "double recommendation solution" has something pharisaic about it, because it seeks to achieve the prescribed goal of providing "soft" information to all (genetic) family members (Damm 2011: 865), so that the initiators no longer appear responsible for this (in this sense see Duttge 2010: 36 and Duttge 2015: 86; on the lack of analogy to predispositions to incurable diseases OLG Koblenz, judgment of 31.7.2013—5 U 1427/12—MedR 2014, 168, 171: against family-related "counselling automatism" also Damm 2014: 143). In addition, granting freedom of decision to those examined tends to overburden them, as well as delegating responsibility (Heidenreich 2019: 322; Schroeder 2015: 165). In truth, however, even with such "privatization of the information conflict", the human geneticist cannot free themselves from responsibility for the imposition of the findings that has been set in motion, especially since communicating an already existing examination finding leaves any relative alarmed by the subtext of the 'recommendation' with no freedom of choice.

Equally important is their informational right of defense. Similarly to the solution in the case of chance discoveries, they would have to be asked, even before the genetic examination is carried out, whether they would also like to be informed in the event of a positive finding and their involvement; the loss of impartiality would be far less than in the case of existing findings. A possible need for secrecy on the part of the person willing to be examined would be of secondary importance because a claim to secrecy can be justifiably established in the case of a necessary involvement of others (Lindner 2007: 286, 294) (Consequently, the BMBF *Right not to know* project group grants medical personnel the right to offer information before genetic diagnostics is carried out in selected case groups ["treatable diseases" or "special solidarity obligations"], if a person willing to undergo the examination refuses it: MedR 2016: 402–403; affirmative Hahn 2019: 202; critical Wehling 2019: 246.Wehling affirms that within families "too much rather than too little genetic risk knowledge is communicated and the right of family members not to know is … marginalized"). Conversely, however, relatives would of course not have the right of veto (also Wollenschläger 2013: 184ff.), because the claim by others to the (equally important) right to knowledge falls within their freedom of action and decision.

An essential, for some even the basic problem of the right not to know per se (Taupitz 1998: 597) lies within the question of how an autonomous decision can be justified without knowledge of the relevant facts. If informed consent is a necessary condition for self-determined action, a right not to know appears almost self-contradictory. However, as the Fribourg (Switzerland) moral theologian and medical ethicist Markus Zimmermann-Acklin rightly points out, this apparent paradox refers to the presupposed concept of autonomy. As long as law and ethics are exposed to the empirical misunderstanding that the individual's autonomy or rather right of self-determination is subject to a "cognitive reservation of performance" (Baranzke 2021), a way out inevitably involving a "dilution" of the knowledge that is then indispensable ("about the possibility of knowledge": Fündling 2015: 260–261) must be sought. It remains puzzling, however, how such consent, which according to its own guiding premise is actually defective, can nevertheless be justified as a sufficient manifestation of "patient autonomy" (Duttge 2015: 88). Obviously, a more careful conceptual differentiation is needed between the autonomy status of each person as a moral/legal reason for the respectful empowerment of (every) person to self-determination, which when actually exercised by real people is to be understood far more context specifically within real-life situations remote from "cognitive one-sidedness" (Steinfath and Pindur 2013: 38). Thus, the attitude of a generally consenting person who does not to want to deal with the opportunities and risks of (predictive) genetic diagnostics from the outset (and thus also not with the "risks of not knowing") can hardly be denied the dignity of a "self-determined" decision. The Frankfurt sociologist Peter Wehling is right to insist that the right to not know can be claimed in very different ways and for very different motives – only after "informed" consideration of the available possibilities of knowledge or generally based on biographical attitude or moral conviction: "It is unfounded ... to privilege one of these practices of wanting not to know ... as the only true and self-determined form—and thus to delegitimise all others" (Wehling 2019: 239–240). This is another example of cultural bias in favour of knowledge.

6.6 Perspectives

For this reason, the legal recognition of a right not to know is only one—although an important—building block in the necessary protection of people from the temptations and constraints of a "geneticised society" (Bühl 2009: 87ff.; Oduncu 2002: 245ff.; see also Lenk/Frommeld 2019: 49, 62 f.: "freedom from stima"). On the one hand, there is the immense task of educating society as a whole about the opportunities and risks of (predictive) genetic diagnostics and, on the other hand, the no less challenging task of sensitizing medicine to the fact that the greatest risk to the self-determination of those affected lies in routinization of procedures (which is why the Swiss Centre for Technology Assessment strongly recommends "individualization" of the education and counselling procedures: TA-SWISS 2016, 339 and 349). At a time of increasing digitization using algorithms, more attention will have to be paid to this (Hahn 2019: 197ff.). All at once, the dynamics of the expansion of modern technologies, as exemplified by expanded asset carrier screenings (Wehling 2019: 241ff.), throw the danger of marginalizing very personal decision-making into sharp relief, also and especially contrary to the mainstream activities of the society as a whole. The answer to a risk of illness, which is necessarily an individual one, should also be found and given individually.

References

Andorno R (2019) Foundations and implications of the right not to know. In: Duttge G, Lenk C (eds) Das sogenannte Recht auf Nichtwissen. Normatives fundament und anwendungsprak-tische Geltungskraft. mentis, Leiden/Boston/Paderborn, pp 69–81

Aristotle (1994) Metaphysics, translated by H. Bonitz, republished by U. Wolf, Rowohlt, Reinbek

Arntz K (2019) Das Recht auf Nichtwissen im Kontext prädiktiver Medizin. Anmerkungen aus ethischer Sicht. In: Duttge G, Lenk C (eds) Das sogenannte Recht auf Nichtwissen. Normatives fundament und anwendungspraktische Geltungskraft. Mentis Verlag, Leiden, Boston, Paderborn, pp 117–129

Baranzke H (2021) Person-zentrierte Pflege als beziehungsassistierte Selbstbestimmung bei Menschen mit Demenz. Ethische Sondierungen in einem komplexen Spannungsfeld unter besonderer Berücksichtigung der professionellen stationären Langzeitpflege. In: Riedel A, Lehmeyer S (eds) Ethik im Pflege- und Gesundheitswesen. Springer

Barbehön M, Folberth A (2019) Die Temporalität der Biopolitik – Eine systemtheoretische Perspektive auf die Regierung "systemfreier Kranker." In: Gerhards H, Braun K (eds) Biopoli-tiken – Regierungen des Lebens heute. Springer, Wiesbaden, pp 97–120

Beauchamp TL, Childress JF (2009) Principles of biomedical ethics, 5th edn. Oxford University Press, New York

BMBF-Projektgruppe Recht auf Nichtwissen (2016) Empfehlungen zum anwendungspraktischen Umgang mit dem "Recht auf Nichtwissen". Medizinrecht 34:399–405

Bobbert M (2012) Krankheitsbegriff und prädiktive Gentests. In: Rothhaar M, Frewer A (eds) Das Gesunde, das Kranke und die Medizinethik. Franz Steiner Verlag, Stuttgart, pp 167–194

Brand A, Dabrock P, Paul N, Schröder P (2004) Gesundheitssicherung im Zeitalter der Genomforschung. Friedrich-Ebert-Stiftung, Berlin

Brownsword R, Wale J (2017) The right to know and the right not to know revisited. Asian Bioeth Rev 9:3–18

Bühl A (2009) Von der Eugenik zur Gattaca-Gesellschaft? In: Bühl A (ed) Auf dem Weg zur biomächtigen Gesellschaft? Verlag für Sozialwissenschaften (VS), Wiesbaden, Chancen und Risiken der Gentechnik, pp 29–96

Bundesministerium für Bildung und Forschung – BMBF (2019) Gemeinsame Erklärung. Nationale Dekade gegen Krebs 2019–2029. https://www.bmbf.de/files/2_GemeinsameErklaerung_BMBF_NDK_Pressekit_2020.pdf

Damm R (2006) Informed Consent und informationelle Selbstbestimmung in der Genmedizin. In: Kern B-R, Wadle E, Schröder K-P, Katzenmeier C (eds) Humaniora. Medizin – Recht – Geschichte. Festschrift für Adolf Laufs zum 70. Geburtstag, Springer, Berlin, Heidelberg, New York, pp 725–751

Damm R (2011) Prädiktive Gesundheitsinformationen in der modernen Medizin. Datenschutz Und Datensicherheit (DuD) 35:859–866

Damm R (2012) Prädiktive Gendiagnostik im Familienverband und Haftungsrecht. Medizinrecht (MedR) 30:705–710

Damm R (2014) Prädiktive Gendiagnostik, Familienverband und Haftungsrecht. Medizinrecht (MedR) 32:139–147

Deutscher Ethikrat (2013) Stellungnahme: Die Zukunft der genetischen Diagnostik – von der Forschung in die klinische Anwendung. Berlin

Di Fabio U (2020) Kommentierung von Art. 2 Abs. 1 GG. In: Maunz T, Dürig G et al (eds) Grundgesetz. Kommentar, Stand: 90. Erg.Lfg., Beck-Verlag, München

Duttge G (2010) Das Recht auf Nichtwissen in der Medizin. Datenschutz Und Datensicherheit 34:34–38

Duttge G (2014) Begrenzung der ärztlichen Aufklärungspflicht aus therapeutischen Gründen? Renaissance eines alten Themas im neuen Patientenrechtegesetz. In: Yamanaka K, Schorkopf F, Jehle J-M (eds) Präventive Tendenzen in Staat und Gesellschaft zwischen Sicherheit und Freiheit. Universitätsverlag Göttingen, Göttingen, pp 143–159

Duttge G (2015) Rechtlich-normative Implikationen des Rechts auf Nichtwissen in der Medizin. In: Wehling P (ed) Vom Nutzen des Nichtwissens. Sozial- und kulturwissenschaftliche Perspektiven. transcript, Bielefeld, pp 75–92

Duttge G (2016) Das Recht auf Nichtwissen in einer informationell vernetzten Gesundheitsversorgung. Medizinrecht 34:664–669

Duttge G, Sax U, Schweda M, Umbach N (2019) Next-generation medicine. Ethische, rechtliche und technologische Fragen genomischer Hochdurchsatzdaten in der klinischen Praxis. Mohr Siebeck, Tübingen

Eißing T (2015) Vorbeugen und Verhindern. Über den vereindeutigenden Umgang mit Unsicherheit bei Frauen mit einer BRCA-Mutation. In: Lemke T, Liebsch K (eds) Die Regierung der Gene. Diskriminierung und Verantwortung im Kontext genetischen Wissens. Springer, Wiesbaden, pp 57–82

Fenger H (2018) Kommentierung des § 11 GenDG. In: Spickhoff A (ed) Medizinrecht. Kommentar, 3rd edn. Beck, München

Feuerstein G (2011) Der Wille zum Wissen – der Drang zum Handeln. Zur Verschränkung von Genetik und Public Health, über den Wissensbetrag der Gesundheitsökonomie und die Kosten einer missratenen Symbiose. In: Moos T, Niewöhner J, Tanner K (eds) Genetisches Wissen. Röhrig Universitätsverlag, St. Ingbert, pp 141–176

Feuerstein G, Kollek R (2001) Vom genetischen Wissen zum sozialen Risiko: Gendiagnostik als Instrument der Biopolitik. Aus Politik Und Zeitgeschichte B 27:26–33

Flatau L, Schulze GS (2019) Zur Methodik der empirischen Begleitstudie im Rahmen des Göttinger BMBF-Projekts "Recht auf Nichtwissen." In: Duttge G, Lenk C (eds) Das sogenannte Recht auf Nichtwissen. Normatives anwendungspraktische Geltungskraft. Mentis Verlag, Leiden, Boston, Paderborn, pp 148–154

Fündling C (2015) Recht auf Wissen vs. Recht auf Nichtwissen in der Gendiagnostik. Nomos Verlagsgesellschaft, Baden-Baden

Griesinger F (2020) Genetische Tumordiagnostik – Basis für die Präzisionsmedizin. Frankfurter Allgemeine Zeitung 16 June 2020, Special Edition: Zukunft der Krebsmedizin: V6

Guttmann J (2007) Wie viel wissen darf der Staat? Die Verwendung prädiktiver Gesundheitsinformationen bei der Einstellung von Beamten. Tectum Verlag, Marburg

Hahn E (2019) Das „Recht auf Nichtwissen" des Patienten bei algorithmengesteuerter Auswertung von Big Data. Medizinrecht (MedR) 37:197–202

Harmann L (2010) Das Recht des Patienten auf Aufklärungsverzicht. Neue Juristische Online-Zeitschrift (NJOZ) 10:819–825

Harris J, Keywood K (2001) Ignorance, information and autonomy. Theor Med 22:415–436

Heidenreich KS (2019) Medizinische Zufallsbefunde in der Diagnostik und Forschung. Peter Lang, Berlin

Heinrichs B (2006) Ethische Aspekte. In: Propping P, Aretz S, Schumacher J, Taupitz J, Guttmann J, Heinrichs B (eds) Prädiktive genetische Testverfahren. Naturwissenschaftliche, rechtliche und ethische Aspekte. Karl Alber, Freiburg, München, pp 112–175

Henn W (2008) Predictive diagnosis and genetic screening: manipulation of fate? Perspect Biol Med 41:282–289

Henn W (2009) Medizinische und ethische Kategorien genetischer Information. In: Hildt E, Kovács L (eds) Was bedeutet genetische information? Walter de Gruyter, New York, pp 19–29

Herdegen M (2000) Die Erforschung des Humangenoms als Herausforderung für das Recht. Juristenzeitung (JZ) 55:633–640

Hildt E (2009) Was ist das Besondere an genetischer Information? In: Hildt E, Kovács L (eds) Was bedeutet genetische information? Walter de Gruyter, New York, pp 7–18

Hodgson SV, Morrison PJ, Irving M (2004) Breast cancer genetics: unsolved questions and open perspectives in an expanding clinical practice. Am J Med Genet (Part C) 129C:56–64

Kant I (1784) Beantwortung der Frage: Was ist Aufklärung? Berlinische Monatsschrift, pp 481–494

Katzenmeier C (2006) Mammographie-screening: Rechtsfragen weitgehend ungeklärt. Deutsches Ärzteblatt 103:A-1054–1058

Kern B-R (2012) Kommentierung des § 11 GenDG. In: Kern B-R (ed) Gendiagnostikgesetz. Kommentar. Beck, München

Kiesel J (2012) Was ist krank? Was ist gesund? Zum Diskurs über Prävention und Gesundheitsförderung. Campus Verlag, Frankfurt, New York

Kraft T, Rott H (2019) Was ist Nichtwissen? In: Duttge G, Lenk C (eds) Das sogenannte Recht auf Nichtwissen Normatives fundament und anwendungspraktische Geltungskraft. mentis Verlag, Leiden, Boston, Paderborn, pp 21–48

Lemke T, Liebsch K (eds) (2015) Die Regierung der Gene. Diskriminierung und Verantwortung im Kontext genetischen Wissens. Springer, Wiesbaden

Lenk C (2019) Normative Schlussfolgerungen aus ethischer Perspektive. In: Duttge G, Lenk C (eds) Das sogenannte Recht auf Nichtwissen. Normatives fundament und anwendungspraktische Geltungskraft. mentis Verlag, Leiden, Boston, Paderborn, pp 168–172

Lenk C, Frommeld D (2019) Ethische und soziologische Aspekte des Rechts auf Nichtwissen. In: Duttge G, Lenk C (eds) Das sogenannte Recht auf Nichtwissen. Normatives fundament und anwendungspraktische Geltungskraft. mentis Verlag, Leiden, Boston, Paderborn, pp 49–68

Leopoldina (Deutsche Akademie der Naturforscher Leopoldina) – Nationale Akademie der Wissenschaften, acatech – Deutsche Akademie der Technikwissenschaften,

Berlin-Brandenburgische Akademie der Wissenschaften (2010) Stellungnahme: Prädiktive genetische Diagnostik als Instrument der Krankheitsprävention. Berlin. https://www. leopoldina.org/uploads/tx_leopublication/201011_natEmpf_praedikative-DE.pdf

Lindner JF (2007) Grundrechtsfragen prädiktiver Gendiagnostik. Medizinrecht 25:286–295

Maio G (2012) Mittelpunkt Mensch: Ethik in der Medizin. Schattauer, Stuttgart

Maio G (2012b) Chancen und Grenzen der personalisierten Medizin – eine ethische Betrachtung. G + G Wissenschaft 12:15–19

Mieth D (2001) Die Diktatur der Gene. Biotechnik zwischen Machbarkeit und Menschenwürde. Herder, Freiburg i.Br

Molnár-Gábor F (2012) Die Herausforderung der medizinischen Entwicklung für das internationale soft law am Beispiel der Totalsequenzierung des menschlichen Genoms. Zeitschrift Für Ausländisches Öffentliches Recht Und Völkerrecht (ZaöRV) 72:695–737

Molnár-Gábor F (2019) Das Recht auf Nichtwissen. Fragen der Verrechtlichung im Kontext von Big Data in der modernen Medizin. In: Duttge G, Lenk C (eds) Das sogenannte Recht auf Nichtwissen. Normatives fundament und anwendungspraktische Geltungskraft. mentis Verlag, Leiden, Boston, Paderborn, pp 83–116

Oduncu FS (2002) Molekulare Medizin. Stimmen Der Zeit 127:245–253

Poser W (2019) Zum Noceboeffekt in Krankenbehandlung und Probanden-experiment. Kann Aufklärung schaden? In: Duttge G, Lenk C (eds) Das sogenannte Recht auf Nichtwissen. Normatives fundament und anwendungspraktische Geltungskraft. mentis, Leiden, Boston, Paderborn, pp 197–210

Propping P (2009) Genetische Krebsdiagnostik. Fluch oder Segen für die Patienten? Der Onkologe 15:1015–1020

Rahner N, Steinke V (2008) Erbliche Krebserkrankungen. Deutsches Ärzteblatt 105:A-706–713

Rehmann-Sutter C (2019) Gibt es eine Pflicht, seine Gene zu kennen? Moralische Kontextualisierung des Rechts auf Nichtwissen. In: Duttge G, Lenk C (eds) Das sogenannte Recht auf Nichtwissen. Normatives Fundament und anwendungspraktische Geltungskraft. mentis, Leiden, Boston, Paderborn, pp 131–145

Renz G (2011) Psychologische Aspekte genetischen Wissens. In: Moos T, Niewöhner J, Tanner K (eds) Genetisches Wissen. Röhrig Universitätsverlag, St. Ingbert, pp 93–114

Retzko K (2006) Prädiktive Medizin versus ein (Grund-)Recht auf Nichtwissen. Shaker, Aachen

Robert-Koch-Institut – RKI (2020) Epidemiologisches Bulletin 6/2020:3–7. https://www.rki.de/ DE/Content/Infekt/EpidBull/Archiv/2020/Ausgaben/06_20.pdf?__blob=publicationFile

Rose N, Novas C (2000) Genetic risk and the birth of the somatic individual. Econ Soc 29:485–513

Sass H-M (1994) Der Mensch im Zeitalter von genetischer Diagnostik und Manipulation. Kultur, Wissen und Verantwortung. In: Fischer EP, Geißler E (eds) Wieviel Genetik braucht der Mensch? Universitätsverlag Konstanz, pp 339–353

Schmücker R (2013) Wieviel Probandenautonomie verträgt die medizinische Forschung. In: Ach JS (ed) Grenzen der Selbstbestimmung in der Medizin. mentis, Münster, pp 209–230

Schreiber H-L (1984) Kontraindikation und Verzicht bei der ärztlichen Aufklärung aus Sicht des Juristen. In: Heim W (ed) Ärztliche Aufklärungspflicht. Deutscher Ärzteverlag, Köln, pp 71–79

Schroeder A (2015) Das Recht auf Nichtwissen im Kontext prädiktiver Gendiagnostik. Springer, Wiesbaden

Solhdju K (2017) Rätselhafte Zukunft. Medizinische Prädiktionen zwischen Wissen und Nichtwissen. In: Friedrich A, Gehring P, Hubig C, Kaminski A, Nordmann A (eds) Technisches Nichtwissen (Jahrbuch Technikphilosophie, 3rd edn). Nomos Verlagsgesellschaft, Baden-Baden, pp 147–168

Solhdju K (2018) Die Versuchung des Wissens. Vorschläge für einen gemeinschaftlichen Umgang mit prädiktiver Gen-Diagnostik. transcript Verlag, Bielefeld

Spickhoff A (2018) Kommentierung des § 630e BGB. In: Spickhoff A (ed.) Medizinrecht. Kommentar. 3rd edn, Beck, München

Steinfath H, Pindur A-M (2013) Patientenautonomie im Spannungsfeld philosophischer Konzeptionen von Autonomie. In: Wiesemann C, Simon A (eds) Patientenautonomie. Theoretische Grundlagen – Praktische Anwendungen. mentis, Münster, pp 27–41

Sternberg-Lieben D (1987) "Genetischer Fingerabdruck" und § 81a StPO. Neue Juristische Wochenschrift (NJW) 40:1242–1247

Stockter U (2011) Wissen als Option, nicht als Obliegenheit – Aufklärung, Einwilligung und Datenschutz in der Gendiagnostik. In: Duttge G, Engel W, Zoll B (eds) Das Gendiagnostikgesetz im Spannungsfeld von Humangenetik und Recht. Göttinger Universitätsverlag, Göttingen, pp 27–51

Swiss Centre for Technology Assessment (TA-SWISS): Brauer S, Strub J-D, Zimmermann M et al (eds) Wissen können, dürfen, wollen? Genetische Untersuchungen während der Schwangerschaft (TA-SWISS 63/2016). Vdf Hochschulverlag, Zürich

Taupitz J (1998) Das Recht auf Nichtwissen. In: Hanau P, Lorenz E, Matthes H (eds) Festschrift für Günther Wiese zum 70. Geburtstag, Luchterhand, Neuwied/Kriftel, pp 583–602

Taupitz J, Guttmann J (2006) Rechtliche Aspekte. In: Propping P, Aretz S, Schumacher J, Taupitz J, Guttmann J, Heinrichs B (eds) Prädiktive genetische Testverfahren. Naturwissenschaftliche, rechtliche und ethische Aspekte. Karl Alber, Freiburg, München, pp 59–110

Wehling P (2009) Nichtwissen: Bestimmungen, Abgrenzungen, Bewertungen. Erwägen – Wissen – Ethik (EWE – Streitforum für Erwägungskultur) 20:95–106

Wehling P (2015) Vom Nutzen des Nichtwissens, vom Nachteil des Wissens. In: Wehling P (ed) Vom Nutzen des Nichtwissens. Sozial- und kulturwissenschaftliche Perspektiven. transcript, Bielefeld, pp 9–50

Wehling P (2019) Die letzte Rettung? Das Recht auf Nichtwissen in Zeiten von Anlageträger-Screening und Genom-Sequenzierung. In: Duttge G, Lenk C (eds) Das sogenannte Recht auf Nichtwissen. Normatives Fundament und anwendungspraktische Geltungskraft. mentis, Leiden, Boston, Paderborn, pp 233–251

Wollenschläger F (2013) Der Drittbezug prädiktiver Gendiagnostik im Spannungsfeld der Grundrechte auf Wissen, Nichtwissen und Geheimhaltung. Krankheitsveranlagung im Familienverbund und das neue Gendiagnostikgesetz. Archiv Des Öffentlichen Rechts (AöR) 138:161–203

Wojtukiewicz MZ, Politynska B, Skalij P, Tokajuk P, Wojtukiewicz AM, Honn KV (2019) It is not just the drugs that matter: the nocebo effect. Cancer Metas Rev 38:315–326

Zerres K (2006) Prädiktive Medizin: Der gesunde Kranke. In: Schumpelick V, Vogel B (eds) Arzt und patient. Eine Beziehung im Wandel. Herder, Freiburg, pp 554–564

Zimmermann-Acklin M (2002) Ethische Überlegungen zur genetischen Diagnostik an kranken Menschen. Zeitschrift Für Medizinische Ethik (ZfmE) 48:369–381

Zylka-Menhorn V (2017) Wie neue Brustkrebsgene zu bewerten sind. Deutsches Ärzteblatt 114: A-894–895

Harms and Benefits of Cancer Screening

7

Bernt-Peter Robra

7.1 Introduction

7.1.1 Early Detection: Clinical Narrative and Public Health Evidence

Clinical practitioners worry about patients with final-stage cancer whom they can only attend to palliatively. On the other hand, they see patients with localized cancer who have been treated successfully and survived for many years without recurrence. Given the (by definition) progressive tendency of malignant growth and the iceberg model (Kramer and Croswell 2009) of as yet symptomless disease in a detectable pre-clinical phase, they join the dots to derive a potent narrative: early detection of cancer protects against late-stage suffering and cancer death. Generalizing normatively, health systems must provide early detection measures. The higher the attendance rate and the higher the number of small cancers detected, the better.

The general public understands this elementary tactic of early detection directed against a dreaded disease. However, clinical experience is flawed by selection biases (selective attendance, preferential detection of slow-growing lesions), lead time (i.e., the time it takes for the diagnosis to be brought forward by screening), and overdiagnosis (see below). Therefore detection rates, a stage shift and a higher proportion of patients surviving for five years are inappropriate measures of the harms and benefits of screening and insufficient for both policy making and individual counselling (Cole and Morrison 1980; Morrison 1982).

B.-P. Robra (✉)
Institute for Social Medicine and Health Services Research, Otto-von-Guericke-University Magdeburg, Leipziger Str. 44, D-39140 Magdeburg, Germany
e-mail: bernt-peter.robra@med.ovgu.de

© Springer Nature Switzerland AG 2021
A. W. Bauer et al. (eds.), *Ethical Challenges in Cancer Diagnosis and Therapy*,
Recent Results in Cancer Research 218,
https://doi.org/10.1007/978-3-030-63749-1_7

The clinical model was consequently replaced by a paradigm of public health and evidence-based medicine (avant la lettre). This posits that early detection is at best an intermediate step and that the efficacy of early intervention must be demonstrated by evidence of benefit in terms of improved outcomes. In their landmark publication *Principles and Practice of Screening for Disease*, Wilson und Jungner stress the importance of prognosis: "…it is clearly vital to determine by experimental surveys whether a better prognosis is given by treating the conditions found at an earlier stage than was previously the practice" (Wilson and Jungner 1968: 27–28). The appropriate experimental methodology is the RCT to be analyzed on the basis of intention to screen (Feinleib and Zelen 1969).

7.1.2 Screening—A Health Claim

The following definition of screening underscores the outcome orientation:

> Medical screening is the systematic application of a test or inquiry to identify individuals at sufficient risk of a specific disorder to benefit from further investigation or direct preventive action (these individuals not having sought medical attention on account of symptoms of that disorder). Key to this definition is that the early detection of disease is not an end in itself; bringing forward a diagnosis without altering the prognosis is useless and may be harmful. (Wald and Law 2015)

The definition does not explicitly state that benefits must outweigh harms, which is a minimum requirement for medical intervention. It also misses out a second ethical point. Screening is a service induced by the physician or the health system. In offering screening, they are making a health claim ('it's good for you') direct to 'consumers' who would not (at the moment) seek medical care. Hence the relation of the physician to (presumptive) screening participants differs from their relation to patients asking for advice or relief. This position of the physician is a major distinction between screening and other forms of medical practice (McKeown 1976). In ethical terms, making a health claim requires that the screening programme offered must be presented with all expected harms and benefits accurately and clearly to the target population at large and to specific individuals considering participation.

This chapter considers the ethical aspects of planning, communicating and evaluating cancer screening programmes. It examines the process of establishing the case for screening, building a service programme, monitoring its operation, maintaining its quality and integrating it with medical progress. In this dynamic process, the harms and benefits of a particular screening modality are shaped and managed by decision makers, which precludes any one-dimensional aggregation of harms and benefits.

7.2 Efficacy—Screening Trials

Screening is a complex technology, more than just the application of a test. Efficacy studies are controlled trials to test the incremental effect of offering a defined screening strategy vs. usual care. In 1963, the Health Insurance Plan of Greater New York (HIP) started a randomized trial on breast cancer screening. 31,000 women aged 40–64 years in the intervention group (IG) were offered annual mammography and physical breast examination; 31,000 women in the control group (CG) followed their usual care. 65% of the invited group attended for the first round. Interim results (Shapiro et al. 1971) counted 246 breast cancer cases in the IG (of which 127 were detected due to screening) and 199 in the CG (+23.6%). With 31 breast cancer deaths in the IG versus 52 in the CG the investigators saw "grounds for cautious optimism". The impressive relative mortality reduction of 40%, however, corresponds to a less impressive 1.4 deaths avoided per 10,000 person-years of observation (more for those attending). Framed the other way, specific mortality over one year does not change for 9998.6 out of 10,000 women invited. 624 breast biopsies were performed based on screening findings, of which 127 resulted in histologically confirmed breast cancers. 497 negative biopsies are iatrogenic harms: 4 per additional cancer detected and 24 per breast cancer death avoided.

Efficacy trials are conducted under the assumption of equipoise—does the intervention work in principle? *Ex ante* no certain benefit can be promised to participants. With informed consent they donate their health and time to a scientific endeavour. This is no longer the case in service-level screening.

The primary outcome of an efficacy trial is the reduction of cause-specific mortality from the target cancer. This is considered a 'hard' outcome if deaths are completely ascertained and the cause of death reliably classified. Cervical and colorectal screening can also reduce cancer incidence, an additional benefit. All-cause mortality, however, is not seen as a primary outcome because target lesions are rare, even efficacious screening intervention only partly reduces cause-specific mortality and competing causes of death can result in total mortality trends quite unrelated to screening. In fact, no cancer screening trial so far has demonstrated a reduction in total mortality, and only a small decline can be expected (Heijnsdijk et al. 2019; Prasad et al. 2016). Even efficacious cancer screening would not be a matter of urgency to individuals at average risk, a point that is rarely stressed in the public discourse.

Additional information useful for understanding the 'mechanism' of screening, building preferences and later extending the efficacy study to full service screening can be collected in trials: determinants of the attendance rate, detection rates by age or other population characteristics, frequency and determinants of false-positive cases or the costs of operating the trial screening service. If the trial population is followed closely (e.g., by means of a cancer registry), the frequency and biological properties of interval cancers detected between screening rounds will be ascertained, some of which will be shown to have been overlooked. Composite indicators can be derived, such as the number of participants needed to screen in order to detect one case, the number of cancers detected through a positive screening result (e.g., a biopsy recommendation), the number needed to screen or to biopsy in order to avoid one specific cancer death or to save one life year in a defined period of time. Costs can be allocated similarly. As screening is applied repetitively, the first screening round (prevalence round) will be compared to subsequent screening rounds when the pool of easily detectable pre-clinical cases has already been exhausted and only the smaller number of newly surfacing cases are detectable and managed (incidence rounds). After several years of follow-up, the cancer incidence and mortality trajectories in the intervention and control groups can be compared, taking account of losses to follow-up and unequal person times of observation.

After the screening test and the diagnostic work-up the screenee will be in one of the four cells of Table 7.1. The probabilities of being screened into one of the four states are a function of the point prevalence of the target lesion in the detectable pre-clinical phase (Pr) and the validity of the screening test. Pr is typically very low. Screenees with a negative screening test will not normally be worked up diagnostically. But sensitivity can be estimated in special studies or by means of interval cases arising between screening rounds. Specificity can be estimated with low bias and error margins from the proportion of screen positive cases and the detection rate (Brecht and Robra 1987).

The probabilities of the respective health states then need to be given values (utility or preference weights, $NU_{T.D.}$) by the relevant decision maker, which may be, for example, a regulatory agency, a medical association, a health insurance fund or the individual screenee. Screening tests per se may not be very invasive, such as the faecal occult blood test or the PSA test. But screening mammography is associated with a dose of radiation and screening colonoscopy is usually carried out with sedation and carries a small iatrogenic risk of perforation (Mansmann et al. 2008). In order for screening to be acceptable, $NU_{T_+ D_+}$ must obviously be assessed as positive, i.e., early detection with its sequelae of early treatment effects (such as life years gained) minus test application, cancers over-diagnosed and overtreated and other side effects of early intervention such as loss of quality of life due to lead

Table 7.1 Expected utility of screening—result of the screening test, presence or absence of the target lesion and net utility of the four possible states

		Target lesion	
		Yes	No
Test	Positive	$Pr \cdot Se \cdot NU_{T_+ D_+}$	$(1 - Pr) \cdot (1 - Sp) \cdot NU_{T_+ D_-}$
	Negative	$Pr \cdot (1 - Se) \cdot NU_{T_- D_+}$	$(1 - Pr) \cdot Sp \cdot NU_{T_- D_-}$

Source Adapted from Robra and Schmacke (2019)
Pr is the point prevalence of the target lesion in the detectable pre-clinical phase, or the a priori risk of disease of an individual screening participant; *Se* sensitivity and *Sp* specificity are parameters of test validity; *NU* stands for net utility or value of the four states and is indexed by subscripts: D_+ and D_- indicate the true state of the target lesion or disease, T_+ and T_- indicate the test result

time. $NU_{T_+D_-}$, the value of false-positive test outcomes, will be negative. It includes consequences such as invasive biopsies, anxiety (Brewer et al. 2007; Brodersen and Siersma 2013) or delay in obtaining subsequent screening (Dabbous et al. 2017). A negative diagnosis following a positive test is often greeted with relief, but false alarm is a harm to the individual it affects. False-negative tests miss the stated objective of early detection (the health claim); they may lead to false reassurance with a delay in diagnosing symptoms. Hence, $NU_{T_-D_+}$ is negative. $NU_{T_-D_-}$ will also be negative, as futile efforts have been undertaken and the reassurance value of being 'confirmed cancer free' is at best minute because the probability $(1-Pr)$ is very high a priori (see the example of the HIP study discussed above). In repetitive screening, the table will include more states. But the first screening is the one that matters most.

The overall value of screening, the balance of harms and benefits, is the sum of the four cells. Risk-based screening (via age brackets, intervals, risk markers) will modify Pr. Quality assurance measures will safeguard Se and Sp. The preferences of the decision makers determine the net utilities or values (Kelly et al. 2015) attributed to the four states. Though $NU_{T_+D_+}$ may be high, this state is a rare event. The sum of all cells may nevertheless well be negative. Hence all harms and benefits must be presented in such a way that each relevant decision maker can set up their own multi-attribute assessment. While economists and epidemiologists struggle to base health-state valuation (Dolan et al. 2005; Dolan and Edlin 2002; Dolan and Kahneman 2008) and preference building for complex scenarios (Fagerlin et al. 2013; Ghanouni et al. 2013; Pignone et al. 2013) on stringent methodology, it is unlikely that different decision makers will give the same weight to all outcomes. NUs will have distributions which can hardly be simplified to aggregate parameters such as QALYs. On the other hand, decisions in individual health care do balance health states that are incommensurable on a daily basis, for example, the probabilistic benefits of anticoagulation in reducing the risk of cardiac events at the cost of an increased risk of cerebral bleeding.

The most important harm caused by screening is overdiagnosis (Gøtzsche and Jørgensen 2011; Independent UK Panel on Breast Cancer Screening 2012). Overdiagnosis means that a cancer detected by screening would not have become clinically relevant during the remaining lifetime of the individual. Overdiagnosis was first mentioned in association with cervical pathology (Spriggs and Boddington 1980) and mammography (Lundgren and Helleberg 1982). Overdiagnosis is a function of tumour biology (growth rate), sensitivity and the patient's competing all-cause mortality risk (Welch and Black 2010). It is an epidemiological concept which can be quantified in controlled studies that compare incidence and mortality with and without screening over many years. Clinicians and pathologists cannot possibly assess overdiagnosis: they see and (over-)treat a case of cancer. The term *pseudodisease* (e.g., Kramer and Croswell 2009) is thus misleading.

The Canadian Task Force on Preventive Health Care provides estimates of overdiagnosis (see Table 7.2).

Table 7.2 Proportion of breast cancers over-diagnosed from screening by age at initial screen, time since first screening, and stage (estimated by Canadian Task Force on Preventive Health Care)

Age of women at initial screen (years)	Breast cancers estimated as over-diagnosed (%)[a]		
	Years after screening	Invasive and in situ cancers (%)	Invasive cancers (%)
40–49	5	41	32
	20	55	48
50–59	5	25	16
	20	16	5

Source Klarenbach et al. (2018); data on age groups 60+ not provided
[a]Overdiagnosis by age was estimated using the following calculation: the numerator is the difference in numbers of cancers in the mammography arm less those in the control arm; and the denominator is the number of screen-detected cancers in the mammography arm. Only the findings from the estimate on overdiagnosis from a Canadian randomized controlled trial are included because it provided an estimate by age and was appraised as being at moderate risk of bias

The Independent UK Panel on Breast Cancer Screening framed overdiagnosis differently: "Therefore, for every breast cancer death prevented, about three over-diagnosed cases will be identified and treated. Of the approximately 307,000 women aged 50–52 years who are invited to screening every year, just over 1% would have an overdiagnosed cancer during the next 20 years. In view of the uncertainties that surround the estimates, the figures cited give a false impression of accuracy" (Independent UK Panel on Breast Cancer Screening 2012). There are more favourable estimates (EUROSCREEN Working Group 2012) and a continuing methodological debate (Carter et al. 2015; Etzioni et al. 2013; Jørgensen et al. 2017), but relations in this order of magnitude are clearly not negligible. The proportion of over-diagnosed cancers in all screen-detected cancers is relatively high in prostate cancer screening and also not negligible in colorectal cancer screening (Brenner et al. 2015; Draisma et al. 2009; Gulati et al. 2014).

The epidemiologic concept of overdiagnosis in screening should not be confused with false-positive screening test results, a problem of specificity and quality assurance (e.g., Carlsson et al. 2016), nor with disease mongering in terms of widening definitions of disease (Moynihan et al. 2012). Clearly, the rate of screen-detected cancers (i.e., the clinical perspective) by far overestimates the likelihood that an individual with screen-detected cancer has their life saved by that screening (Welch and Frankel 2011). In ethical terms, overdiagnosis violates the principle of non-maleficence.

Heleno et al. (2013) assessed how often harm was specified in randomized trials of cancer screening. Of 57 cancer screening trials examined, the most important harms of screening—overdiagnosis and false-positive findings—were quantified in only four and two trials, respectively.

7.3 Effectiveness—Screening Programmes

The step from screening trial to service screening programme requires the relevant decision maker to assess the evidence, establish a case for action and issue a policy recommendation or regulations according to their allocation standards. According to the European Commission (European Commission 2017: 14): "To qualify as a programme there should be a public screening policy documented in a law, or an official regulation, decision, directive or recommendation. The policy should define, as a minimum, the screening test, the examination intervals and the group of persons eligible to be screened; and the screening examinations should be financed by public sources (apart from a possible co-payment)."

The illustrative data in Table 7.3 was prepared from the results of between two and eight (depending on age) screening trials for the 2018 Canadian recommendations for breast cancer screening in women not at increased risk of breast cancer (Klarenbach et al. 2018).

Table 7.3 Breast cancer mortality, absolute effect of screening using mammography with or without clinical breast examination, false positives and unnecessary biopsies from an estimated cohort of women in a breast screening programme for 7 years of screening

	Age range (years)			
	40–49	50–59	60–69	70–74
Women who are not screened: risk of dying of breast cancer per 1000	3.85	5.00	6.15	10.31
Women who are screened: risk of dying from breast cancer, absolute effect per 1000 screened for a median of 7 years (95% CI)	0.58 fewer (0.27–0.85)	0.75 fewer (0.35–1.10)	0.92 fewer (0.43–1.35)	1.55 fewer (0.72–2.27)
Number needed to screen (NNS) to prevent 1 death from breast cancer (95% CI)	1724 (1176–3704)	1333 (909–2857)	1087 (741–2326)	645 (441–1389)
GRADE rating of certainty of evidence	Low	Very low	Low	Very low
FP mammography per 1000 women screened	294	294	256	219
Biopsies on FP per 1000 women screened	43	37	35	30
FP mammography per 1 breast cancer death prevented (based on 3 cycles of screening)[a]	508	392 (M)	278	141
Biopsies on FP per 1 breast cancer death prevented (based on 3 cycles of screening)[a]	74	50 (M)	38	19

Source Klarenbach et al. (2018, Tables 1 and 3 condensed); see original for further annotations
Notes (i) the median duration of screening trials was 7 years (range 3–12 years) and the impact of this duration of screening on benefits and harms was used; (ii) the data are used to approximate a cohort of women entering the screening programme; (iii) the proportion of cancers over-diagnosed must also be considered (see Table 7.2)
FP = false positive, *M* = calculated using the moderate baseline risk for this age group
[a]Three cycles of screening for which women are screened every 2–3 years, for a total of 6–9 years of a screening period. Calculation: Initial screening cycle + 2 (subsequent screening cycle) to estimate harms occurring with 7 years of screening

Available screening recommendations or regulations differ depending on the evidence base considered (RCTs, observational studies), the scope of harms and benefits taken into account, and the respective weights given to them. This methodological challenge is shared with other medical practice guidelines (Brawley et al. 2011; Elmore and Lee 2019; Jørgensen et al. 2017; Qaseem et al. 2012b, 2019a, b).

More consequential than guidelines are the screening programmes operational at the service level. In a policy document unanimously adopted by the Health Ministers of the European Union (The Council of the European Union 2003) the Council asserts (respective text numbers):

(8) Evidence exists concerning the efficacy of screening for breast cancer and colorectal cancer, derived from randomized trials, and for cervical cancer, derived from observational studies. (9) Screening is, however, the testing for diseases of people for which no symptoms have been detected. In addition to its beneficial effect on the disease-specific mortality, screening can also have negative side effects for the screened population. Healthcare providers should be aware of all the potential benefits and risks of screening for a given cancer site before embarking on new population-based cancer screening programmes. Furthermore, for the informed public of today, these benefits and risks need to be presented in a way that allows individual citizens to decide on participation in the screening programmes for themselves. (10) Ethical, legal, social, medical, organizational and economic aspects have to be considered before decisions can be made on the implementation of cancer screening programmes.

The Council recommends that member states "offer evidence-based cancer screening through a systematic population-based approach with quality assurance at all appropriate levels" for three target lesions—cervical cancer precursors, breast cancer and colorectal cancer—based, respectively, on pap smears starting not before the age of 20 and not later than the age of 30, mammography for women aged 50–69 and faecal occult blood screening in men and women aged 50–74. This Council document can be seen as a turning point from efficacy assessment to organized service screening aimed at population-level effectiveness and autonomy for the three target cancers mentioned. Evidence in favour of screening for other cancers was considered insufficient at that time.

Table 7.4 summarizes structural characteristics of screening programmes in the EU28 (European Commission 2017). They are heterogeneous despite a common evidence base and high-level political consensus. They also achieve heterogeneous examination and detection rates. The health prospects of European citizens therefore differ. On the other hand, a common system of reporting and evaluation is in place and guidelines continue to be updated in a methodological way (Anttila et al. 2015; Schünemann et al. 2019a, b).

Public choice can and must be well-informed choice, with decision makers committed to the common weal and free from conflicts of interest (Rasmussen et al. 2013). Heterogeneity in screening programmes does not (necessarily) signal a deficit in policy making if the relevant decision makers—in revealing their public preferences or values—follow public health ethics procedures (Childress et al. 2002). In accordance with the context and scope of their responsibility, the relevant

Table 7.4 Service screening in the European Union EU28 (up to 2016)

	Recommended age range (years)	Lower age limit	Upper age limit	Interval (years)
Breast cancer screening	50–69	40–50	64–74	1.5–3
Cervical cancer screening[a]	25 or 30–64 or 69	20–30	59–70	3–5
Colorectal cancer screening[b]	50–74	40–50	74–80	gFOBT, FIT: 1–2; endoscopy: once in a lifetime, 5–10

Source Collated from European Commission (2017), Tables 3.1.1, 4.7, 4.14.1 and 7.1
[a]HPV test as the primary screening test by some programmes (as stand-alone screening test or co-testing with cytology); in non-population-based cytology testing the screening interval was often much shorter than the recommend interval of 3 or 5 years
[b]Most EU member states are adopting narrower age ranges than 50–74, based on cost-effectiveness considerations and availability of resources

decision makers will try to minimize harms, maximize beneficial effects, and provide a sustainable infrastructure with efficient programme operation and transparent documentation and monitoring. Data from international controlled trials need to be amalgamated with regional risk distributions, resources and competing public health priorities (opportunity costs), as screening and the (inconsequential) work-up of symptomless individuals crowd out other medical services for which the decision makers are accountable and which may be of higher value to them or their clients (Qaseem et al. 2012a). In other words, each policy decision is context dependent.

An organized screening programme can be seen as a public good (Anomaly 2011) to strengthen control of cancer and also as an opportunity to improve cancer diagnosis and treatment in the health system at large. In this, fair and transparent procedures (Daniels 2000), considerations of distributional justice (Deding et al. 2019) and consumer participation (as opposed to expert advice) should be followed from the start (Marckmann and in der Schmitten 2014; Parker et al. 2017; Rychetnik et al. 2013).

As real-world health policy is prognostically extrapolated from trial results, periodic reassessment and updates of the policy are indicated as experience is accumulated from further research and ongoing service evaluation. Model predictions generate insight and can be helpful in checking assumptions and determining options (e.g., Callender et al. 2019; Habbema et al. 2014; Mandelblatt et al. 2016; Rutter et al. 2016). In Germany, it took from 1971 to 2018 for the annual cervical screening recommendation to be relaxed to three-yearly for the age group 35 + (in association with HPV co-testing), although there had been convincing evidence at least since 1985 demonstrating that a three-year interval would suffice (Hakama et al. 1986). Switzerland has disinvested in mammographic screening (Biller-Andorno and Juni 2014).

7.4 Autonomy—Back to the Citizen

Armstrong and Eborall (2012) reduce public screening logic to a patronizing power scheme: "One of the central tenets of public health strategies, such as population-based screening, is that non-symptomatic individuals should make their bodies available to health professionals for regular inspection, and that this process needs to be routinised if it is to protect the health of citizens". Individuals who benefit from screening, however, are distinct from individuals who are affected by harms in terms of false-positive tests or overdiagnosis. In proposing a screening policy, the regulator (implicitly) determines how much benefit for a few is worth how much harm for many others (Marckmann and in der Schmitten 2014)—a utilitarian perspective. The presumptive screenee must decide ex ante whether to take part in this screening lottery (Kramer and Croswell 2009) or opt out of a publicly recommended ("nudged", Ploug et al. 2012) scheme. For this decision to be a fully informed one, however, the presumptive screenee needs more than a quantified summary table of harms and benefits such as Table 7.3—they must also (first) clarify their own value judgements or ordered preferences vis-à-vis screening procedures and outcomes in the context of their priorities in life.

Caverly et al. examined how US guidelines presented the harms and benefits of recommended cancer prevention and screening interventions (Caverly et al. 2016). Of 55 positive recommendations in 32 guidelines for breast, prostate, colorectal, cervical and lung cancer, only 17 presented absolute effect information on both harms and benefits. The others presented harms and benefits asymmetrically or were incomplete. None complied with GRADE recommendations for tables summarizing findings (Guyatt et al. 2013). The key EU recommendation quoted above would be rated 'incomplete', as both harms and benefits were mentioned, but neither was quantified.

Educational materials to inform the target groups of screening are also mostly incomplete and asymmetrical (Beck et al. 2019; Gummersbach et al. 2010; Seidel et al. 2014). So it is hardly surprising that people are not well informed when asked about screening matters (Dreier et al. 2012; Gigerenzer et al. 2009; Gummersbach et al. 2010; Leyva et al. 2016)—the less educated even less so (Berens et al. 2019). Doctors are also not well informed (Anderson et al. 2013; Wegwarth and Gigerenzer 2018).

Invitation letters to organized screening programmes are intersections of public and individual choice. Values, legitimate preferences and opportunity costs are, however, not identical on these two levels. How individuals react to the contents and media of decision aids can be tested (e.g., Gummersbach et al. 2015; Hersch et al. 2015; Kim et al. 2018; Smith et al. 2010; Weiner et al. 2018). Evidence-based decision aids have become increasingly available in the context of shared decision making (Hersch et al. 2017; Lenz et al. 2012; Stacey et al. 2017; Woloshin et al. 2012). A Cochrane Review found "growing evidence that decision aids may improve values-congruent choices"; in prostate-specific antigen screening this reduced the number of people choosing PSA screening (Stacey et al. 2017). Raffle (2001) clearly described the trade-off between high screening uptake and informed choice. In the framework of the German National Cancer Plan, the Federal Parliament ruled in 2013 that an individually informed decision for or against attendance (opt-in) is the first public priority, even if public uptake targets are compromised or individuals may forego possible benefits (Helou 2014).

Empowering citizens (not 'patients') for self-determination needs preference-sensitive, autonomy-enhancing materials tailored to what they need and want to know, including qualitative aspects such as pain or practical alternatives to screening such as watchful waiting or primary prevention; these do not figure prominently in quantitative evidence-based guidelines (Dreier et al. 2018; Hersch et al. 2013; Schröer-Günther et al. 2019; Wood et al. 2018). The ubiquitous social gradient must also be tackled (Deding et al. 2019; Lutz et al. 2019).

Empowering will become more important, with guidelines starting to delegate evaluation of low-certainty evidence back to the presumptive screenee as 'conditional recommendations' or 'discretionary screening'. For instance, the Canadian recommendations based on the evidence tabulated above read: "For women aged 40 —49 years, we recommend not screening with mammography; the decision to undergo screening is conditional on the relative value a woman places on possible benefits and harms from screening (conditional recommendation; low-certainty evidence)" (i.e., opt-in) and "For women aged 70–74 years, we recommend screening with mammography every 2—3 years; the decision to undergo screening is conditional on the relative value that a woman places on possible benefits and harms from screening (conditional recommendation; very low-certainty evidence)" (i.e., opt-out) (Klarenbach et al. 2018; see also Laine et al. 2016; Schünemann et al. 2019a; Siu et al. 2016; Siu 2016; Wolf et al. 2018). Probably more helpful for the perplexed is recent guidance on colorectal screening which comes with a risk calculator and is stratified by 15-year colorectal cancer risk (threshold: 3%) (Helsingen et al. 2019). Other possible cutpoints would define an acceptability region for the presumptive screenee. The German College of General Practitioners and Family Physicians (DEGAM) recommend an opt-in strategy for PSA screening which is not currently part of the German cancer screening programme: "Men who don't explicitly ask for prostate cancer early detection should not be informed proactively. Men who ask for prostate cancer early detection should be informed about advantages and disadvantages. Benefits and risks should be explained using natural numbers and graphics." (Kötter 2016). DEGAM's stance is in explicit contradiction of the German Inter-disciplinary Guidelines (Leitlinienprogramm Onkologie 2019) which recommends providing information about prostate cancer screening to men aged 45 and over as a matter of principle.

7.5   The Learning Health System

Since the 2003 EU recommendations, evidence on available technologies has needed updating as new protocols for established target cancers became available and had to be incorporated into routine service (European Commission 2017; Faden et al. 2013). The principal steps were:

- the replacement of film with digital mammography (Nelson et al. 2016; Pisano et al. 2005; Stout et al. 2014). Mammographic screening has been contested (Gøtzsche 2015; Laine et al. 2016).
- the change from guaiac-based occult blood testing to immunochemical testing (iFOBT or FIT) for colorectal cancer (Brenner and Tao 2013; Lee et al. 2014; Lew et al. 2018), and the increase of endoscopic screening for colorectal cancer (Helsingen et al. 2019; Holme et al. 2018; Lauby-Secretan et al. 2018).
- the implementation of testing for human papilloma virus (HPV), an aetiologic factor and incidence marker, in cervical cancer screening (Kitchener et al. 2014; Ronco et al. 2010) and the vaccination of girls (and boys) against HPV (Drolet et al. 2019).

Stratifying screening by a priori risk with upcoming molecular risk and progression markers will certainly be investigated further (Autier 2019; Pashayan et al. 2018) given the key function of Pr in the harm–benefit balance. Risk-based screening stratifies the target population more and more finely until it may be called targeted or even individualized screening.

For cancers not yet endorsed by the EU28, further developments might be slow. The investigators of the major European efficacy study on prostate cancer screening (ERSPC) consider further quantification of harms and their reduction a prerequisite for the introduction of population-based screening (Schröder et al. 2014). Opportunistic testing of older people should be reduced and feasibility studies of high-quality PSA screening should be started for men aged 55–59 years (Heijnsdijk et al. 2018). In the meantime, it will be hard to keep medical professionals from screening (Ransohoff et al. 2002).

For lung cancer screening, a European position statement recommends implementation of low-dose CT screening throughout Europe as soon as possible but lists a number of preconditions to be met first (Oudkerk et al. 2017). Skin cancer screening is part of the German cancer screening programme but the level of evidence is low and more evaluation is necessary (Hübner et al. 2018).

Screening is a half-way technology. Progress in therapy as well as progress in prevention will change the distribution of harms and benefits (Birnbaum et al. 2016). Further advances will continue to be evaluated in treatment and primary prevention, including lifestyle changes, vaccination and chemoprevention (Colditz and Peterson 2018; Cuzick et al. 2019; Maas et al. 2016; Nelson et al. 2019).

7.6 Conclusion

The evaluation of cancer screening has moved from clinical judgement to quantified evidence based on controlled trials. Reduction of specific mortality, not all-cause mortality, is the main benefit. Overdiagnosis and false-positive tests are the main harms. Harms were found to be underrepresented in trial reports, guidelines and information to presumptive participants. Overdiagnosis was suspected early. But medical professionals cannot clinically recognize over-diagnosed cases, and quantification of excess cases due to screening had to await the long-term results of controlled studies. It took time for overdiagnosis to be considered in the quantitative harm–benefit discourse.

The most important shortcoming of guidelines and health services decisions, however, is the opacity of value judgements exercised by public decision makers when designing programmes and inviting citizens to take part in the screening lottery. This lottery would require explicit justification in terms of a superior public health goal. But cancer screening is, by all accounts, an elective medical service. A public decision maker should not persuade individuals into participating (Woloshin et al. 2012), make participation mandatory or enforce attendance targets, e.g., by incentives to GPs (Austoker 1999).

Some health services refrain from making screening attendance a moral obligation and have started to explicitly respect and enhance the autonomy of the individual. At the service level, there are good reasons to structure publicly accountable screening programmes. But this very structure makes it difficult to inform individuals about their options in an open-ended way. In fact, the individual will need to accept or to opt out of a higher-level consensus. An opt-in strategy reduces public pressure. But in an unstructured, de-programmed situation the individual can fall victim to unfettered professional dominance and the old clinical model could return through the back door. The same caveat applies to finely stratified risk-based screening.

Supporting individual choice in screening and probability-based rather than paternalistic counselling would need to include citizen-centred research on values and preferences in a qualitative research agenda. Ultimately, the only way of finding out whether and how a screening programme really works is to commit the health system to embarking on it—cautiously.

References

Anderson BL, Williams S, Schulkin J (2013) Statistical literacy of obstetrics-gynecology residents. J Grad Med Educ 5:272–275. https://doi.org/10.4300/JGME-D-12-00161.1

Anomaly J (2011) Public health and public goods. Public Health Ethics 4:251–259. https://doi.org/10.1093/phe/phr027

Anttila A, Lönnberg S, Ponti A et al (2015) Towards better implementation of cancer screening in Europe through improved monitoring and evaluation and greater engagement of cancer registries. Eur J Cancer 51:241–251. https://doi.org/10.1016/j.ejca.2014.10.022

Armstrong N, Eborall H (2012) The sociology of medical screening: past, present and future. Sociol Health Illn 34:161–176. https://doi.org/10.1111/j.1467-9566.2011.01441.x

Austoker J (1999) Gaining informed consent for screening. Is difficult—but many misconceptions need to be undone. BMJ 319:722–723

Autier P (2019) Personalised and risk based cancer screening. BMJ, l5558. https://doi.org/10.1136/bmj.l5558

Beck S, Borutta B, Walter U et al (2019) Systematic evaluation of written health information on PSA based screening in Germany. PLoS ONE 14:e0220745. https://doi.org/10.1371/journal.pone.0220745

Berens E-M, Kaucher S, van Eckert S et al (2019) Knowledge about mammography screening in Germany by education and migrant status—results of a cross-sectional study (InEMa). Appl Cancer Res 39:288. https://doi.org/10.1186/s41241-019-0076-1

Biller-Andorno N, Juni P (2014) Abolishing mammography screening programs? A view from the Swiss Medical Board. N Engl J Med 370:1965–1967. https://doi.org/10.1056/NEJMp1401875

Birnbaum J, Gadi VK, Markowitz E et al (2016) The effect of treatment advances on the mortality results of breast cancer screening trials: a microsimulation model. Ann Intern Med 164:236–243. https://doi.org/10.7326/M15-0754

Brawley O, Byers T, Chen A et al (2011) New American cancer society process for creating trustworthy cancer screening guidelines. JAMA 306:2495–2499. https://doi.org/10.1001/jama.2011.1800

Brecht JG, Robra BP (1987) A graphic method of estimating the specificity of screening programmes from incomplete follow-up data. Methods Inf Med 26:53–58. https://doi.org/10.1055/s-0038-1635479

Brenner H, Tao S (2013) Superior diagnostic performance of faecal immunochemical tests for haemoglobin in a head-to-head comparison with guaiac based faecal occult blood test among 2235 participants of screening colonoscopy. Eur J Cancer 49:3049–3054. https://doi.org/10.1016/j.ejca.2013.04.023

Brenner H, Altenhofen L, Stock C et al (2015) Prevention, early detection, and overdiagnosis of colorectal cancer within 10 years of screening colonoscopy in Germany. Clin Gastroenterol Hepatol 13:717–723. https://doi.org/10.1016/j.cgh.2014.08.036

Brewer NT, Salz T, Lillie SE (2007) Systematic review: The long-term effects of false-positive mammograms. Ann Intern Med 146:502–510. https://doi.org/10.7326/0003-4819-146-7-200704030-00006

Brodersen J, Siersma VD (2013) Long-term psychosocial consequences of false-positive screening mammography. Ann Fam Med 11:106–115. https://doi.org/10.1370/afm.1466

Callender T, Emberton M, Morris S et al (2019) Polygenic risk-tailored screening for prostate cancer: a benefit-harm and cost-effectiveness modelling study. PLoS Med 16:e1002998. https://doi.org/10.1371/journal.pmed.1002998

Carlsson SV, de Carvalho TM, Roobol MJ et al (2016) Estimating the harms and benefits of prostate cancer screening as used in common practice versus recommended good practice: a microsimulation screening analysis. Cancer 122:3386–3393. https://doi.org/10.1002/cncr.30192

Carter JL, Coletti RJ, Harris RP (2015) Quantifying and monitoring overdiagnosis in cancer screening: a systematic review of methods. BMJ 350:g7773. https://doi.org/10.1136/bmj.g7773

Caverly TJ, Hayward RA, Reamer E et al (2016) Presentation of benefits and harms in US cancer screening and prevention guidelines: systematic review. J Natl Cancer Inst 108:djv436. https://doi.org/10.1093/jnci/djv436

Childress JF, Faden RR, Gaare RD et al (2002) Public health ethics: mapping the terrain. J Law Med Ethics 30:170–178. https://doi.org/10.1111/j.1748-720x.2002.tb00384.x

Colditz GA, Peterson LL (2018) Obesity and cancer: evidence, impact, and future directions. Clin Chem 64:154–162. https://doi.org/10.1373/clinchem.2017.277376

Cole P, Morrison AS (1980) Basic issues in population screening for cancer. J Natl Cancer Inst 64:1263–1272

Cuzick J, Sestak I, Forbes JF et al (2019) Use of anastrozole for breast cancer prevention (IBIS-II): long-term results of a randomised controlled trial. Lancet. https://doi.org/10.1016/S0140-6736 (19)32955-1

Dabbous FM, Dolecek TA, Berbaum ML et al (2017) Impact of a false-positive screening mammogram on subsequent screening behavior and stage at breast cancer diagnosis. Cancer Epidemiol Biomarkers Prev 26:397–403. https://doi.org/10.1158/1055-9965.EPI-16-0524

Daniels N (2000) Accountability for reasonableness. BMJ 321:1300–1301. https://doi.org/10.1136/bmj.321.7272.1300

Deding U, Henig AS, Hindersson P et al (2019) Determinants of non-participation in colon examination following positive stool sample in colorectal cancer screening. Eur J Public Health 29:1118–1124. https://doi.org/10.1093/eurpub/ckz072

Dolan P, Edlin R (2002) Is it really possible to build a bridge between cost-benefit analysis and cost-effectiveness analysis? J Health Econ 21:827–843

Dolan P, Kahneman D (2008) Interpretations of utility and their implications for the valuation of health. Econ J 118:215–234

Dolan P, Shaw R, Tsuchiya A et al (2005) QALY maximisation and people's preferences: a methodological review of the literature. Health Econ 14:197–208

Draisma G, Etzioni R, Tsodikov A et al (2009) Lead time and overdiagnosis in prostate-specific antigen screening: importance of methods and context. J Natl Cancer Inst 101:374–383. https://doi.org/10.1093/jnci/djp001

Dreier M, Borutta B, Töppich J et al (2012) Mammography and cervical cancer screening—a systematic review about women's knowledge, attitudes and participation in Germany. Gesundheitswesen 74:722–735. https://doi.org/10.1055/s-0031-1286271

Dreier M, Krueger K, Walter U (2018) Patient-rated importance of key information on screening colonoscopy in Germany: a survey of statutory health insurance members. BMJ Open 8: e019127. https://doi.org/10.1136/bmjopen-2017-019127

Drolet M, Bénard É, Pérez N et al (2019) Population-level impact and herd effects following the introduction of human papillomavirus vaccination programmes: updated systematic review and meta-analysis. Lancet 394:497–509. https://doi.org/10.1016/S0140-6736(19)30298-3

Elmore JG, Lee CI (2019) A guide to a guidance statement on screening guidelines. Ann Intern Med 170:573–574. https://doi.org/10.7326/M19-0726

Etzioni R, Gulati R, Mallinger L et al (2013) Influence of study features and methods on overdiagnosis estimates in breast and prostate cancer screening. Ann Intern Med 158:831–838. https://doi.org/10.7326/0003-4819-158-11-201306040-00008

European Commission (2017) Cancer screening in the European union: report on the implementation of the council recommendation on cancer screening. International Agency for Research on Cancer, Lyon, France

EUROSCREEN Working Group (2012) Summary of the evidence of breast cancer service screening outcomes in Europe and first estimate of the benefit and harm balance sheet. J Med Screen 19(Suppl 1):5–13. https://doi.org/10.1258/jms.2012.012077

Faden RR, Kass NE, Goodman SN et al (2013) An ethics framework for a learning health care system: a departure from traditional research ethics and clinical ethics. Hastings Cent Rep Spec 43:S16–S27. https://doi.org/10.1002/hast.134

Fagerlin A, Pignone M, Abhyankar P et al (2013) Clarifying values: an updated review. BMC Med Inform Decis Mak 13(Suppl 2):S8. https://doi.org/10.1186/1472-6947-13-S2-S8

Feinleib M, Zelen M (1969) Some pitfalls in the evaluation of screening programs. Arch Environ Health 19:412–415. https://doi.org/10.1080/00039896.1969.10666863

Ghanouni A, Smith SG, Halligan S et al (2013) Public preferences for colorectal cancer screening tests: a review of conjoint analysis studies. Expert Rev Med Devices 10:489–499. https://doi.org/10.1586/17434440.2013.811867

Gigerenzer G, Mata J, Frank R (2009) Public knowledge of benefits of breast and prostate cancer screening in Europe. J. Natl. Cancer Inst. 101:1216–1220. https://doi.org/10.1093/jnci/djp237

Gøtzsche PC (2015) Mammography screening is harmful and should be abandoned. J R Soc Med 108:341–345. https://doi.org/10.1177/0141076815602452

Gøtzsche PC, Jørgensen KJ (2011) The breast screening programme and misinforming the public. J R Soc Med 104:361–369. https://doi.org/10.1258/jrsm.2011.110078

Gulati R, Inoue LYT, Gore JL et al (2014) Individualized estimates of overdiagnosis in screen-detected prostate cancer. J Natl Cancer Inst 106:djt367. https://doi.org/10.1093/jnci/djt367

Gummersbach E, Piccoliori G, Zerbe CO et al (2010) Are women getting relevant information about mammography screening for an informed consent: a critical appraisal of information brochures used for screening invitation in Germany, Italy, Spain and France. Eur J Public Health 20:409–414. https://doi.org/10.1093/eurpub/ckp174

Gummersbach E, in der Schmitten J, Mortsiefer A, et al (2015) Willingness to participate in mammography screening—a randomized controlled questionnaire study of responses to two patient information leaflets with different factual content. Dtsch Arztebl Int 112:61–68. https://doi.org/10.3238/arztebl.2015.0061

Guyatt GH, Oxman AD, Santesso N et al (2013) GRADE guidelines: 12. Preparing summary of findings tables—binary outcomes. J Clin Epidemiol 66:158–172. https://doi.org/10.1016/j.jclinepi.2012.01.012

Habbema JDF, Wilt TJ, Etzioni R et al (2014) Models in the development of clinical practice guidelines. Ann Intern Med 161:812–818. https://doi.org/10.7326/M14-0845

Hakama M, Miller AB, Day NE (eds) (1986) Screening for cancer of the uterine cervix, vol 76. IARC Scientific Publications. IARC, Lyon

Heijnsdijk EAM, Bangma CH, Borras JM et al (2018) Summary statement on screening for prostate cancer in Europe. Int J Cancer 142:741–746. https://doi.org/10.1002/ijc.31102

Heijnsdijk EAM, Csanádi M, Gini A et al (2019) All-cause mortality versus cancer-specific mortality as outcome in cancer screening trials: a review and modeling study. Cancer Med 8:6127–6138. https://doi.org/10.1002/cam4.2476

Heleno B, Thomsen MF, Rodrigues DS et al (2013) Quantification of harms in cancer screening trials: literature review. BMJ 347:f5334. https://doi.org/10.1136/bmj.f5334

Helou A (2014) Early detection of cancer in the German national cancer plan: health policy and legal regulations. Bundesgesundheitsblatt Gesundheitsforschung Gesundheitsschutz 57:288–293. https://doi.org/10.1007/s00103-103-1902-3

Helsingen LM, Vandvik PO, Jodal HC et al (2019) Colorectal cancer screening with faecal immunochemical testing, sigmoidoscopy or colonoscopy: a clinical practice guideline. BMJ 367:l5515. https://doi.org/10.1136/bmj.l5515

Hersch J, Jansen J, Barratt A et al (2013) Women's views on overdiagnosis in breast cancer screening: a qualitative study. BMJ 346:f158

Hersch J, Barratt A, Jansen J et al (2015) Use of a decision aid including information on overdetection to support informed choice about breast cancer screening: a randomised controlled trial. Lancet 385:P1642-1652. https://doi.org/10.1016/S0140-6736(15)60123-4

Hersch JK, Nickel BL, Ghanouni A et al (2017) Improving communication about cancer screening: moving towards informed decision making. Public Health Res Pract 27:e2731728. https://doi.org/10.17061/phrp2731728

Holme Ø, Løberg M, Kalager M et al (2018) Long-term effectiveness of sigmoidoscopy screening on colorectal cancer incidence and mortality in women and men. Ann Intern Med 168:775–782. https://doi.org/10.7326/M17-1441

Hübner J, Eisemann N, Brunßen A et al (2018) Skin cancer screening in Germany: review after ten years. Bundesgesundheitsblatt Gesundheitsforschung Gesundheitsschutz 61:1536–1543. https://doi.org/10.1007/s00103-018-2836-6

Independent UK Panel on Breast Cancer Screening (2012) The benefits and harms of breast cancer screening: an independent review. Lancet 380:1778–1786. https://doi.org/10.1016/S0140-6736 (12)61611-0

Jørgensen KJ, Kalager M, Barratt A et al (2017) Overview of guidelines on breast screening: why recommendations differ and what to do about it. Breast 31:261–269. https://doi.org/10.1016/j. breast.2016.08.002

Kelly MP, Heath I, Howick J et al (2015) The importance of values in evidence-based medicine. BMC Med Ethics 16:69. https://doi.org/10.1186/s12910-015-0063-3

Kim GY, Walker JG, Bickerstaffe A et al (2018) The CRISP-Q study: communicating the risks and benefits of colorectal cancer screening. Aust J Gen Pract 47:139–145. https://doi.org/10. 31128/AFP-04-17-4195

Kitchener HC, Canfell K, Gilham C et al (2014) The clinical effectiveness and cost-effectiveness of primary human papillomavirus cervical screening in England: extended follow-up of the ARTISTIC randomised trial cohort through three screening rounds. Health Technol Assess 18:1–196. https://doi.org/10.3310/hta18230

Klarenbach S, Sims-Jones N, Lewin G et al (2018) Recommendations on screening for breast cancer in women aged 40–74 years who are not at increased risk for breast cancer. CMAJ 190: E1441–E1451. https://doi.org/10.1503/cmaj.180463

Kötter T (2016) Family practioners' counseling regarding PSA screening: practice recommendation of the German College of general practitioners and family physicians (DEGAM). Z Allg Med 92:495–499. https://doi.org/10.3238/zfa.2016.0495-0499

Kramer BS, Croswell JM (2009) Cancer screening: the clash of science and intuition. Annu Rev Med 60:125–137. https://doi.org/10.1146/annurev.med.60.101107.134802

Laine C, Dickersin K, Mulrow C (2016) Time to douse the firestorm around breast cancer screening. Ann Intern Med 164:303–304. https://doi.org/10.7326/M15-2978

Lauby-Secretan B, Vilahur N, Bianchini F et al (2018) The IARC perspective on colorectal cancer screening. N Engl J Med 378:1734–1740. https://doi.org/10.1056/NEJMsr1714643

Lee JK, Liles EG, Bent S et al (2014) Accuracy of fecal immunochemical tests for colorectal cancer: systematic review and meta-analysis. Ann Intern Med 160:171. https://doi.org/10.7326/ M13-1484

Leitlinienprogramm Onkologie (ed) (2019) Interdisziplinäre Leitlinie der Qualität S3 zur Früherkennung, Diagnose und Therapie der verschiedenen Stadien des Prostatakarzinoms: S3-Leitlinie Prostatakarzinom, version 5.1, May 2019, AWMF-Register no. 043/022OL. https://www.leitlinienprogramm-onkologie.de/leitlinien/prostatakarzinom/

Lenz M, Buhse S, Kasper J et al (2012) Decision aids for patients. Dtsch Arztebl Int 109:401–408. https://doi.org/10.3238/arztebl.2012.0401

Lew J-B, St John D, James B, Macrae FA et al (2018) Evaluation of the benefits, harms and cost-effectiveness of potential alternatives to iFOBT testing for colorectal cancer screening in Australia. Int J Cancer 143:269–282. https://doi.org/10.1002/ijc.31314

Leyva B, Persoskie A, Ottenbacher A et al (2016) Do men receive information required for shared decision making about PSA testing? Results from a national survey. J Cancer Educ 31:693–701. https://doi.org/10.1007/s13187-015-0870-8

Lundgren B, Helleberg A (1982) Single oblique-view mammography for periodic screening for breast cancer in women. J Natl Cancer Inst 68:351–355

Lutz A, Zuercher K, Nanchen D et al (2019) Towards proportionate universalism in health promotion and prevention: reflections and courses of action. Rev Med Suisse 15:1987–1990

Maas P, Barrdahl M, Joshi AD et al (2016) Breast cancer risk from modifiable and nonmodifiable risk factors among white women in the United States. JAMA Oncol 2:1295–1302. https://doi. org/10.1001/jamaoncol.2016.1025

Mandelblatt JS, Stout NK, Schechter CB et al (2016) Collaborative modeling of the benefits and harms associated with different U.S. breast cancer screening strategies. Ann Intern Med 164:215–225. https://doi.org/10.7326/M15-1536

Mansmann U, Crispin A, Henschel V et al (2008) Epidemiology and quality control of 245 000 outpatient colonoscopies. Dtsch Arztebl Int 105:434–440. https://doi.org/10.3238/arztebl.2008. 0434

Marckmann G, in der Schmitten J, (2014) Krebsfrüherkennung aus Sicht der Public-Health-Ethik. Bundesgesundheitsbl. 57:327–333. https://doi.org/10.1007/s00103-013-1913-0

McKeown T (1976) An approach to screening policies. J R Coll Physicians Lond 10:145–152

Morrison AS (1982) The effects of early treatment, lead time and length bias on the mortality experienced by cases detected by screening. Int J Epidemiol 11:261–267. https://doi.org/10. 1093/ije/11.3.261

Moynihan R, Doust J, Henry D (2012) Preventing overdiagnosis: how to stop harming the healthy. BMJ 344:e3502. https://doi.org/10.1136/bmj.e3502

Nelson HD, O'Meara ES, Kerlikowske K et al (2016) Factors associated with rates of false-positive and false-negative results from digital mammography screening: an analysis of registry data. Ann Intern Med 164:226–235. https://doi.org/10.7326/M15-0971

Nelson HD, Fu R, Zakher B et al (2019) Medication use for the risk reduction of primary breast cancer in women: updated evidence report and systematic review for the US preventive services task force. JAMA 322:868–886. https://doi.org/10.1001/jama.2019.5780

Oudkerk M, Devaraj A, Vliegenthart R et al (2017) European position statement on lung cancer screening. Lancet Oncol 18:e754–e766. https://doi.org/10.1016/S1470-2045(17)30861-6

Parker L, Carter S, Williams J et al (2017) Avoiding harm and supporting autonomy are under-prioritised in cancer-screening policies and practices. Eur J Cancer 85:1–5. https://doi. org/10.1016/j.ejca.2017.07.056

Pashayan N, Morris S, Gilbert FJ et al (2018) Cost-effectiveness and benefit-to-harm ratio of risk-stratified screening for breast cancer: a life-table model. JAMA Oncol 4:1504–1510. https://doi.org/10.1001/jamaoncol.2018.1901

Pignone MP, Howard K, Brenner AT et al (2013) Comparing 3 techniques for eliciting patient values for decision making about prostate-specific antigen screening: a randomized controlled trial. JAMA Intern Med 173:362–368. https://doi.org/10.1001/jamainternmed.2013.2651

Pisano ED, Gatsonis C, Hendrick E et al (2005) Diagnostic performance of digital versus film mammography for breast-cancer screening. N Engl J Med 353:1773–1783. https://doi.org/10. 1056/NEJMoa052911

Ploug T, Holm S, Brodersen J (2012) To nudge or not to nudge: cancer screening programmes and the limits of libertarian paternalism. J Epidemiol Community Health 66:1193–1196. https://doi. org/10.1136/jech-2012-201194

Prasad V, Lenzer J, Newman DH (2016) Why cancer screening has never been shown to "save lives"—and what we can do about it. BMJ 352:h6080. https://doi.org/10.1136/bmj.h6080

Qaseem A, Alguire P, Dallas P et al (2012a) Appropriate use of screening and diagnostic tests to foster high-value, cost-conscious care. Ann Intern Med 156:147–149. https://doi.org/10.7326/ 0003-4819-156-2-201201170-00011

Qaseem A, Forland F, Macbeth F et al (2012b) Guidelines International Network: toward international standards for clinical practice guidelines. Ann Intern Med 156:525–531. https:// doi.org/10.7326/0003-4819-156-7-201204030-00009

Qaseem A, Lin JS, Mustafa RA et al (2019) Screening for breast cancer in average-risk women: a guidance statement from the American College of Physicians. Ann Intern Med 170:547–560. https://doi.org/10.7326/M18-2147

Qaseem A, Crandall CJ, Mustafa RA et al (2019) Screening for colorectal cancer in asymptomatic average-risk adults: a guidance statement from the American College of Physicians. Ann Intern Med 171:643–654. https://doi.org/10.7326/M19-0642

Raffle AE (2001) Information about screening—is it to achieve high uptake or to ensure informed choice? Health Expect 4:92–98. https://doi.org/10.1046/j.1369-6513.2001.00138.x

Ransohoff DF, McNaughton Collins M, Fowler FJ (2002) Why is prostate cancer screening so common when the evidence is so uncertain? A system without negative feedback. Am J Med 113:663–667. https://doi.org/10.1016/s0002-9343(02)01235-4

Rasmussen K, Jørgensen KJ, Gøtzsche PC (2013) Citations of scientific results and conflicts of interest: the case of mammography screening. Evid Based Med 18:83–89. https://doi.org/10.1136/eb-2012-101216

Robra BP, Schmacke N (2019) Prinzipien und Methoden von Früherkennungsuntersuchungen. In: Günster C, Klauber J, Robra BP, Schmacke N, Schmuker C (eds) Versorgungs-report Früherkennung. MWV Medizinisch Wissenschaftliche Verlagsgesellschaft, Berlin, pp 9–29. https://doi.org/10.32745/9783954664023-1

Ronco G, Giorgi-Rossi P, Carozzi F et al (2010) Efficacy of human papillomavirus testing for the detection of invasive cervical cancers and cervical intraepithelial neoplasia: a randomised controlled trial. Lancet Oncol 11:249–257. https://doi.org/10.1016/S1470-2045(09)70360-2

Rutter CM, Knudsen AB, Marsh TL et al (2016) Validation of models used to inform colorectal cancer screening guidelines: accuracy and implications. Med Decis Making 36:604–614. https://doi.org/10.1177/0272989X15622642

Rychetnik L, Carter SM, Abelson J et al (2013) Enhancing citizen engagement in cancer screening through deliberative democracy. J Natl Cancer Inst 105:380–386. https://doi.org/10.1093/jnci/djs649

Schröder FH, Hugosson J, Roobol MJ et al (2014) Screening and prostate cancer mortality: results of the european randomised study of screening for prostate cancer (ERSPC) at 13 years of follow-up. Lancet 384:2027–2035. https://doi.org/10.1016/S0140-6736(14)60525-0

Schröer-Günther M, Fechtelpeter D, Zschorlich B et al (2019) Development of decision aids for organized cervical carcinoma screening in Germany. Gesundheitswesen. https://doi.org/10.1055/a-1028-7283

Schünemann HJ, Lerda D, Quinn C et al (2019a) Breast cancer screening and diagnosis: a synopsis of the European Breast Guidelines. Ann Intern Med. https://doi.org/10.7326/M19-2125

Schünemann HJ, Lerda D, Dimitrova N et al (2019b) Methods for development of the European commission initiative on breast cancer guidelines: recommendations in the era of guideline transparency. Ann Intern Med. https://doi.org/10.7326/M18-3445

Seidel G, Münch I, Dreier M et al (2014) Are German information materials on colorectal cancer screening understandable or do they fail? Rating of health information by users with different educational backgrounds. Bundesgesundheitsblatt Gesundheitsforschung Gesundheitsschutz 57:366–379. https://doi.org/10.1007/s00103-013-1908-x

Shapiro S, Strax P, Venet L (1971) Periodic breast cancer screening in reducing mortality from breast cancer. JAMA 215:1777–1785. https://doi.org/10.1001/jama.1971.03180240027005

Siu AL (2016) Screening for breast cancer: U.S. preventive services task force recommendation statement. Ann Intern Med 164:279–296. https://doi.org/10.7326/M15-2886

Siu AL, Bibbins-Domingo K, Grossman DC et al (2016) Convergence and divergence around breast cancer screening. Ann Intern Med 164:301–302. https://doi.org/10.7326/M15-3065

Smith SK, Trevena L, Simpson JM et al (2010) A decision aid to support informed choices about bowel cancer screening among adults with low education: randomised controlled trial. BMJ 341:c5370. https://doi.org/10.1136/bmj.c5370

Spriggs AI, Boddington MM (1980) Progression and regression of cervical lesions. Review of smears from women followed without initial biopsy or treatment. J Clin Pathol 33:517–522. https://doi.org/10.1136/jcp.33.6.517

Stacey D, Légaré F, Lewis K et al (2017) Decision aids for people facing health treatment or screening decisions. Cochrane Database Syst Rev 4:CD001431. https://doi.org/10.1002/14651858.CD001431.pub5

Stout NK, Lee SJ, Schechter CB et al (2014) Benefits, harms, and costs for breast cancer screening after US implementation of digital mammography. J Natl Cancer Inst 106:dju092. https://doi.org/10.1093/jnci/dju092

The Council of the European Union (2003) Council recommendation of 2 December 2003 on cancer screening (2003/878/EC). Off J Eur Union L 327/34–L 327/38

Wald N, Law M (2015) Medical screening. In: Warrell DA, Cox TM, Firth JD (eds) Oxford textbook of medicine. Oxford University Press, pp 95–108

Wegwarth O, Gigerenzer G (2018) The barrier to informed choice in cancer screening: statistical illiteracy in physicians and patients. Recent Results Cancer Res 210:207–221. https://doi.org/10.1007/978-3-319-64310-6_13

Weiner AB, Tsai KP, Keeter M-K et al (2018) The influence of decision aids on prostate cancer screening preferences: a randomized survey study. J Urol 200:1048–1055. https://doi.org/10.1016/j.juro.2018.05.093

Welch HG, Black WC (2010) Overdiagnosis in cancer. J Natl Cancer Inst 102:605–613. https://doi.org/10.1093/jnci/djq099

Welch HG, Frankel BA (2011) Likelihood that a woman with screen-detected breast cancer has had her "life saved" by that screening. Arch Intern Med 171:2043–2046. https://doi.org/10.1001/archinternmed.2011.476

Wilson JMG, Jungner G (1968) Principles and practice of screening for disease. In: Public health papers, vol 34. World Health Organization, Geneva

Wolf AMD, Fontham ETH, Church TR et al (2018) Colorectal cancer screening for average-risk adults: 2018 guideline update from the American cancer society. CA Cancer J Clin 68:250–281. https://doi.org/10.3322/caac.21457

Woloshin S, Schwartz LM, Black WC et al (2012) Cancer screening campaigns—getting past uninformative persuasion. N Engl J Med 367:1677–1679. https://doi.org/10.1056/NEJMp1209407

Wood B, Russell VL, El-Khatib Z et al (2018) "They should be asking us": a qualitative decisional needs assessment for women considering cervical cancer screening. Glob Qual Nurs Res 5:2333393618783632. https://doi.org/10.1177/2333393618783632

Cancer, the Media and Dealing with Knowledge

8

Florian Steger and Maximilian Schochow

8.1 Introduction

The functions of the mass media are to provide information, entertain and help to shape public opinion. Their primary function is to convey knowledge by expanding the subjective understanding of the recipient citizen. The information function leads to various demands on the mass media. They should strive for completeness, and report objectively and comprehensibly. The aim is to present events and problems in a way that is also accessible to citizens who are not experts. However, many misunderstandings can arise in the communication of knowledge. Journalists can convey information incorrectly. People may not understand the message. Important content is lost during the process of transferring information. A special challenge is the mediation of medical knowledge. In addition to pure factual content, it often involves subjective experiences, hopes and desires (Beck 2020).

One example of this is media reports about cancer therapies. Almost every day, new developments in cancer research are reported in the media. Reports of new diagnostic procedures and therapeutic approaches in cancer research are published on television, radio and the internet. There are also articles in daily and weekly newspapers, especially in the numerous medical journals. Articles on research approaches and clinical trials in cancer research can be found mainly in medical journals read and discussed by a specialist audience. Some of those new diagnostic procedures and therapeutic approaches are also taken up by the mass media and

F. Steger (✉) · M. Schochow
Institut für Geschichte, Theorie und Ethik der Medizin,
Universität Ulm, Parkstraße 11, 89073 Ulm, Germany
e-mail: florian.steger@uni-ulm.de

M. Schochow
e-mail: maximilian.schochow@uni-ulm.de

© Springer Nature Switzerland AG 2021
A. W. Bauer et al. (eds.), *Ethical Challenges in Cancer Diagnosis and Therapy*,
Recent Results in Cancer Research 218,
https://doi.org/10.1007/978-3-030-63749-1_8

discussed by a broader audience. This applies in particular to cancer research, which is strongly influenced by the hopes and expectations of the public.

An example of mass media reporting is the liquid biopsy case. In 2015 the German weekly magazine *Der Spiegel* reported on this method, which searches for conspicuous molecules in the blood of patients (Heinrich 2015). Two years later the radio station *Deutschlandfunk* broadcast "Cancer diagnostics. Liquid Biopsy Alternative Approach" (Schmude 2017). In 2018, the *Deutsches Ärzteblatt International* published a clinical trial on liquid biopsy in tumour genetic diagnosis (Jung and Kirchner 2018). In 2019, with reports on this topic finally becoming more frequent, Heidelberg University Hospital issued a press release presenting a new blood test that was a "milestone in breast cancer diagnostics" (Press Release 2019). Television, radio, the internet, and daily and weekly newspapers reported a scientific breakthrough in early cancer detection. The *Frankfurter Allgemeine Zeitung* printed more than ten articles in 2019 on this topic. A few weeks after the press release, however, it became clear that the blood test was not a breakthrough in the early detection of cancer after all. The 'milestone' turned into a cancer diagnostics scandal (Hackenbroch 2019).

The various promises of a cure produced by cancer research do not all quickly become discredited. A recent example is a therapeutic approach against cancer. Since 2017, several reports have appeared on television (Cichy 2017a, b; Stern TV 2017), in newspapers (Gießelmann 2017a; Schweitzer and Kuhrt 2017) and on the radio (Keller 2018) about the curative use of methadone in cancer therapy. In these media reports, a scientist and several doctors—a palliative care doctor, a general practitioner and an oncologist—reported that methadone had great potential in cancer therapy. The painkiller, which is a well-known heroin substitute, supposedly showed positive results on the cell model and in the treatment of patients. It had reduced the number of cancer cells in vitro and in some cases almost completely destroyed cancer cells (Cichy 2017a, b).

Apart from the scientists' and doctors' accounts, the media also reported statements from patients whose tumours or metastases had shrunk as a result of the combined administration of methadone and chemotherapy. Both doctors and patients commented on the positive effect of methadone. It was even claimed that methadone had cured patients for whom chemotherapy alone had ceased to be effective. Television reports in particular presented the curative use of methadone in cancer therapy as a new therapeutic perspective for oncology (Cichy 2017a, b; Stern TV 2017). The background to these reports was two sources that claimed to provide evidence of the effectiveness of methadone as a cancer treatment. The first source includes three in vitro studies on glioblastoma and leukaemia cells (Friesen et al. 2008, 2013, 2014). These studies show that methadone improves the efficacy of chemotherapeutic agents, kills cancer cells and overcomes their chemoresistance. The second source is a retrospective overview of 27 individual treatment trials of the effect of methadone (Onken et al. 2017).

Critics pointed out that the results of experiments on the cell model as well as anecdotal evidence from individual cases are insufficient to draw conclusions on the effectiveness of methadone in cancer therapy. Therefore, there is no empirical evidence for a successful therapy with methadone (Hübner et al. 2017; Steger et al. 2018). The debate on the use of methadone in cancer therapy is ongoing, and involves doctors, patients and ethicists as well as bioscientists. From an ethical perspective, several aspects need to be considered. In addition to questions of patient autonomy, the requirements of non-harm, well-being and justice are pivotal (Beauchamp and Childress 2013).

This chapter analyzes this debate. First, we question the role of the media and their responsibility regarding the issue of methadone as a cancer drug. Next, we examine empirical evidence presented for the use of methadone in cancer treatment, then discuss the use of methadone in cancer patients based on the four principles of biomedical ethics. The main arguments are summarized in the final section.

8.2   Media

8.2.1   Television and Newspapers

The topic of methadone as a therapeutic agent against cancer has become a public issue mainly due to extensive coverage in the mass media. Three programmes that were broadcast on national television deserve special mention here. The first was a report by Christiane Cichy entitled "Methadone as a cancer drug", which was shown on 12 April 2017 on the German TV programme *Plusminus* (Cichy 2017a). This was quickly followed by a documentary "Methadone against cancer?", broadcast on 21 June 2017 with subsequent discussion on the *Stern TV* programme on the RTL channel (Stern TV 2017) and the report "Methadone as a cancer drug— the reactions" on *Plusminus* on 16 August 2017 (Cichy 2017b). At the time, the subject was also widely discussed in daily and weekly newspapers: in the *Süd-deutsche Zeitung*, journalist Felix Hütten asked "Methadone—miracle cure for cancer?" (Hütten 2017) and the weekly newspaper *Die Zeit* reported on the hype about heroin substitutes against cancer (Schweitzer and Kuhrt 2017).

Although critical views were also being presented by the media—among others the daily newspaper *Bild* commented that "Methadone is not a miracle cure!" (Majorczyk 2017)—the demand for methadone-based cancer therapy increased rapidly. Jutta Hübner, Professor of Integrative Oncology at the University of Jena, describes the effect of the media reports in an interview with *Deutschlandfunk* radio as follows: "The really important point was that a television channel that is otherwise considered to be very serious was able to do this. It is the first time that we … have such media attention for a topic and such high pressure from the patients" (Keller 2018). This anecdotal impression was confirmed by an online survey of approximately 500 haemato-oncologists in Germany, more than 80% of whom were often or very often asked about methadone by their patients (Winkler 2017).

8.2.2   The *Plusminus* Report "Methadone as a Cancer Drug"

The presentation, especially in the TV programmes, was highly tendentious. In the nationwide report on *Plusminus* on 12 April 2017, the presenter introduced the topic with a clear criticism of the pharmaceutical industry. He said that pharmaceutical companies invest billions of euros every year in research into new active substances to combat cancer and are constantly launching new drugs. The industry is therefore not interested in a substance that offers hope for thousands of patients but yields hardly any profit (Cichy 2017a). This set the tone for the entire media debate: "big pharma" is trying to prevent methadone-based therapy in order to continue making substantial profits from chemotherapeutic drugs (Gießelmann 2017b). Later in the show, patients were interviewed. A glioblastoma patient described how she was given 12–15 months to live following an operation. At the time of the broadcast she had already survived this prognosis by one year, and even three years after the diagnosis, she is still doing well. The patient attributes this miracle to methadone. In addition to chemotherapy, she took 35 drops twice daily (Cichy 2017a). What the viewer does not learn is that about 8% of glioblastoma patients are still alive five years after the tumour is first discovered. The report went on to present research by a scientist at the University Hospital in Ulm, who has made a discovery from which many cancer patients might benefit (Cichy 2017a).

At this point in time, the audience does not know how well this remedy works or whether it is effective at all. Nevertheless, such statements create 'facts' and are reinforced by suggestive comments and music, thus a single case leads to conclusions about a whole group of patients. The researcher shows further examples of patients, for example, two X-rays of a patient's head, in one of which a tumour appears as a white ball in the head, while in the second image, the white ball has disappeared. The statement is clear—even large tumours such as those in the brain that no longer respond to therapy have disappeared (Cichy 2017a). At this point, it is clearly suggested that the use of methadone leads to the disappearance of tumours. What is not mentioned, however, is that these tumours are surgically removed as standard. In a patient with this type of glioblastoma, any X-ray after surgery looks like this, because the tumour has been removed. As the report continues, further patients are interviewed, specialists in palliative medicine are asked about their experiences with methadone and diagrams are shown suggesting that methadone therapy is almost 100% effective. Critics of methadone administration, on the other hand, are framed as lobbyists for the pharmaceutical industry, supposedly sponsored, whether directly or indirectly, by the industry itself. It is also claimed that the pharmaceutical industry is blocking clinical research on methadone as a cancer drug because it does not want to support such research projects (Cichy 2017a). The television programmes "Methadone as a cancer drug", "Methadone as a cancer drug—the reactions" and the *Stern TV* documentary "Methadone against cancer?" left the audience with the impression that a promising therapy against cancer is being suppressed due to financial interests.

8.2.3   Fake News and Facts

A media-ethical analysis of the report on *Plusminus,* "Methadone as a cancer drug", classified it as ethically harmless (Dernbach 2017). At the same time, an increasing number of voices were criticizing the programme (Gießelmann 2017b; Hübner et al. 2017; Steger et al. 2018). In the public media, the one-sided and suggestive presentation style, sometimes bordering on fake news, was also criticized (Keller 2018). In particular, the narrative that the pharmaceutical industry is preventing research contains several pieces of misinformation, according to majority opinion.

In the television programmes, editorial offices suggested that methadone is effective as a cancer treatment (Cichy 2017a, b; Stern TV 2017). However, none of the scientific supporters interviewed proposed the use of methadone independently of or instead of chemotherapy. Research on the cell culture model also assumed that in order to be effective, methadone needs to be used as part of chemotherapy (Friesen et al. 2008, 2013, 2014). Furthermore, the programmes did not sufficiently emphasize that in vitro studies and anecdotal evidence from individual cases are not adequate proof of the efficacy of a drug. In the television programmes, evidence-based medicine standards were explained either extremely inadequately or not at all. Nor was the validity of the available studies critically questioned. Finally, these programmes suggested that the pharmaceutical industry was actively undermining research efforts (Cichy 2017a, b; Stern TV 2017).

There would have to be some kind of evidence to justify talk of active obstruction of research. However, no such proof was provided. The impression was also created that funding by the pharmaceutical industry was the only way to finance such research. The promotion of research into methadone as a cancer treatment is possible independently of funding by the pharmaceutical industry. For example, German Cancer Aid, a foundation for the promotion of cancer research, has indicated that the financing of clinical research on methadone-based cancer therapy is in principle possible (Hübner et al. 2017). Furthermore, the German Federal Ministry of Education and Research (*Bundesministerium für Bildung und Forschung*, BMBF) established a funding initiative in 2013 that supports clinical studies of high relevance to patient care (BMBF 2019). This means that for many years there have been funding opportunities from outside the pharmaceutical industry. A declaration of intent to conduct a phase I/II study with methadone in patients was given as early as 2015 (Güthle et al. 2015).

In the meantime, German Cancer Aid has approved €1.6 million for a clinical study on methadone in cancer therapy. The study of 70 patients at the University Hospital in Ulm, due to start in 2020, will investigate the effect of methadone in advanced colon cancer therapy in a scientific and open-ended manner (Kotlorz 2020). Media reporting on methadone as a cancer treatment tends to present fake news, with facts taken out of context or simply ignored. Personal opinions and anecdotal evidence are presented as scientific evidence. The media have a special obligation towards the public when it comes to health issues. In a digital age characterized by an unmanageable mass of information, it is difficult for the lay person to separate reliable information from fake news (Steger et al. 2018). These media institutions have failed to adequately discharge their responsibility towards the public regarding methadone as a cancer therapy.

8.3 Dealing with Knowledge

8.3.1 Methadone as Heroin Substitute and Painkiller

Methadone is a synthetic opioid. The drug is widely known to the general public from its use in heroin substitution therapy. It is also a powerful painkiller and can be administered in neuropathic pain therapy (Hübner et al. 2017). When methadone is used as a heroin substitute or as an analgesic, its main pharmacological mechanism of action—the activation of μ opioid receptors—is identical to the mechanisms of action of other opioids, such as morphine. In heroin substitution therapy, drug uptake and excretion with a constant blood level is kept much slower than with heroin in order to avoid concentration peaks (euphoria) and concentration valleys (withdrawal symptoms), as Chou and his team explain (Chou et al. 2014). Like other representatives of this drug group (e.g., morphine), methadone has strong side effects, which include respiratory depression, sedation and nausea. In oncology, methadone has been used for palliative pain management. According to the standards of evidence-based medicine, the clinical use of a drug requires empirical evidence of its effectiveness and risks. This also applies to what is known as off-label use. The term 'off-label use' means that a drug is administered for an indication for which it is not officially approved, meaning that there is little empirical evidence of its efficacy. According to a statement by the German Society for Palliative Medicine on off-label use, these practices are permissible if there is a minimum of empirical evidence of efficacy (Rémi and Bausewein 2016). In order to assess the off-label application of methadone in cancer therapy, the available empirical evidence must therefore be examined.

8.3.2 Evidence Test 1: Methadone in the Cell Culture Model

In 2008, a research team at Ulm University Hospital started in vitro studies on glioblastoma and leukaemia cells (Friesen et al. 2008, 2013, 2014). These studies show that D,L-methadone improves the effectiveness of chemotherapeutic drugs, kills cancer cells and overcomes the chemoresistance of these cells. It should be noted that these results are based on studies with a cell culture model. They provide information about the effects of D,L-methadone at the cellular level. To date there are no prospective clinical studies on the anti-tumour effects of methadone. This means that, so far, there is no research proving the effect of methadone as a cancer treatment in actual patients.

Other studies (Friesen et al. 2008, 2013, 2014) essentially concentrated on doxorubicin as the chemotherapeutic agent whose effect is enhanced by D,

L-methadone. Doxorubicin is a naturally produced anthracycline, which leads to programmed cell death via various molecular mechanisms. It is often used in combination with other chemotherapeutic agents in some cases of leukaemia or lymphoma and in various solid tumours. Doxorubicin may cause severe local toxicity in irradiated tissues. Long-term administration may lead to irreversible cardiomyopathy with cardiac arrhythmia and fatal heart failure (Wellstein et al. 2018). It should also be considered that pharmacodynamic and pharmacokinetic drug interactions often have a distinct specificity for the chemical structure of the drugs involved (Erickson and Penning 2018). This means that an interaction between D,L-methadone and doxorubicin cannot be arbitrarily extended to other drugs used in combination with D,L-methadone.

A research team from the German Cancer Research Centre (DKFZ) in Heidelberg has also conducted an in vitro study on the effect of methadone on cultured glioblastoma cell lines (Latzer et al. 2018). The aim of this study was to replicate the results of the aforementioned in vitro studies on methadone. The results of this study do not demonstrate any effect of methadone on the glioblastoma cells investigated (Latzer et al. 2018). Thus, transferability from one line to another, as well as to the highly complex, genetically unique constellation that marks each individual patient, is questionable. In another recent study on cell cultures, a research team led by Landgraf et al. (2019) demonstrated that the effect of D, L-methadone on cancer cells depended strongly on the respective chemotherapeutic agent. According to Landgraf et al. (2019), the increase in toxicity of chemotherapeutic agents caused by D,L-methadone is determined by the drug and the cell line used. Similarly, Oppermann et al. (2019) were able to prove an effect of D, L-methadone in principle. However, they concluded that the viability of glioblastoma cells is only reduced if the concentration of D,L-methadone is so high that it has a toxic effect on the patient. Then again, no interactions could be observed in combination with the standard therapy. Accordingly, Oppermann et al. (2019) could not recommend use of D,L-methadone in glioblastoma therapy. Whether these findings can be generalized to entire groups of patients with the same tumour type is therefore questionable.

8.3.3 Evidence Test 2: Methadone in Retrospective Studies

Another source of evidence for the effectiveness of methadone as a cancer treatment is a retrospective study documenting the administration of methadone in 27 individual treatment trials (Onken et al. 2017). The study examined the safety and toxicity of methadone in cancer therapy. It is important to note that this retrospective study did not seek to examine the palliative use of methadone; rather, the aim was to clarify questions regarding side effects and tolerability of a possible curative use of methadone in cancer therapy. It references the studies on the cell model already mentioned. As Hübner et al. (2017) showed, this study has considerable deficiencies. The information on dosage regimes, patient data and survival times is incomplete or deficient, therefore, the reliability of this study is questionable. An evaluation of the available evidence base shows that the efficacy of methadone as a cancer therapeutic is insufficiently proven. In fact, large cohort studies would be necessary to provide adequate proof of efficacy.

Proof of the anti-tumoural effect of methadone in a cell culture model is not sufficient to prove its efficacy. In addition, the results of some in vitro studies have not yet been replicated. A retrospective study on the safety and toxicity of methadone in a possible curative application has considerable shortcomings and should not be considered meaningful. Accordingly, to date there is no sufficient or reliable scientific evidence base for the efficacy of methadone as a cancer treatment. Thus, scientists or doctors who promote methadone as an effective means to fight cancer find themselves in conflict with the principles of good scientific practice.

8.4 Ethics

8.4.1 Good Scientific Practice

Initially we have to investigate whether the use of methadone as a cancer treatment violates the rules of good scientific practice. In 1998, the German Research Foundation (*Deutsche Forschungsgemeinschaft*, DFG) published the Safeguarding Good Scientific Practice guidelines, further revised in 2013 (DFG 2013). The DFG recommends a number of general principles that should be taken into account when drawing up rules of good scientific practice: "Adherence to the general principles of scientific work, for example: to work lege artis, document results, consistently question all results yourself, maintain strict honesty with regard to the contributions of partners, competitors and predecessors". In addition, the paper provides guidelines on "cooperation and leadership responsibility in working groups ..., the supervision of young researchers ..., the securing and storage of primary data ... and scientific publications ..." (DFG 2013).

In 1998, the German Rectors' Conference (*Hochschulrektorenkonferenz*, HRK) recommended the establishment of ombudsmen and standing commissions (HRK 1998). These committees were to investigate allegations of academic misconduct at the universities and, if necessary, to take action. The designation of ombudsmen as 'confidants' is to be taken literally, as all information is treated confidentially. In order to guarantee the independence of the ombudsmen, these positions should not be held by vice-rectors, deans or others with management functions in their respective institution. In summer 2018, the DFG decided to revise the Safeguarding Good Scientific Practice guidelines in the light of changes in research practice brought about by the digital turn and new developments in publishing, the structure of research institutions and forms of cooperation. The new Code of Conduct. Guidelines for Safeguarding Good Research Practice (*Kodex. Leitlinien zur Sicherung guter wissenschaftlicher Praxis*) has been in force since 2019. The Code of Conduct requires all universities and non-university research institutions to implement 19 guidelines in a legally binding manner in order to be able to receive DFG funding (DFG 2019).

Against this background, we should examine whether the use of methadone as a cancer treatment agent is a violation of good scientific practice. A fundamental component of good scientific practice is working *lege artis*. This would require empirical evidence that methadone has any effect as a therapeutic agent. To date, however, there is no evidence of the effect of methadone against cancer. Therefore, the use of methadone as a cancer therapeutic agent is barred, as it would be a violation of good scientific practice. In addition, the requirement for transparency in the communication of scientific results was violated. The abridged presentation created the public perception that methadone is a cancer therapeutic and gave the impression that scientific studies in the form of clinical trials support this result. Communication to the public should have covered the fact that the effect of methadone has not yet been proven in clinical studies and, explicitly, that to date only laboratory research has taken place, that there is no clinical evidence and that the risks are difficult to assess. Such scientific misinformation violated scientific integrity.

8.4.2   Patient–Doctor Relationship

The use of methadone as a cancer therapeutic, especially in the care of terminally ill patients, has been discussed in the media. Many of these patients see possible methadone therapy as their last hope (Hübner et al. 2017). This results in a high demand for methadone therapy. There have already been reports of patients discontinuing chemotherapy if doctors have not complied with their request for methadone administration (Hübner et al. 2017). Other patients have had methadone prescribed by another doctor without consulting the oncologist responsible for treatment. The use of methadone without the knowledge of the treating oncologist has even led to one documented death (Hübner et al. 2017). It has been shown that the promotion of methadone as a cancer therapeutic has a considerable influence on the relationship between patient and doctor. We now need to examine how the four principles of Beauchamp and Childress (2013) are to be weighted—patient autonomy, non-harm, well-being and justice.

8.4.2.1   Patient Autonomy Versus Non-Harm

Patients demand treatment with methadone because they have learned of its alleged effectiveness through media reports. On the one hand, doctors are obliged to respect patient autonomy; on the other, they have an obligation to prevent harm to their patients. With regard to patient autonomy, education is of crucial importance. Only an evidence-based and comprehensive education enables the patient to make self-determined decisions. Informed consent—the instrument for achieving patient autonomy—depends on the successful communication of relevant information by the doctor.

Two aspects must be taken into account in regard to information about the use of methadone in cancer therapy. First, it is an off-label use of methadone. Off-label use places special demands on doctors in terms of patient education (Lenk and Duttge 2014). Doctors must inform their patients that there is no authorization for this specific use of the drug, which means that there are particular risks. In the case of methadone, there are also serious side effects. As an opioid, methadone has considerable undesirable effects on the human organism and, like other representatives of this group of substances, can cause fatal respiratory arrest. In addition, methadone has considerable potential for interaction with other drugs that are also administered simultaneously in tumour therapy, and is excreted at different rates in each individual. If administered repeatedly, this can lead to underdosage and, more dangerously, to overdoses causing the corresponding adverse drug effects (Fredheim et al. 2008). Ultimately, methadone entails a high risk of dependence (Kosten and George 2002).

Second, doctors must inform their patients that there is no reliable evidence base, i.e., no proof of the effectiveness of methadone therapy for cancer. This information is more difficult to convey because patients feel well informed by media coverage. Doctors must therefore not only impart knowledge, but also correct existing misinformation. Educating patients about methadone administration for cancer therapy presents doctors with serious challenges. The already difficult educational process in oncology is made more difficult by patients' presumed prior knowledge stemming from dubious media reports. The situation is further aggravated by the fact that patients with advanced disease in particular are demanding treatment with methadone. These patients are usually in an emotionally tense state and see a glimmer of hope in the possibility of methadone therapy. This means that the information process regarding methadone as a cancer therapy takes more time and brings with it a high potential for conflict. There is a danger that doctors will comply with the patient's request for methadone in order to maintain patient compliance. In addition, media coverage can lead to the patient no longer being open to evidence-based education by the doctor. Thus the propagation of methadone as a potential cure for cancer endangers both patient autonomy and well-being.

8.4.2.2 Benevolence Versus Justice

Media reports often point out that methadone is a cheap drug from which pharmaceutical companies cannot make a large profit. New cancer drugs, on the other hand, are very expensive and hence very profitable. Consequently, the question of allocation is often discussed in the media. According to the media, it would be fairer to spend the scarce resources of the healthcare system on a cheap drug, from which many patients would benefit, than on expensive therapies that only help a few patients.

Meanwhile, several medical professional bodies have supported the medical education process, speaking out against the hasty acceptance of methadone in cancer therapy and demanding empirical evidence from clinical research as a condition of its use. These include the German Society for Haematology and

Medical Oncology (DGHO) (Schuler et al. 2017) and the German Society for Palliative Medicine (Deutsche Gesellschaft für Palliativmedizin, DGP) (DGP 2017).

In accordance with the principles of evidence-based medicine, a hierarchy of medical knowledge must be assumed (Evidence-Based Medicine Working Group 1992; Hadorn et al. 1996; Montori and Guyatt 2008). Empirical evidence from systematic reviews and randomized control studies forms the top of this hierarchy. At the lower end is the opinion of medical experts. Through the work of the Grades of Recommendation Assessment, Development, and Evaluation Working Group (GRADE), it is now possible to formulate therapeutic guidelines based on the relevant evidence (Guyatt et al. 2011). As there is currently no empirical evidence from clinical studies for the therapeutic benefit of methadone in cancer, treating doctors are often confronted with recommendations based on a low level of evidence. When benefits and risks of particular therapies are being considered, the use of a drug without empirical evidence is associated with a very high risk. The administration of methadone as a therapeutic agent against cancer is neither medically indicated nor does it correspond to the standard of medical specialists. It is therefore ethically justifiable to reject this form of treatment.

8.5 Conclusion

The media have a special responsibility when they convey medical knowledge. They must distinguish between confirmed and non-confirmed knowledge in medical research and care. They must deal with the dilemma of hope and expectation on the one hand and evidence-based knowledge on the other. To do this, it is necessary to handle knowledge with great care. They should not stir up unfounded hopes in the recipients. Rather, the media must critically accompany the recipient and provide them with comprehensive information, explaining the opportunities but also the risks. According to the current state of affairs, there is no sufficiently reliable evidence base for methadone-based cancer therapy, and its promotion therefore runs counter to good scientific practice. The standards of evidence-based medicine require research in the form of clinical studies. As long as clinical studies have not provided proof of the effectiveness of methadone in cancer therapy, it is ethically unacceptable for the media to raise the hopes of patients with advanced illnesses. The inadmissible promotion of methadone-based cancer therapy also influences the relationship between patient and doctor. Doctors are being increasingly pressurized by patients demanding methadone-based cancer therapy. This creates a conflict between the autonomy of the patient and the doctor's obligation to do no harm. Ostensible knowledge of patients based on dubious media coverage further complicates the already demanding educational process in oncology. To deal with these challenges, doctors need support from two sources. The first is the professional authority of medical societies, and here support is already being provided by many medical associations in Germany. The second consists of balanced, objective and transparent reporting in the media. Here, there is a clear deficit. A change is needed in the way this subject is presented by the media. Public media institutions in particular are called upon to fulfil their responsibility towards society in this case and to set an example.

References

Beauchamp TL, Childress JF (2013) Principles of biomedical ethics, 7th edn. Oxford University Press, New York
Beck K (2020) Kommunikationswissenschaft. 6th edn. UTB–UVK, Stuttgart
Chou R, Cruciani RA, Fiellin DA, Compton C, Farrar JT, Haigney MC, Inturrisi C, Knight JR, Otis-Green S, Marcus SM, Mehta D, Meyer MC, Portenoy R, Savage S, Strain E, Walsh S, Zeltzer L (2014) Methadone safety: a clinical practice guideline from the American pain society and college on problems of drug dependence, in collaboration with the heart rhythm society. J Pain 15:321–337
Cichy C (2017a) Plusminus. Methadon als Krebsmittel. Report, 12 Apr 2017. https://www.youtube.com/watch?v=rcedV2gQ1V8. Accessed 25 Feb 2020
Cichy C (2017b) Plusminus. Methadon als Krebsmittel—Die Reaktionen. Report, 18 Aug 2017. https://www.youtube.com/watch?v=-7OeXoqdqDE. Accessed 25 Feb 2020
Dernbach B (2017) Medienethischer Kommentar zum Fall: „Methadon zur Tumourtherapie". Ethik Med 29:330–333
Erickson MA, Penning TM (2018) Drug Toxicity and Poisoning. In: Brunton LL, Hilal-Dandan R, Knollmann BC (eds) Goodman & Gilman's. The pharmacological basis of therapeutics. McGraw-Hill, New York, pp 55–64
Evidence-Based Medicine Working Group (1992) Evidence-based medicine. A new approach to teaching the practice of medicine. JAMA 268:2420–2425
Fredheim OMS, Moksnes K, Borchgrevink PC, Kaasa S, Dale O (2008) Clinical pharmacology of methadone for pain. Acta Anaesthesiol Scand 52:879–889
Friesen C, Roscher M, Alt A, Miltner E (2008) Methadone, commonly used as maintenance medication for outpatient treatment of opioid dependence, Kills Leukemia cells and overcomes chemoresistance. Can Res 68:6059–6064
Friesen C, Roscher M, Hormann I, Fichtner I, Alt A, Hilger RA, Debatin KM, Miltner E (2013) Cell death sensitization of leukemia cells by opioid receptor activation. Oncotarget 4:677–690
Friesen C, Hormann I, Roscher M, Fichtner I, Alt A, Hilger R, Debatin KM, Miltner E (2014) Opioid receptor activation triggering downregulation of cAMP improves effectiveness of anti-cancer drugs in treatment of glioblastoma. Cell Cycle 13:1560–1570
German Federal Ministry of Education and Research (Bundesministerium für Bildung und Forschung, BMBF) (2019) Bekanntmachung: Richtlinie zur Förderung klinischer Studienmit hoher Relevanz für die Patientenversorgung. Bundeszeiger vom 27 Feb 2018. https://www.bmbf.de/foerderungen/bekanntmachung-1609.html. Accessed 25 Feb 2020
German Rectors' Conference (Hochschulrektorenkonferenz, HRK) (1998) Empfehlung des 185. Plenums am 6. Juli 1998 in Bonn. Zum Umgang mit wissenschaftlichem Fehlverhalten in den Hochschulen. https://www.hrk.de/uploads/tx_szconvention/Empfehlung_Zum_Umgang_mit_wissenschaftlichem_Fehlverhalten_in_den_Hochschulen_06071998.pdf. Accessed 25 Feb 2020
German Research Foundation (Deutsche Forschungsgemeinschaft, DFG) (2013) Proposals for safeguarding good scientific practice. Recommendations of the commission on professional self-regulation in science. https://www.dfg.de/download/pdf/dfg_im_profil/reden_stellungnahmen/download/empfehlung_wiss_praxis_1310.pdf. Accessed 25 Feb 2020

German Research Foundation (Deutsche Forschungsgemeinschaft, DFG) (2019) Code of conduct. Guidelines for safeguarding good research practice. https://www.dfg.de/download/pdf/foerderung/rechtliche_rahmenbedingungen/gute_wissenschaftliche_praxis/kodex_gwp_en.pdf. Accessed 25 Feb 2020

German Society for Palliative Medicine (Deutsche Gesellschaft für Palliativmedizin, DGP) (2017) Stellungnahme der Deutschen Gesellschaft für Palliativmedizin zum Einsatz von D, L-Methadon zur Tumortherapie. https://www.dgpalliativmedizin.de/images/20170705_DGP_Stellungnahme_Methadon.pdf. Accessed 25 Feb 2020

Gießelmann K (2017a) Methadon in der Krebstherapie: Nicht ohne Absprache mit dem Onkologen. aerzteblatt.de. https://www.aerzteblatt.de/treffer?mode=s&wo=49&s=methadon&typ=1&nid=77415. Accessed 25 Feb 2020

Gießelmann K (2017b) Diskussion um potenzielle Anti-Tumour-Wirkung von Methadon. aertzteblatt.de. https://www.aerzteblatt.de/nachrichten/75734/Diskussion-um-potenzielle-Anti-Tumour-Wirkung-von-Methadon. Accessed 25 Feb 2020

Güthle M, Friesen C, Hofheinz RD, Muche R, Ettrich TJ, Perkhofer L, Berger A, Seufferlein T (2015) Eine Phase I/II-Studie zur Therapie mit D,L-Methadon in der Behandlung von Patienten mit histologisch gesicherten chemorefraktären kolorektalen Karzinomen. Zeitschrift für Gastroenterologie 53:KG214

Guyatt G, Oxman AD, Akl EA, Kunz R, Vist G, Brozek J, Norris S, Falck-Ytter Y, Glasziou P, de Beer H, Jaeschke R, Rind D, Meerpohl J, Dahm P, Schünemann HJ (2011) GRADE guidelines: 1. Introduction—GRADE evidence profiles and summary of findings tables. J Clin Epidemiol 64:383–394

Hackenbroch V (2019) Das Märchen vom Wundertest aus Heidelberg. Der Spiegel, 29 March 2019. https://www.spiegel.de/wissenschaft/brustkrebs-das-maerchen-vom-wundertest-aus-heidelberg-a-00000000-0002-0001-0000-000163155878. Accessed 25 Feb 2020

Hadorn DC, Baker D, Hodges JS, Hick N (1996) Rating the quality of evidence for clinical practice guidelines. J Clin Epidemiol 49:749–754

Heinrich C (2015) Medizin-Innovation. Zur Krebsdiagnose reicht ein Blutstropfen. Der Spiegel,14 June 2015. https://www.spiegel.de/gesundheit/diagnose/liquid-biopsy-den-krebs-durchs-blut-aufspueren-a-1036738.html. Accessed 25 Feb 2020

Hübner J, Hartmann M, Wedding U, Gießler W, Schuler U, Hochhaus A (2017) Methadon in der Onkologie: „Strohhalmfunktion" ohne Evidenz. Deut Ärzteblatt 114:A-1530–A-1538

Hütten F (2017) Methadon—Wundermittel gegen Krebs? Süddeutsche Zeitung, 24 July 2017. https://www.sueddeutsche.de/gesundheit/medizin-methadon-wundermittel-gegen-krebs-1.3597694. Accessed 25 Feb 2020

Jung A, Kirchner T (2018) Liquid biopsy in tumour genetic diagnosis. Deut Ärzteblatt Int 115:169–174

Keller M (2018) Über Krebs und Hoffnung. Der Fall Methadon. Deutschlandfunk. https://www.deutschlandfunk.de/ueber-krebs-und-hoffnung-der-fall-methadon.740.de.html?dram:article_id=414968. Accessed 25 Feb 2020

Kosten TR, George TP (2002) The neurobiology of opioid dependence: implications for treatment. Sci Pract Perspect 1:13–20

Kotlorz T (2020) Erstmals klinische Studie zu Methadon in Krebstherapie. Pressemitteilung des Universitätsklinikums Ulm. https://www.uniklinik-ulm.de/aktuelles/detailansicht/news/erstmals-klinische-studie-zu-methadon-in-krebstherapie.html?tx_news_pi1%5Bcontroller%5D=News&tx_news_pi1%5Baction%5D=detail&cHash=0b46497db07dfeca0181d278636d43ef. Accessed 25 Feb 2020

Landgraf V, Griessmann M, Roller J, Polednik C, Schmidt M (2019) DL-methadone as an enhancer of chemotherapeutic drugs in head and neck cancer cell lines. Anticancer Res 39:3633–3639

Latzer P, Kessler T, Sahm F, Rübmann P, Hielscher T, Platten M (2018) Methadone does not increase toxicity of temozolomide in glioblastoma cells. Neuro Oncol 20(Suppl 3):285

Lenk C, Duttge G (2014) Ethical and legal framework and regulation for off-label use: European perspective. Ther Clin Risk Manag 10:537–546

Majorczyk S (2017) Methadon ist kein Wundermittel! Die Bild, 29 June 2017. https://www.bild.de/ratgeber/gesundheit/methadon/kommentar-methadon-in-der-krebstherapie-52381960.bild.html. Accessed 25 Feb 2020

Montori VM, Guyatt GH (2008) Progress in evidence-based medicine. JAMA 300:1814–1816

Onken J, Friesen C, Vajkoczy P, Misch M (2017) Safety and tolerance of D,L-methadone in combination with chemotherapy in patients with glioma. Anticancer Res 37:1227–1235

Oppermann H, Matusova M, Glasow A, Dietterle J, Baran-Schmidt R, Neumann K, Meixensberger J, Gaunitz F (2019) d, l-methadone does not improve radio- and chemotherapy in glioblastoma in vitro. Cancer Chemother Pharmacol 83:1017–1024

Press Release (2019) Forscher des Universitätsklinikums Heidelberg entwickeln ersten marktfähigen Bluttest für Brustkrebs. https://www.klinikum.uni-heidelberg.de/newsroom/forscher-des-universitatsklinikums-heidelberg-entwickeln-ersten-marktfahigen-bluttest-fur-brustkrebs/. Accessed 25 Feb 2020

Rémi C, Bausewein C (2016) Zum Umgang mit Off-Label-Use in der Palliativmedizin. https://www.dgpalliativmedizin.de/images/161212_Offlabel_online.pdf. Accessed 25 Feb 2020

Schmude M (2017) Krebs-Diagnostik. Alternativ-Ansatz liquid biopsy. Deutschlandfunk, 15 Aug 2017. https://www.deutschlandfunk.de/krebs-diagnostik-alternativ-ansatz-liquid-biopsy.676.de.html?dram:article_id=393537. Accessed 25 Feb 2020

Schuler U, Wörmann B, Arbeitskreis Palliativmedizin (2017) Methadon bei Krebspatienten: Zweifel an Wirksamkeit und Sicherheit. Hämatologie und Onkologie. Mitglieder-Rundschreiben der DGHO 2:17–18

Schweitzer J, Kuhrt N (2017) Heroinersatz gegen Krebs. Die Zeit, 25 Sept 2017. https://www.zeit.de/suche/index?q=methadon+krebs. Accessed 25 Feb 2020

Steger F, Gierschik P, Rubeis G (2018) Methadon gegen Krebs. Ethische Aspekte. Der Onkologe 24:915–920

Stern TV (2017) Methadon gegen Krebs?—Die ganze reportage. Broadcast 21 June 2017. https://www.youtube.com/watch?v=Gc_9wdodz68. Accessed 25 Feb 2020

Wellstein A, Giaccone G, Atkins MB, Sausville EA (2018) Cytotoxic drugs. In: Brunton LL, Hilal-Dandan R, Knollmann BC (eds) Goodman & Gilman's. The pharmacological basis of therapeutics. McGraw-Hill, New York, pp 1167–1201

Winkler E (2017) Methadon gegen Krebs—auch eine Frage für die Ethik und Theorie der Medizin. Ethik Med 29:269–272

Ethical Aspects of Regulating Oncology Products

9

Lorenzo Guizzaro, Spyridon Drosos, Ulrik Kihlbom, and Francesco Pignatti

9.1 Introduction

Medicines, including medicines for cancer, are subject to a very tight set of rules. Such rules are enforced by regulators such as the European Medicines Agency in the European Union or the Food and Drugs Administration in the US, in their role of "gatekeepers". To complement their role as gatekeepers, regulators have been considered as exercising "directive" and "conceptual" powers (Carpenter 2014). "Directive" power manifests itself in the ability to write guidelines that instruct manufacturers and researchers regarding the expectations to be met for regulatory submissions. The "conceptual" power is defined as the "capacity to shape patterns and terms of thought and learning". In addition, regulators are increasingly adopting the role of enablers (Ehmann et al. 2013), by developing themselves innovative methods or by providing scientific advice to developers.

In this chapter, we elaborate on key ethical considerations related to such functions that regulate exercise. In the first part, we explore the arguments around the fact that medicinal products should indeed be regulated. In the second part of our chapter, we investigate pressing ethical dilemmas that regulators have to grapple with. The chapter is written from a Western (namely European) point of

Lorenzo Guizzaro and Spyridon Drosos are equal contribution.

L. Guizzaro (✉) · S. Drosos · F. Pignatti
Human Medicines Division, European Medicines Agency, Domenico Scarlattilaan 6, 1083 HS Amsterdam, The Netherlands
e-mail: lorenzo.guizzaro@ema.europa.eu

U. Kihlbom
Centre for Research Ethics and Bioethics, Uppsala University, Uppsala, Sweden

© Springer Nature Switzerland AG 2021
A. W. Bauer et al. (eds.), *Ethical Challenges in Cancer Diagnosis and Therapy*,
Recent Results in Cancer Research 218,
https://doi.org/10.1007/978-3-030-63749-1_9

view, and does not claim a universal, one-size response to the discussed ethical dilemmas; it cannot be excluded that the same dilemmas might be resolved in different ways in other countries.

9.2 Ethical Justifications for Regulating Oncology Products as Opposed to not Regulating Them

Medicines have not always been tightly regulated. In the past, manufacturers could introduce new substances to the market—claiming beneficial effects on diseases—with very little characterisation of their safety and efficacy. More regulation was progressively imposed after health disasters. The requirement to file a new drug application to the FDA before marketing a medicine in the US (in 1938) followed the 1937 Elixir Sulphanilamide disaster when the diethylene glycol—used as a solvent—claimed over one hundred lives after exposure to this untested antibiotic in the US (Wax 1995). A further strengthening of the requirements followed the (mostly European) thalidomide disaster. But are there solid reasons—setting aside the reaction to extreme events—to regulate medicines?

In proposing elements towards addressing this question, we will adopt the well-known four principles (Beauchamp and Childress 2001): beneficence, doing good to patients; non-maleficence, the abstention from doing harm to patients; and the ideals of distributional justice and patients' autonomy. While we acknowledge that these principles have been formulated in a different context, we believe that they still provide a useful framework for our discussion.

Beneficence and non-maleficence are translated in practice in the requirements to demonstrate efficacy and safety of treatments, respectively. The role of regulators can be also easily seen as supporting distributional justice. In particular, regulators are capable of dedicating sufficient resources to the assessment of complex evidence. By contrast, most health care centres do not have the capacity to carry out such resource-intensive assessment on their own. Accordingly, by centralising the assessment of medicines, regulators reduce the heterogeneity in the quality of care that would otherwise be provided by health care centres. The centralised assessment of medicines ensures that access to safe and efficacious medicines will be made available to most patients regardless of the health care centre at which they receive treatment. This could be challenged, however, considering a current phenomenon whereby medicines are imported privately by patients in what is sometimes called *buyer clubs*. In some of those clubs, patients may collaborate with healthcare professionals to access a medicine that is unapproved in their own country. Individual patients, healthcare professionals or their organisations cannot be expected to have the capacity to assess relevant scientific evidence.

The discussion on autonomy has not been less controversial. On the one hand, the gatekeeping role of regulators might be seen—at a first glance—to be at odds with John Stuart Mill's (1806–1873) principle of autonomy: "The only purpose for which power can be rightfully exercised over any member of a civilised community, against his will, is to prevent harm to others" (Mill 1859, 21–22). There are at least two ways of relating Mill's principle to our discussion. In the first scenario, we can take the "member of a civilised community" to be a pharmaceutical company, seeking the right—according to their will—to introduce a medicine to the market. In this case, it should be easy to accept that an assessment of (at least) the risk of harm to patients is fully compatible with the principle. In the second scenario, the "member of a civilised community" is an individual patient. In this case, preventing the availability and use of a medicine might at first appear not to pass the test of Mill's "harm principle", at least in the context of anti-cancer medicines (arguably, different considerations might apply to transmittable diseases).

We maintain that in the absence of the support offered by regulators, the conditions for autonomous decision-making would not be met. A temperate understanding of the requirements for patients' autonomous choice, in the context of (negative) informed consent, would include the patients' justified belief, that their doctor understands the properties of the available treatment options (Kihlbom 2008). However, assessing the data from clinical and non-clinical studies and translating this wealth of evidence into likely effects in patients in clinical practice requires a time-investment and a wide range of expertise that cannot be realistically expected from treating physicians. The regulatory agencies employ specialised teams that take the responsibility to carry out such assessments and to communicate their results in the summary of products characteristics and other documents. Pharmaceutical companies can claim to have the same capability. However, their assessment and communication cannot be assumed to be unbiased. Due to financial interest (Resnik 2000) and to a genuine belief in the theory that they developed and/or decided to pursue (Brewer and Chinn 1994; Allen 2011), the company's assessment of their own results need to be complemented by the one of financially disinterested regulators.

A similar point has been made by Shorr (1992): In the context of pressure to ease regulation for AIDS-targeting products, Shorr argues that future (AIDS) sufferers would be affected because—without pressure from gate-keeping regulators—medicines' developers would likely characterise the (positive and negative) effects of their products to a lesser extent. This would be "harm for others" and is further support for the compatibility of medicines' regulators with autonomy, even in Mill's sense.

In making the case that patients' interests are not always reflected in their behaviour in an ideally unregulated market, Abraham (2008) raises a related similar point. Abraham suggests that the possible disconnect between actions and interests is due to the imperfect knowledge of which means are best to achieve the desired outcomes. This is not in contrast with the presumption of global competence for all adults, if the presumption is understood to apply to adults receiving unbiased and understandable information regarding their options. This condition should not be assumed to be fulfilled by the flow of information between pharmaceutical companies, prescribers and patients.

In this section—and in most of this chapter—we discuss the regulation of oncology products in terms of approving their commercial use. However, use of (new) products has also occurred in clinical studies (see relevant chapter) and in expanded access schemes, such as the "compassionate use" in the European Union (EMA 2007) and the "right to try" in the US (Darrow et al. 2015). These schemes respond to the principle that—in absence of other satisfactory options—patients with life-threatening conditions should be allowed a course of action that presents significant uncertainties. The understanding that the burden of data interpretation is partially shifted to the individual level in such cases is reflected by the imposed conditions of use of medicines authorised under such schemes (reported for example in EMA 2013, 2014), according to which the prescription is made by clinicians who are "skilled" or "experienced" in the specific setting.

The arguments put forward above justify the need for an unbiased regulator to ascertain the characteristics of candidate medicines. However, a further step is the decision-making of approving or not approving a medicine. A completely libertarian approach would be limiting the activity of regulators to a descriptive approach cataloguing risks and benefits of medicines. At the opposite end of the spectrum, a strongly paternalistic approach would be to decide—solely on the basis of regulators' preferences—which medicines access the market. A more nuanced approach will be discussed in Sect. 9.3.4.

9.3 Ethical Dilemmas Explored

9.3.1 Research in Animals

In this section, we discuss the response of regulators to the use of animal models in biomedical research. For the purpose of this discussion, we outline the use of animals in the different phases of the development of a medicinal product, including oncology products; we identify the two key ethical discourses to their use; and we explore how legislators and regulators have sought to respond to the ethical dilemma of the use of animals for biomedical research. For the purpose of our inquiry, we refer primarily to the preferences of the European Union legislator and regulator.

At the outset, it bears clarifying that animals (live animals, as well as cells and tissues derived from animals) are used mainly in the preclinical phase of the development of a medicine. Typically, the preclinical development of a medicinal product involves the phases of identifying the so-called hit compounds, the so-called lead compounds and toxicity studies (Nuffield Council on Bioethics 2005). The first stage in the preclinical phase is that of discovery and selection of potential new medicines; in this context, researchers aim to identify the so-called hit compounds. Those are the compounds that are found to be of most interest for a specific therapeutic condition. In the next stage, that of the characterisation of promising medicinal products, researchers aim at narrowing down to the so-called lead compounds. For the purpose of that assessment, researchers will study the physicochemical, pharmacokinetic, and toxicological properties of the lead compounds in order to better evaluate their potential clinical usefulness. Most of the animals used by the pharmaceutical industry are involved in this second phase of medicine development. Once the most promising compound has been selected, researchers will carry out toxicity studies in animals in order to generate data on the safety of that compound. If promising, the generated data will be used by researchers seeking to gain regulatory approval for the conduct of a trial in humans.

The use of live animals in the above-mentioned phases of preclinical development exposes them to a wide array of contingent and direct harms (Hubrecht 2014). Direct harms are those that are unavoidable consequences of the research. Those harms vary widely in terms of their magnitude and depend on the particular research protocol. Accordingly, the harm may relate to the adverse effect from the administered substance(s), the genetic alteration of the animal, any surgery performed, or exposure to certain stressors (e.g. pain, fatigue). By contrast, contingent harms are those that result as an unintended consequence of using animals. Such harms include the adverse effects on the animals from transport to and keeping in the research facilities.

The question then arises as to whether the exposure of animals to a wide array of direct and contingent harms is justified or not. Two discourses have arisen in response to this ethical quandary (Nuffield Council on Bioethics 2005). The first discourse, premised on consequentialist considerations, weighs the benefits derived from the use of animals in research against the harms to which those animals are exposed. In terms of benefits, consideration shall also be given to the type and aims of the research. On the one hand, animals may be used for the purpose of basic research, which is intended to enhance our knowledge of how animals develop and function at the behavioural, cellular and molecular levels, without anticipating any immediate benefits from such new knowledge. On the other hand, there is applied research, intended at directly improving medical practice by developing, for instance, new medicinal products. In view of its more direct effect on the lives of people, the latter is more easily justified. According to certain convincing accounts (Greek and Greek 2010), basic research in sentient animals is societally not justified.

The second discourse is motivated by deontological/rights-based considerations. According to this school of thought, any sentient being has a right to not be used as a means to an end of others, in particular if such use would cause it pain or suffering. This position would exclude all research that would expose animals to pain. It is clear that the above two positions are not fully reconcilable. The former subjects the use of animals to a calculation of estimated benefits and harms, while the latter precludes any such research regardless of the anticipated benefits.

Further to the above preliminary considerations, we would like to submit that the current legislative and regulatory frameworks in the European Union for research in animals is based primarily on consequentialist considerations, while also incorporating outcomes arrived at to a certain extent through deontological views. The legislative framework in the European Union is set out in Directive 2010/63/EU on the protection of animals used for scientific purposes. Directive 2010/63/EU is an advancement over the previous regime for the use of animals for research purposes, as was set forth in the now-repealed Directive 86/609/EC (Hartung 2010).

An example of deontic-driven thinking is reflected in Article 5(3) of Directive 2010/63/EU, which practically outlaws research in great apes, as the closest species to human beings with the most advanced social and behavioural skills. A Member State (of the European Union) may allow such use, only exceptionally, on a provisional basis, "in relation to an unexpected outbreak of a life-threatening or debilitating clinical condition in human beings". This exception, however, is subject to very strict conditions, involving among others: a justification that the research aim cannot be fulfilled through use of other species other than the great apes or by the use or alternative methods; and a prior approval by the Member States (acting in the context of the Committee of Article 56(1) of the same Directive). This exception may not be relied upon to allow basic research in great apes. In accordance with the first Report of the European Commission on the implementation of Directive 2010/63/EU, there was neither basic nor applied research in great apes in the European Union in the reported period 2015–2017.

By and large, however, Directive 2010/63/EU is premised on consequentialist considerations. It is structured around the formal implementation in the European Union of the 3Rs (Replacement, Reduction and Refinement of animal tests), as articulated by Russell and Burch more than 60 years ago (Russell and Burch 1992). In the context of the Directive, the principle of replacement refers to the non-use of higher living vertebrates and cephalopods when other methods exist for the same research purpose. Generally speaking, replacement is either absolute (complete) or relative (incomplete). Absolute replacement refers to methods that require no animal-derived biological materials. An example of absolute replacement is in silico analyses, which refer to the computer-performed modelling studies of the biological activity of substances, and the modelling of biochemical, physiological, pharmacological and toxicological processes. Currently, results from in silico analyses still require results from in vivo and in vitro studies. However, it is expected that, in the long run, integrative approaches incorporating in silico analyses will reduce laboratory work and effectively succeed in the 3Rs (Jean-Quartier et al. 2018). In contrast, relative replacement refers to the use of cells and tissues derived from living or humanely killed animals for studying in vitro.

The principle of reduction aims at ensuring that the number of animals used in a research project is reduced to a minimum without compromising the objectives of the project. Generally speaking, the principle of reduction is twofold. First, it sets out to reduce the number of animals used within a project by seeking to ensure that the number of animals needed for a given project is determined correctly. One way of ensuring this is by improving the statistical design of the project in order to correctly ascertain the number of animals needed to sufficiently power the study. As reported (Hubrecht 2014), the number of animals needed is usually over-estimated due to the fact that the research protocol is not robustly informed by statistical considerations. Second, the principle of reduction seeks to reduce the number of projects undertaken, by eliminating, as much as possible, duplication of experiments. One way of reducing such duplication is through the more effective dissemination of animal studies. If there is sufficient scientific literature, it may be possible for a pharmaceutical company to decide to not conduct an additional needless study by relying instead on published literature. Even if it is not possible to rely on the published results of previous animal studies, it may be possible to improve future study designs by ascertaining, for instance, through the review of the available studies that fewer animals may suffice for the purpose of the research.

The principle of refinement requires that the use of live animals in research projects should eliminate or reduce, as much as possible, any possible pain, suffering, distress or lasting harm caused to the animals. This principle aims at reducing both direct and contingent harms. Ideally, it should be implemented in a dynamic manner, with the researchers refraining from assuming that the current practices are the best practices; instead, they should regularly review the ways in which an animal is used, in order to further reduce its suffering.

One important refinement method, with potentially far-reaching implications for animal welfare, relates to the use of humane endpoints. This method requires indicators of likely suffering to be detected as early as possible. For instance, if a specific clinical sign (e.g., abnormally low body temperature; or signs of coma; or a severely reduced body weight) is known to lead inevitably to painful death, it will be preferable, instead of allowing the suffering of the animal to increase prior to its death, to euthanise it at an earlier point in time in a humane way. Humane endpoints can also be used to provide an upper limit to the permissible suffering of the animals used. When the suffering exceeds a certain threshold, it may no longer be justifiable to continue using the particular animal.

Further to the above considerations, it is submitted that the European Union legislator has adopted a primarily consequentialist regulatory paradigm, in which the use and suffering of animals is accepted but should be limited as much as possible.

9.3.2 Use of Unethically Collected Data

In this section of the chapter, we investigate the regulators' response to data that was collected unethically, namely in deviation from the standards that apply to the conduct of clinical trials. For the purpose of our inquiry, we turn to the experience in the European Union to identify ways in which the competent authorities have tried to navigate the dilemma of using potentially useful data that has nonetheless being collected unethically. In addition, we seek to gauge what ethical considerations underpin the approach of the regulator in the European Union to the use of unethically collected data.

This section of the chapter is situated at the intersection of clinical research and ethics. It was after the passage in 1938 of the United States (U.S.) Food, Drug and Cosmetic Act, which required the submission of evidence on the safety of a medicinal product as a pre-requisite for its marketing authorisation, that research on human participants started being practiced on a scale that was unprecedented until then. In parallel, different responses to the ethical validity of such research started emerging. The evolution has been traced of those responses from research paternalism, which placed the physician at the centre of human experimentation without any need for consent from the patient, to a model of collaborative partnership which placed more actors, such as patients and patients' organisations, at the heart of the enterprise of planning, conducting and disseminating clinical research (Emanuel et al. 2008).

The evolution of the ethics of biomedical research has been incremental, catalysed at times by abject failures in the treatment of persons by physicians. Most famously, the foundational Nuremberg Code was laid down in 1957, by the International Military Tribunal, as part of the trial of the Nazi doctors that committed murder and torture under the guise of medical research (Annas and Grodin 2008). Numerous guidance documents, both legally-binding and not, have been informed by and written since the Nuremberg Code, including among others: the 1964 Declaration of Helsinki of the World Medical Association (most recently revised in 2013); the 1979 Belmont Report of the U.S. National Commission for the Protection of Human Subjects of Biomedical and Behavioural Research; the 1982 International Ethical Guidelines for Biomedical Research Involving Human Subjects of the Council for International Organisations of Medical Sciences in collaboration with the World Health Organisation; the 1996 Good Clinical Practice: Consolidated Guidance of the International Conference on Harmonisation (ICH) of Technical Requirements for Registration of Pharmaceuticals for Human Use; the 1997 Convention on Human Rights and Biomedicine (most recently revised in 2005) (Emanuel et al. 2008).

In the European Union, the conduct of clinical trials is specifically regulated under Directive 2001/20/EC and Commission Directive 2005/28/EC (Beyleveld and Sethe 2008). Those two instruments acknowledge their debt to the previous guidance documents. In particular, Recital 8 of Directive 2005/28/EC provides that decisions related to the authorisation of medicinal products in the European Union should take account of the ICH Guidance on Good Clinical Practice, while Article 3 of this Directive expressly incorporates the Declaration of Helsinki into the EU legal order, by stating that "Clinical trials shall be conducted in accordance with the Declaration of Helsinki on Ethical Principles for Medical Research Involving Human Subjects, adopted by the General Assembly of the World Medical Association". Similarly, Recital 2 of Directive 2001/20/EC highlights that "the accepted basis for the conduct of clinical trials in humans is founded in the protection of human rights and the dignity of the human being with regard to the application of biology and medicine, as for instance reflected in the 1996 version of the Helsinki Declaration".

The two Directives establish a framework aimed at safeguarding the rights, safety and well-being of trial participants, and that the results of clinical trials are credible. To that end, the two Directives lay down rules related to the conditions that must be fulfilled for the lawful conduct of a clinical trial (prior favourable opinion by the Ethics Committee(s) in the respective Member State; observance of the rights of trial participants such as the right to informed consent, the right to physical and mental integrity, and the right to privacy and protection of personal data).

The question then arises as to whether the data collected in violation of the rules laid down by the two Directives may be assessed and relied upon for the approval of a medicinal product. This question might be easier to address, from an ethical standpoint, when dealing with a medicinal product that offers no advantage over authorised treatments. The question, however, becomes more pressing in the case of medicinal products intended for an unmet medical need. In the latter scenario, the rejection of the unethically collected data entails a delay in the authorisation of a much-needed treatment.

The relevant legal provisions and regulatory guidance appear to take a strong stance for the rejection of such data. In this respect, the first point of reference is Article 1(4) of Directive 2001/83/EC which provides that "All clinical trials, including bioavailability and bioequivalence studies, shall be designed, conducted and reported in accordance with the principles of good clinical practice [GCP]". The second point of reference is Directive 2001/83/EC, the legislative instrument that sets out, among others, the rules for the authorisation of medicinal products for human use. Annex I to Directive 2001/83/EC foresees that "All clinical trials, conducted within the European Community, must comply with the requirements of Directive 2001/20/EC of the European Parliament and of the Council on the approximation of the laws, regulations and administrative provisions of the Member States relating to the implementation of good clinical practice in the conduct of clinical trials on medicinal products for human use. To be taken into account during the assessment of an application, clinical trials, conducted outside the European Community, which relate to medicinal products intended to be used in the European Community, shall be designed, implemented and reported on what good clinical practice and ethical principles are concerned, on the basis of principles, which are equivalent to the provisions of Directive 2001/20/EC. They shall be carried out in accordance with the ethical principles that are reflected, for example, in the Declaration of Helsinki".

The regulatory guidance is equally explicit in making the assessment of clinical trial data contingent on their GCP compliance. The Committee for Medicinal Products for Human Use (CHMP)—the scientific committee of the EMA that is the main decision-maker on medicines in the European Union—released in 2015 a "Position paper on the non-acceptability of replacement of pivotal clinical trials in cases of GCP non-compliance in the context of marketing authorisation applications" which provides in this respect the following: "In case a study is found to be GCP non-compliant during an inspection, the applicant/MAH [Marketing Authorisation Holder] may comment on the inspection findings, provide a re-analysis of the data (excluding the non-GCP compliant data) and/or present a justification why, in their view, the data can be relied upon. The CHMP will formulate their opinion on the benefit/risk taking into account the data from the remaining studies included in the same application as well as the applicant's/MAH's response, as applicable and detailed above.

In case the application contains only one pivotal study which is found to be GCP non-compliant and reanalysis is not provided or not possible, this means that the application no longer contains any pivotal clinical data that can be used to support the safety and efficacy of the medicinal product in the context of the application in question". The CHMP indicates in its reflection paper that an applicant/MAH will have the opportunity to either submit a re-analysis of the data (excluding the data found to be non-GCP compliant) or will have the opportunity to explain the reasons for which the data should still be relied upon despite their GCP shortcomings. These two opportunities of the applicant/MAH reflect the right of the applicant/MAH to be heard and support the granting of the sought of marketing authorisation. They do not however detract from the key point, which is that non-GCP compliant data may not be taken into account by the regulator. Notably, in both the legislation and the regulatory guidance, no distinction is made between medicinal products intended for an unmet need and other medicinal products. The requirement for GCP compliance applies equally to all types of products.

In this strict approach, one can identify a rejection of purely utilitarian considerations. From a purely utilitarian perspective, one could argue that the infringement of GCP standards, through for instance the violation of the trial participants' right to their mental/physical integrity, should not render unusable any clinical data that could potentially be useful. The interference of the trial sponsor with the mental/physical integrity of the trial participants, even if detestable, could be argued to belong to the past. Accordingly, it could be argued that this past act, this *fait accompli*, should not preclude the future usefulness of the data that was collected on the basis of the past act. It could be further argued that the GCP non-compliant data should be used in case that the weighing up of the suffering of the trial participants versus and the benefits to patients that would use the product under review would come out in favour of the latter.

The applicable legal and regulatory guidance do not make any room for such purely utilitarian considerations. On the contrary, it is understood that the GCP standards, formed over many decades of reflecting on the ethical experimentation on humans, take precedence. In that priority-setting, one could be tempted to identify both rule-utilitarian and deontological considerations.

The above strict framework, which rejects clinical data collected in contravention of the applicable GCP standards, should be seen against the backdrop of regulatory mechanisms that still allow patients to access an unauthorised product. In this respect, it bears noting that patients may be granted exceptional access to an unauthorised medicinal product on the basis of compassionate use, specifically when there are no satisfactory authorised therapies for their particular condition. In addition, if the medicine has already been authorised, but not for their condition, then patients may still be using this medicine off label.

9.3.3 Decision-Making Under Uncertainty

Clinical studies that form the basis of regulatory decisions are primarily analysed to establish that a medicine influences an outcome (for example, survival) and to quantify how big this influence is. This measurement is subject to errors, such as concluding that there is an influence when there is not one ("false positive") or concluding that there is no effect when there is ("false negative"). Beyond these two errors, several other uncertainties are present when assessing a medicine (Janssens et al. 2019), in particular in relation to its safety. Reducing all uncertainties to negligible levels is theoretically possible; however, it would require larger studies and result in an increase in the burden on study participants and a systematic delaying in the time when new medicine would reach the public.

As discussed in the previous chapter, the inclusion of participants in clinical studies is justified as long as equipoise is maintained. Extending a study until the point where all uncertainties are resolved would not comply with this standard. Furthermore, even from a societal perspective, the principle of beneficence supports allowing the public to access a medicine that can (very likely) be useful to patients rather than withholding it until perfect knowledge is reached. With any reasonable study size, there is a trade-off between minimising the time and patients required during the development and maximising the level of certainty available at the time of marketing authorisation. As this has most widely been studied for efficacy, this translates into balancing the risk of false positives and the risk of false negatives.

It has been argued that the trade-off should be adapted depending on the consequences of each type of error. In indications where patients can already be treated satisfactorily with available options, then any risk of approving an alternative that might not be efficacious would be difficult to justify. On the other hand, for some cancer indications with a poor prognosis and not effective treatments, the chance of granting patients access to a life-saving treatments (and to minimise patients that in trials are assigned to other, less efficacious options) might be worth accepting a comparatively higher risk of approving a non-efficacious treatment. Along these lines, Isakov et al. (2019) have proposed a formal way of determining on a case-by-case basis the thresholds of risk-acceptance, taking into account the "in-trial costs" (the participants enrolled) and the "post-trial costs", which are the negative health consequences of the two possible "errors" (false positive and false negative). The application of their method would lead to accepting a risk of false-positive decisions of 27.8% for pancreatic cancer and 1.5% for prostate cancer.

Regulatory decisions, however, do not only rely on a statistical test for efficacy, but also take into account the safety information arising from the trial and from all the clinical and preclinical studies conducted as part of a development programme, as well as support for efficacy from other sources (other trials or studies on the mechanism of action) and a clinical judgement regarding the importance of both the desired and undesired effects. While a framework that satisfactorily formalises all these elements has not been validated and adopted to date, regulators have developed means to adapt the level of uncertainty accepted depending on the therapeutic context. In the European Union, medicines intended for life-threatening diseases can obtain a conditional marketing authorisation (CMA) if the benefit to public health of their immediate availability outweighs the risk inherent in the fact that additional data is required (Commission Regulation 2006). This CMA can be renewed as such, converted into a standard marketing authorisation upon completion of further studies, or withdrawn if new information demonstrates that the benefit-risk is negative (as recently described in Harold et al. 2019, for Olaratumab). As shown in a recent review of the first ten years of experience with the CMA scheme (EMA 2017), more than half of the medicines that received CMA are intended to treat cancers. To give a sketch of the type of uncertainties that can be handled through postponing a final decision upon completion of a new study, for nine oncology products, CMA was given on the condition to perform a study demonstrating a benefit in overall survival, where no benefit was conclusively demonstrated at the time of initial evaluation.

9.3.4 The Use of Patients' Preferences and the Handling of Their Heterogeneity

As discussed above, the need for regulating medicines arises in the existence of biases in the ascertainment of facts regarding the properties of medicines and disturbances in the flow of relevant information. However, this does not mean that regulators should decide based on their own preferences. In an ideal scenario, a perfectly informed patient would choose their course of treatment based on the knowledge of the likelihood of benefits and risks, and on the importance that, according to their preference, they would assign to benefits and risks. To be clear, each patient would have a different set of equally legitimate preferences leading to potentially different choices (Postmus et al. 2016, 2018). While this scenario is not realised in practice at an individual level, regulators should aim to recreate it in their decision-making.

Indeed, regulators are increasingly seeking ways to gather the view of patients and to involve them in decision-making (Mavris et al. 2019). This is an extremely important step, but not a sufficient one given the heterogeneity of preferences and the fact that there is no simple way of ensuring that the patients included in the decision-making process are representative of the full range of preferences in the concerned population (Daniels and Sabin 1998).

Take as example the theoretical case of an extremely toxic treatment for a cancer indication with unfavourable prognosis. The treatment might have little or no survival advantage on average, but it would shorten the life-span of some patients due to its toxicity, and significantly increase it for other patients. The decision of taking this medicine would be a complex one involving factors (e.g., age, history of the disease, stage of their lives); however, if one were inclined to reduce decision-making to just one factor, it would ultimately depend on patients' risk-taking propensity.

In such cases, how should regulators decide? Should they rely on the most risk-averse patients? Or perhaps try to "average" preferences, under the assumption (not necessarily correct) that most patients would be satisfied with such a stance? One possible course of action is to understand what characteristics would make patients more or less inclined to accept the risks connected to such treatment. If—for example—available data would support the notion that only (some of the) patients who exhausted all other options would be willing—under the hypothetical scenario of complete and unbiased information of potential benefits and risks—to take a certain medicine, regulators could approve the product in a "last-line" indication. This would satisfy the requirement of maximising autonomy by allowing access to all patients who would potentially choose the treatment, while limiting the risk that patients with different options would receive the treatment due to lack of information or incorrect communication of its efficacy and safety profile. However, systematic information regarding the heterogeneity of patients' preferences (and its possible determinants) is not always available. As regulators' requirements shape the landscape of available data, one might hope that that such data will be more available in the future (Eichler et al. 2012; Postmus et al. 2016, 2018).

9.4   Recent Developments and an Outlook on the Future of Medicines' Regulation

For the reasons mentioned above in Sect. 9.2, and despite ever-present pressures for de-regulation, we believe medicines' regulation is here to stay. The dilemmas explored in Sect. 9.3 have been debated long enough to allow well-developed (even if different) responses by different stakeholders. There should be no doubt that refined, or even completely new, responses will keep emerging in respect of these long-discussed ethical dilemmas. There should also be no doubt that new ethical questions will keep emerging in respect of the regulation of medicines. By way of example, in recent years, there has been a shift towards the idea of generating data for regulatory decision-making in the context of everyday clinical practice, rather than exclusively in the experimental setting of clinical trials. This approach—often referred to as Real-World Evidence—has the potential to speed up the generation of knowledge regarding medicines, and to generate data in a context closer to the final use of the medicines, including the potential to address the problem of under-representation of minorities in clinical studies, which affects the extent to which regulatory actions and healthcare practices are relevant to some individual within societies (Duma et al. 2018). As reviewed more extensively in Eichler et al. (2019), using such data will require solutions to problems both of technical and ethical nature, including privacy concerns. In this sense, it is interesting to see the role that patients' advocacy groups (e.g., Friends of Cancer Research 2016) will play in this conversation.

Another recent trend is the pressure towards Open Science, defined as "the movement to make scientific research, data and dissemination accessible to all levels of an inquiring society" (Pontika et al. 2015). Sharing data on the research done on cancer medicines has numerous potential advantages, but also has to find a way to protect privacy of research participants and reward the researchers for their effort (Bauchner et al. 2016). Regulators have started fostering the potential of data sharing in terms of allowing access to data that informed their decision-making (Bonini et al. 2014; Marino and Drosos 2019) and in terms of facilitating developers to learn from others' experience (Alteri and Guizzaro 2018). This is, however, a fast-moving field, and both the complexities of the dilemmas involved and potential solutions will emerge in the future.

Acknowledgements The authors are grateful to H. G. Eichler and M. Mavris, for their suggestions that greatly improved the quality of this chapter.
Disclaimer The views expressed in this article are the personal views of the author(s) and may not be understood or quoted as being made on behalf of or reflecting the position of the regulatory agency/agencies or organisations by/with which the authors are employed/affiliated.

References

Abraham J (2008) Sociology of pharmaceuticals development and regulation: a realist empirical research programme. Sociol Health Illn 30(6):869–885
Allen M (2011) Theory-led confirmation bias and experimental persona. Res Sci Technol Educ 29 (1):107–127
Alteri E, Guizzaro L (2018) Be open about drug failures to speed up research. Nature 563 (7731):317–319
Annas GJ, Grodin MA (2008) The nuremberg code. In: Emanuel EJ, Grady C, Crouch RA, Lie RK, Miller FG, Wendler D (eds) The Oxford textbook of clinical research ethics. Oxford University Press, Oxford
Bauchner H, Golub RM, Fontanarosa PB (2016) Data sharing: an ethical and scientific imperative. JAMA 315(12):1238–1240
Beauchamp TL, Childress JF (2001) Principles of biomedical ethics. Oxford University Press, USA
Beyleveld D, Sethe S (2008) The european community directives on data protection and clinical trials. In: Emanuel EJ, Grady C, Crouch RA, Lie RK, Miller FG, Wendler D (eds) The Oxford textbook of clinical research ethics. Oxford University Press, Oxford
Bonini S, Eichler HG, Wathion N, Rasi G (2014) Transparency and the European medicines agency—sharing of clinical trial data. N Engl J Med 371(26):2452–2455
Brewer WF, Chinn CA (1994) The theory-ladenness of data: an experimental demonstration. In: Ram A, Eiselt K (eds) Proceedings of the sixteenth annual conference of the cognitive science society. Erlbaum, New Jersey
Carpenter D (2014) Reputation and power, vol 137. Princeton University Press
Commission Regulation. No 507/2006 on the conditional marketing authorisation for medicinal products for human use falling within the scope of Regulation (EC) No 726/2004 of the European Parliament and of the Council 2006. L 92/6
Daniels N, Sabin J (1998) The ethics of accountability in managed care reform: recent efforts at reforming managed care practices have one thing in common: a call for accountability to consumers. Health Aff 17(5):50–64

Darrow JJ, Sarpatwari A, Avorn J, Kesselheim AS (2015) Practical, legal, and ethical issues in
    expanded access to investigational drugs. N Engl J Med 372:279–286
Directive 2010/63/EU (2010) Directive on the protection of animals used for scientific purposes.
    https://eur-lex.europa.eu/legal-content/EN/TXT/?uri=CELEX:02010L0063-20190626
Duma N, Vera Aguilera J, Paludo J et al (2018) Representation of minorities and women in
    oncology clinical trials: review of the past 14 years. J Oncol Pract 14(1):e1–e10
Ehmann F, Papaluca Amati M, Salmonson T, Posch M, Vamvakas S, Hemmings R, Eichler HG,
    Schneider CK (2013) Gatekeepers and enablers: how drug regulators respond to a challenging
    and changing environment by moving toward a proactive attitude. Clin Pharmacol Ther 93
    (5):425–432
Eichler HG, Abadie E, Baker M, Rasi G (2012) Fifty years after thalidomide; what role for drug
    regulators? Br J Clin Pharmacol 74(5):731–733
Eichler HG, Bloechl-Daum B, Broich K, Kyrle PA, Oderkirk J, Rasi G, Santos Ivo R,
    Schuurman A, Senderovitz T, Slawomirski L, Wenzl M (2019) Data rich, information poor:
    can we use electronic health records to create a learning healthcare system for pharmaceuticals?
    Clin Pharmacol Ther 105(4):912–922
EMA (2007) Guideline on compassionate use of medicinal products, pursuant to article 83 of
    regulation (EC) No 726/2004 Available at: https://www.ema.europa.eu/en/documents/
    regulatory-procedural-guideline/guideline-compassionate-use-medicinal-products-pursuant-
    article-83-regulation-ec-no-726/2004_en.pdf. Accessed 07 May 2020
EMA (2013) Conditions of use, conditions for distribution and patients targeted and conditions for
    safety monitoring addressed to member states for Daclatasvir available for compassionate use.
    Available at: https://www.ema.europa.eu/en/documents/other/conditions-use-conditions-distribution-
    patients-targeted-conditions-safety-monitoring-adressed_en-0.pdf. Accessed 07 May 2020
EMA (2014) Conditions of use, conditions for distribution and patients targeted and conditions for
    safety monitoring addressed to member states for Ledipasvir/Sofosbuvir available for
    compassionate use. Available at: https://www.ema.europa.eu/en/documents/other/conditions-
    use-conditions-distribution-patients-targeted-conditions-safety-monitoring-adressed/
    sofosbuvir-available-compassionate-use_en.pdf. Accessed 07 May 2020
EMA (2015) Position paper on the non-acceptability of replacement of pivotal clinical trials
    in cases of GCP non-compliance in the context of marketing authorisation applications.
    Available at https://www.ema.europa.eu/en/documents/other/position-paper-non-acceptability-
    replacement-pivotal-clinical-trials-cases-gcp-non-compliance_en.pdf. Accessed 07 May 2020
EMA (2017) Conditional marketing authorisation. Report on ten years of experience at the
    European Medicines Agency. Available at https://www.ema.europa.eu/en/documents/report/
    conditional-marketing-authorisation-report-ten-years-experience-european-medicines-agency_
    en.pdf. Accessed 24 Nov 2019
Emanuel EJ, Wendler D, Grady JO (2008) An ethical framework for biomedical research. In:
    Emanuel EJ, Grady C, Crouch RA, Lie RK, Miller FG, Wendler D (eds) The Oxford textbook
    of clinical research ethics. Oxford University Press, Oxford
Friends of Cancer Research (2016) https://www.focr.org/events/blueprint-breakthrough-exploring-
    utility-real-world-evidence-rwe. Accessed 07 May 2020
Greek R, Greek J (2010) Is the use of sentient animals in basic research justifiable? Philos Ethics
    Humanit Med 5:14
Hartung T (2010) Comparative analysis of the revised Directive 2010/6106/EU for the protection
    of laboratory animals with its predecessor 86/609/EEEEC—a t4 report. ALTEX Alternat
    Animal Exp 27(4):285–303
Harold R, Camarero J, Melchiorri D, Sebris Z, Enzmann H, Pignatti F (2019) Revocation of the
    conditional marketing authorisation of a cancer medicine: the olaratumab experience. Eur J
    Cancer 123:25–27
Hubrecht R (2014) The welfare of animals used in research. Wiley, Chistester
Isakov L, Lo AW, Montazerhodjat V (2019) Is the FDA too conservative or too aggressive?: a
    Bayesian decision analysis of clinical trial design. J Econ 211(1):117–136

Jean-Quartier C, Jeanquartier F, Jurisica I et al (2018) In silico cancer research towards 3R. BMC Cancer 18:408

Janssens R, Zafiropoulos N, Koenig F, Kouroumalis A, Guizzaro L, Pignatti F, Stevens H, Simoens S, Huys I, Posh M (2019) Improving the transparency of marketing authorisation decisions: towards a framework for managing uncertainties. Value Health 22:S780

Kihlbom U (2008) Autonomy and negatively informed consent. J Med Ethics 34:146–149

Marino S, Drosos S (2019) The European medicines agency's approach to transparency. In: Fernandez Lynch H, Cohen I, Shachar C, Evans B (eds) Transparency in health and health care in the United States: law and ethics. Cambridge University Press, Cambridge, pp 210–226

Mavris M, Helms AF, Bere N (2019) Engaging patients in medicines regulation: a tale of two agencies. Nat Rev Drug Discov 18:885–886

Mill JS (1859) On liberty. Oxford University Press, Oxford

Nuffield Council on Bioethics (2005) The ethics of research involving animals. Nuffield Council on Bioethics, London

Pontika N, Knoth P, Cancellieri M, Pearce S (2015) Fostering open science to research using a taxonomy and an eLearning portal. In: Proceedings of the 15th international conference on knowledge technologies and data-driven business 2015 Oct 21, pp 1–8

Postmus D, Mavris M, Hillege HL, Salmonson T, Ryll B, Plate A, Moulon I, Eichler HG, Bere N, Pignatti F (2016) Incorporating patient preferences into drug development and regulatory decision making: results from a quantitative pilot study with cancer patients, carers, and regulators. Clin Pharmacol Ther 99(5):548–554

Postmus D, Richard S, Bere N, van Valkenhoef G, Galinsky J, Low E, Moulon I, Mavris M, Salmonsson T, Flores B, Hillege H (2018) Individual trade-offs between possible benefits and risks of cancer treatments: results from a stated preference study with patients with multiple myeloma. Oncologist 23(1):44

Resnik DB (2000) Financial interests and research bias. Perspect Sci 8(3):255–285

Russell WMS, Burch RL (1992) The principles of human experimental technique, special. Universities Federation for Animal Welfare, Methuen

Shorr AF (1992) AIDS and the FDA: an ethical case for limiting patient access to new medical therapies. IRB Ethics Hum Res 14(4):1–5

Wax PM (1995) Elixirs, diluents, and the passage of the 1938 federal food, drug and cosmetic act. Ann Intern Med 122(6):456–461

Liver Living Donation for Cancer Patients: Benefits, Risks, Justification

10

Silvio Nadalin, Lara Genedy, and Alfred Königsrainer

10.1 Introduction

Living donor liver transplantation (LDLT) has been an established procedure since the mid-1980 for children and since 1992 for adults (Nadalin et al. 2006). LDLT currently covers all standard indications for liver transplantation (LT), and the results are similar or even better than for standard deceased donor liver transplantation (DDLT). With the prevailing donor shortage, LDLT has become a relevant option for many patients, even with generally accepted indications, but especially for patients with a liver tumor because of the long waiting time associated with a high risk of tumor progression. In this particular context, transplant oncology has become a new main emphasis encompassing multiple disciplines (Hibi et al. 2017; Hibi and Sapisochin 2019).

LDLT covers the standard oncologic indications for DDLT (i.e., hepatocellular carcinoma: HCC, perihilar cholangiocarcinoma: phCCA, neuroendocrine liver metastasis: NELM, and hemangioendothelioma in selected patients) and recently a new and promising indication is given by colorectal liver metastasis (CRLM) (Hagness et al. 2013; Line et al. 2018; Königsrainer et al. 2019). In all these cases, a clear restriction/limit has been reported to guarantee good/acceptable long-term results. In general, international guidelines define a five-year survival rate of almost 50% after LT as a benchmark for tumor indications.

According to the currently used selection criteria, the five-year survival rate after LT for HCC is around 70% (Mazzaferro et al. 2018), for NELM over 80% (Mazzaferro et al. 2016), for phCCA 64% (Ethun et al. 2018), for CRLM 80% (Dueland et al. 2020) and for hemangioendothelioma 81% (Lai et al. 2017a). In this

S. Nadalin · L. Genedy · A. Königsrainer (✉)
Director Department of Surgery and Transplantation, University Hospital,
Hoppe-Seyler-Strasse 3, 72076 Tübingen, Germany
e-mail: alfred.koenigsrainer@med.uni-tuebingen.de

© Springer Nature Switzerland AG 2021
A. W. Bauer et al. (eds.), *Ethical Challenges in Cancer Diagnosis and Therapy*,
Recent Results in Cancer Research 218,
https://doi.org/10.1007/978-3-030-63749-1_10

135

chapter, we will mainly focus on LDLT for HCC and discuss the main ethical aspects in this context and also their application for non-standard oncological indications.

10.2   LDLT for HCC

In general, HCC patients undergoing liver transplantation can be selected according to morphometric and/or biological criteria:

Morphometric Selection Criteria
   The validated criteria most often used for LT in HCC patients are based on morphometric data from CT scan or MRI (i.e., number and size of neoplastic lesions) represented by the Milan criteria with a 5 yr OS probability of 75%. The Milan criteria have been extended by different groups (San Francisco, Tokyo, up to seven criteria), but according to the Metro Ticket concept, the farther you move outside of Milan, the higher the cost of the ticket in terms of reduced OS rates (Mazzaferro et al. 2018).

Biological Selection Criteria
   It has been clearly demonstrated that the long-term results of LT for HCC (i.e., overall survival (OS) and disease-free survival (DFS)) are influenced not only by the above-mentioned "morphometric" criteria, but also and mainly by the biological character of the tumor (i.e., different grades of aggressivity/malignancy).
   In the context of LT for HCC, the biological parameters are mainly represented by:

- Tumor grading
- Alpha fetoprotein (AFP); (absolute value, delta rise, response to downstaging) (Vibert al. 2010; Merani et al. 2011; Hameed et al. 2014; Samoylova et al. 2014; Agopian et al. 2017; Trevisani et al. 2019)
- Protein induced by vitamin K absence or antagonist-II (PIVKA II); des-γ-carboxy prothrombin (DCP)—(surrogate for microvascular invasion) (Kim et al. 2016; Lee et al. 2018)
- Positron emission tomography fluorodeoxyglucose-18 avidity (PET FDG18) (Hsu et al. 2016; Kornberg et al. 2017; Yaprak et al. 2018)
- Response to downstaging treatment (Parikh et al. 2015; Yao et al. 2015)
- Neutrophil/lymphocyte ratio, platelet lymphocyte ratio (Xia et al. 2017)
- The different combinations of all of the above: e.g., the TRAIN Score (Lai et al. 2016), Metro Ticket 2.0 Model (Mazzaferro et al. 2018), or 5–5-500 Rule (Shimamura et al. 2019).

All the above-mentioned studies demonstrate that if positive prognostic biological parameters are met, an extension of the indication beyond morphometric criteria is associated with similar good results as in patients within the standard morphometric criteria.

Accordingly, extension of the actual borders should be allowed. However, if the legal rules do not permit any extension, the only chance we have is to do an evidence-based extension of indications in LDLT settings. During the last ten years, different working groups reported on the role of LDLT in patients affected by HCC (Clavien et al. 2012; Galle et al. 2018, ILTS 2019). The main aspects can be summarized as follows: LDLT is acceptable for HCC patients who have an expected five-year survival similar to that for comparably staged patients receiving a DDLT, which means a minimum recipient overall survival of 60% at five years.

With this in mind, there have also been considerations about the option to expand the standard San Francisco criteria, provided that there is no extra hepatic disease and the following biological selection criteria are fulfilled: AFP < 400 ng/mL, FDG-18 non-avid tumor, DCP < 400, response to LRT, MoRAL, TRAIN, HALT Scores (ILTS 2019). The reliability of the above-mentioned concepts was recently demonstrated in both Eastern and Western studies (Liang et al. 2012; Azoulay et al. 2017).

10.3 LDLT for Non-HCC

In principle, the same criteria should be applied to non-HCC patients with primary (e.g., phCCA) or secondary (e.g., CRM, L-NET) liver tumor, both via the standard DDLT and by means of living donation. However, since the lack of organs is the main problem, certain tumor entities are excluded from LT by societies and authorities. LT for phCCA can currently be performed only as part of a clinical study; CRLM is considered an absolute contraindication even though excellent results have been published for this indication. Recent data show that LT for non-resectable CRLM without extrahepatic metastasis is a viable option in highly selected patients (ILTS 2019; Dueland et al. 2020). To overcome the organ paucity, the Oslo Group proposed the use of segmental DD split grafts using a new technique described by Line et al. as the RAPID procedure (i.e., Resection and Partial Liver segment 2–3 transplantation with Delayed total hepatectomy) (Line et al. 2015). Even though the RAPID concept works, the basic problem of organ scarcity remains. Therefore, we recently proposed the concept of living donor RAPID (LD-RAPID) as a feasible and safe alternative using very small grafts (left lateral segments) with expected very low risks for the donor (Königsrainer et al. 2019).

10.4   Risks of LDLT

Considering that on the LDLT stage there are two main players (i.e., donor and recipient), "LDLT is the only surgical procedure with a potentially 200% risk of mortality" remarked Prof. Christoph E. Broelsch (1944–2019) once in a bon mot.

The donor's risks and burdens must be perceived as the complex assortment of potential physical (fatal risk), social and psychological outcomes (non-fatal risk) (Volk et al. 2006). More precisely, the donor's main risks include the general risks associated with organ procurement surgery and the physical consequences related to loss of a part of the liver. Furthermore, psychological and emotional risks related to recovery and the aftermath of surgery as well as the effects on the relationship between donor, recipient, and others are also involved (Strong and Lynch 1996; Knibbe et al. 2007; Cronin and Millis 2008; Lieber et al. 2018).

10.4.1   Medical and Surgical Complications

The medical risk for the donor includes the general surgical risk and additionally the risk of hepatectomy and increases proportionally with the mass of tissue removed. Altogether they occur in less than 2% of procedures. Typical complications are bleeding, bile leakage, perihepatic abscesses, wound infection, and late bile duct or vascular strictures. Lieber et al. retrospectively analyzed 51,185 LDLT procedures within the timeframe 1991 to 2017 with the following results: biliary fistula in 1.96%, wound infection in 1.33%, pleural effusion in 1.29%, bleeding in 0.92%, infection in 0.88% (Patel et al. 2007; Nadalin et al. 2015; Suh et al. 2015; Lieber et al. 2018).

The mortality risk for the donor is usually very low and decreased significantly with an increase in experience. According to the latest reports, the total risk is 0.1% for the left lateral segments and 0.5% for right hepatectomy (Middleton et al. 2006; Nadalin et al. 2015; Lee et al. 2017).

10.4.2   Non-medical Complications

The long-term non-medical complications are mainly psychological complications and financial burden.

10.4.2.1   Psychological Complications

Other than for their selflessness, the living donors would not be patients and would not be undergoing major abdominal surgery. Their expectations, therefore, are considerably different from those of the typical patient with some form of medical pathology. This alone underscores the importance of comprehensive preoperative patient education and also of careful postoperative observation for depression or other psychiatric/psychological disorders.

Psychological problems have been described before and after living donation. Pre-donation burdens can arise from care of the organ recipient, especially those with very close emotional ties and with acutely life-threatening disease. But a chronic disease of the recipient is also associated with stress for the donor, especially if the donor lives in and/or supports the recipient's household or even participates in the care/medical care of the recipient.

The postoperative period is initially determined by the inpatient hospital stay, the postoperative pain and the convalescence, which usually lasts several months. The restrictions on everyday life and at work (mainly related to reduce physical capacity) are a problem for donors during this time. In addition, there are also concerns for the recipient and for possible lasting negative consequences of the living donation. These worries and fears may persist in the longer term, even if the donor and recipient are in good health.

Some psychosomatic disorders have been reported, however, such as diffuse nonspecific abdominal symptoms and pain (Trotter et al. 2001; Beavers et al. 2002, Fukunishi et al. 2002a), sexual dysfunction (Kim-Schluger et al. 2002), anxious depression, and overall complaints (Walter et al. 2005, Nadalin et al. 2007).

A minority of donors exhibits an enhanced perception of distress and low self-esteem before and after surgery, which can easily be overlooked in the preoperative evaluation or during postoperative care (Walter et al. 2002, Walter et al. 2005a, b). Similarly, it has been reported that for some donors the reported return to normalcy took a significant amount of time, even when no serious medical complications were experienced (Siegler et al. 2004; Hwang et al. 2006; Nadalin et al. 2007).

In the special setting of extended indications, Volk et al. (2006) suggested that autonomy should be paramount only if the donor's decision-making process is logical and informed. For example, in patients with HCC exceeding the Milan criteria, having no other option like DDLT, potential donors are left with the perception that only few other options are available. A qualitative analysis of the donor decision-making process in Japan highlighted how this perceived lack of choice can act as a psychological burden and influence donors' decisions (Fujita et al. 2006). Accordingly, the performance of LDLT in such patients should be individualized and careful consideration of the psychological burden on the donor is highly necessary.

10.4.2.2 Economic Complications

Donors can expect to experience significant financial burdens including a mean recovery period of three months including loss of salary and out-of-pocket costs. Moreover, the donor's ability to obtain life insurance may be compromised (Volk et al. 2006).

10.5 Benefits of LDLT

10.5.1 Benefits for the Recipient

The primary benefits for the organ recipient can be simply summarized as improved health and extension of life or, equally, as the chance to be cured. Moreover, two other aspects have been observed: influence on adherence and possible improvement of social and family relationships.

Influence on adherence: In their first example, Schiano and Rhodes described the case of an adolescent who had issues with non-adherence in prior treatment and the hopes of his parents that a living donation by one of them could positively change this (Schiano and Rhodes 2015). Jain et al. report that in the case of living donor kidney transplantation (LDKT), the self-reported non-adherence was significantly higher in recipients of living-related than of deceased grafts. The differences were associated with younger recipient age and the belief that immunosuppressive drugs are less important for living-related donations. Conversely, LDLT recipients seem to be more adherent than DDLT recipients, as shown in a study by Denhaerynck et al., where DDLT was a determinant of non-adherence in addition to a belief in alternative medications, high regimen complexity, poor knowledge about medications, and cost issues (Denhaerynck et al. 2014).

Possible improvement of social and family relationships: on the one hand, one may think that an intense experience like living donation would necessarily cause stronger emotional and social bonding within a family. On the other hand, one should also take a closer look at the family dynamics, as Erim et al. did (2006). Depending on the relationship between donor and recipient and the role of other family members (e.g., if another member was also a potential donor), tension could appear within the family, which might influence the psychosocial situation after LDLT.

Furthermore, expectations of the donor, like strengthening of the bond to the recipient or with regard to the recipient's adherence to post-transplant care, might have a strong impact on the relationship between donor and recipient, both supportively and destructively (Schiano and Rhodes 2015).

10.5.2 Benefits for the Donor

The benefits to the donor are mainly social and psychological (Lieber et al. 2018).

Indeed, for living donors, the benefit of donation is primarily a psychological and not a medical one since living donors are in perfect or nearly perfect health before surgery. Various studies have analyzed the changes in QoL after donation for LDLT (Beavers et al. 2001; Trotter et al. 2001; Fukunishi et al. 2002a, b; Karliova et al. 2002; Kim-Schluger et al. 2002; Humar et al. 2005; Miyagi et al. 2005; Verbesey et al. 2005; Walter et al. 2005). In general, donors have an increased sense of self-esteem after donation and rarely regret their decision to donate (Nadalin et al. 2007).

Donors whose recipients do well clinically are themselves more likely to do well psychologically (Erim et al. 2003; Miyagi et al. 2005). This suggests an inherent benefit for the donor from the simple act of donation. Interestingly, while the health benefits of donation have not been studied in detail, there is evidence that altruism is associated with improvements in health and longevity (Post 2005; Volk et al. 2006; Nadalin et al. 2007).

10.6 Ethical Aspects and Justification of LDLT for Cancer

In general, two key ethical principles guide the practice of candidate selection and organ allocation: the principle of justice and the principle of utility (Dawwas and Gimson 2009).

(1) *The principle of justice (or equity)*: candidate selection and organ allocation should be dictated by the degree of an individual's *need* for transplant, thereby ensuring that those with equal needs can have equity of access to this scarce resource. The quantification of need for transplant can be accomplished using a variety of scoring systems that therefore prioritize patients according to their projected survival prospects without transplant, irrespective of their post-transplant outcome.

(2) *Principle of utility (or efficiency)*: This principle should prioritize patients with the greatest survival perspective after undergoing transplant, thereby maximizing the overall absolute (rather than net) lifesaving utility of this finite resource. A purely utilitarian system would rank patients according to their anticipated post-transplant outcome, regardless of their survival prospects in the absence of this procedure.

Additionally, in an era of ongoing organ shortage (e.g., in Germany), the allocation of each organ to the recipient with the maximum calculated survival or transplant benefit remains the goal for all transplant systems. Consequently, not the most urgent patient is the first candidate to receive a graft, but rather the patient who is supposed to have the greatest benefit (Otto 2013).

In addition to the above-mentioned key principles, the following goals should be considered in settings of transplant oncology (e.g., HCC) (Pomfret et al. 2011; Lai et al. 2017b):

(1) Maximalize the post-transplant outcome: i.e., reduce post-transplant tumor recurrence and increase overall survival

(2) Minimize the risk of dying on the waiting list: i.e., by adjustment of priority rules including the risk of tumor progression and response to therapy

(3) Avoid futile transplantation: i.e., in patients who may benefit from other non-transplant treatments or who have a high risk of tumor recurrence (see biological marker)

In LDLT, the donor's altruism represents the fundamental ethical principle, which is based on the following four principles of (1) beneficence (doing good), (2) non-maleficence (avoiding harm), (3) respect for autonomy, and (4) respect for justice (promoting fairness) (Petrini 2010; Gordon 2012; Jennings et al. 2013; Panocchia et al. 2013; Venkat and Eshelman 2014; Gordon et al. 2015; Lieber et al. 2018).

All these things put together can be summarized in the concept of double equipoise of living organ donation, which evaluates the relationship between the recipient's need, the donor's risk, and the recipient's outcome. It considers each donor–recipient pair as a unit, analyzing whether the specific recipient's benefit justifies the specific donor's risk (Akoad 2012).

Therefore, when a double equipoise decision is being made for the donor and the recipient, it is acceptable to include not only mortality and morbidity data but also quality of life, psychological, and social considerations related to the two parties (Pomfret et al. 2011).

Miller (2008) eloquently described the ethical dimensions of equipoise for LDLT with a graphic depiction that incorporates a careful assessment of the recipient need, the donor risk (safety), and the possibility of a good outcome for the recipient. The tension between these fundamental principles results in triangles of differing shapes and proportions that vary with the circumstances of each donor and each recipient. The concept of double equipoise describes the balance between the recipient's survival benefit with or without LDLT and the probability of mortality for the donor (Cronin et al. 2001).

The concept of double equipoise suggests that there clearly exists an area of excessive donor risk and unacceptably low recipient benefit. As physicians, we feel that it is not ethically defensible for a living donor to undergo an operation with a mortality risk greater than the expected rate of 0.5% (as reported by centers around the world). Nor do we feel that it is acceptable for a donor to undertake any risk if the recipient benefit will predictably be very low (e.g., if the recipient has extra-hepatic disease or a tumor with aggressive biology and poor prognostic factors). These situations fall within the zone of ethical unacceptability. Conversely, there are situations of donor–recipient balance that appear to be ethically acceptable. An adult donor who is providing a liver segment to a pediatric recipient is one example that falls within the zone of ethical acceptability. In this situation, the donor risk is well-defined and small, and the recipient benefit is almost always a highly successful and durable transplant. The zone of ethical uncertainty is the most complex area. What are the minimal benefits to a recipient that warrant the use of a living donor, and to what extent must the recipient benefit (e.g., 50% survival at two years) to justify the use of a living donor for extended indications and marginal recipient benefits? In this context, one should take into consideration not only the OS rate, but also the psychosocial benefit (e.g., giving to some young mother the opportunity to live at least three years longer with her small children) (Pomfret et al. 2011).

This is particularly true when we try to apply LDLT beyond the standardized oncological indications (e.g., HCC beyond UCSF, CRLM, CCA). In such cases, the main ethical question is whether a patient who is not eligible for DDLT should be eligible for LDLT (Lieber and Schiano et al. 2018). The main ethical issue is the potential harm to the living donor and the financial burden for society against the potentially uncertain prognosis. If donor risks can be minimized and selection criteria for patients with HCC or other liver tumors optimized, LDLT appears to be justified both from the extended life expectancy and from a cost-effectiveness perspective (Pascher and Neuhaus 2003).

In the context of life expectancy, a five-year OS of 50–70% has been considered a reasonable benchmark in DDLT. But when the potential transplant recipient is deemed to be medically or psychosocially a higher risk than other transplant recipients, should the standard benchmark of a 50–70% chance of recipient five-year survival be used for living donation? Additionally, patients who receive LDLT are not taking an organ from the deceased donor organ pool—a living donor organ would only be donated to a specific recipient because of some special feature of their personal relationship. No one else who needs an organ would be in line for that organ. In that way, LDLT does not involve injustice to other candidates on the transplant list (Lieber et al. 2018).

Therefore, when extending the oncological indication, the transplant community should accept LDLT when the risk–benefit ratio is reasonable and not when it is unreasonable. In this regard, Lieber et al. suggested a 40% likelihood of five-year survival as a cut-off for LDLT (Lieber et al. 2018).

One additional major point of debate is whether it is ethically correct to offer the possibility of a re-transplantation with a DDLT to a patient with early graft failure after LDLT for extended oncological indications. Clavien et al. reported on the international consensus conference on liver transplantation for HCC and concluded that "based on utility, justice, and equity, they did not support re-transplantation for patients who were beyond these (standard eligibility) criteria, because these patients would not have qualified for DDLT in the first place" (Clavien et al. 2012). One could argue that using a deceased organ from the common pool to transplant a patient who was determined to be ineligible for that organ would be unjust to another patient who is entitled to the gift of life because of the great likelihood of deriving a significant benefit from it. Therefore, despite the emotional burden of withholding the opportunity for re-transplantation following organ failure, transplant teams should not offer a deceased organ to a living donor–recipient with acute graft failure given the injustice to others on the transplant list (Lieber et al. 2018).

Consequently, it is essential to perform adequate informed consent focused on risk, benefits and outcome benefits of both donor and recipient (Gordon 2012; Gordon et al. 2015). In any living donor situation, the harms and burdens to the donor are justified by the significant benefit to the recipient. This means that the organ donor needs to have a robust understanding of the risks and burdens involved and the capacity to consider them in the context of the values and priorities that the donor finds most salient (Miller 2014; Hays et al. 2015; Lieber et al. 2018).

Informed consent for live organ donation is an ethical prerequisite, legally obligatory and comprises part of the *Patient's Rights Condition of Medicare Participation* for hospitals (Gordon et al. 2015). It is a process that entails clinician–patient communication to assess patients' competence to make decisions, followed by the disclosure of information, and assurance of patient comprehension of disclosed information. It culminates in a voluntary decision and agreement to undergo the suggested procedure (Sugarman et al. 2005). Obtaining informed consent upholds the principle of self-determination and supports autonomous treatment decisions consistent with the donor's life goals, values and beliefs while also fostering patient-centered care (Gordon et al. 2015).

In this context, the independent living donor advocate (ILDA) role serves as a safeguard for the ethical informed consent process in the care of this special patient population (Hays et al. 2015). Fundamentally, the ILDA helps to ensure that basic ethical principles guiding informed consent have been met: that every living donor proceeds voluntarily, armed with adequate information about risks and benefits, and uninfluenced by coercive pressure. Ideally, the ILDA serves as both reality check and bridge between the prospective donor and the rest of the care team, helping the prospective donor process the pros and cons of the decision to donate, and communicating these wishes to the transplant team.

Ultimately, the transplant team must respect the principle of non-maleficence to the donor by preventing donations that could ultimately do more harm to the donor than is justified for the benefit provided to the recipient. The focus on minimizing donor risks by excluding donors for medical and psychosocial reasons, as well as the employment of strict criteria for the acceptability of LDLT, will help maintain society's trust in organ transplantation (Lieber et al. 2018).

References

Agopian VG, Harlander-Locke MP, Markovic D et al (2017) Evaluation of patients with Hepatocellular Carcinomas that do not produce α-Fetoprotein. JAMA Surg 152(1):55–64

Akoad ME (2012) Living-donor grafts for patients with hepatocellular carcinoma. Virtual Mentor 14(3):215–220

Azoulay D, Audureau E, Bhangui P et al (2017) Living or Brain-dead Donor Liver Transplantation for Hepatocellular Carcinoma: A Multicenter, Western. Intent-To-Treat Cohort Study Ann Surg 266(6):1035–1044

Beavers KL, Sandler RS, Fair JH et al (2001) The living donor experience: donor health assessment and outcomes after living donor liver transplantation. Liver Transpl 7(11):943–947

Beavers KL, Sandler RS, Shrestha R (2002) Donor morbidity associated with right lobectomy for living donor liver transplantation to adult recipients: a systematic review. Liver Transpl 8(2):110–117

Clavien PA, Lesurtel M, Bossuyt PM et al (2012) Recommendations for liver transplantation for hepatocellular carcinoma: an international consensus conference report. Lancet Oncol 13(1):e11-22

Cronin DC, Millis JM (2008) Living donor liver transplantation: The ethics and the practice. Hepatology 47(1):11–13

Cronin DC, Millis JM, Siegler M (2001) Transplantation of liver grafts from living donors into adults–too much, too soon. N Engl J Med 344(21):1633–1637

Dawwas MF, Gimson AE (2009) Candidate selection and organ allocation in liver transplantation. Semin Liver Dis 29(1):40–52

Denhaerynck K, Schmid-Mohler G, Kiss A et al (2014) Differences in Medication Adherence between Living and Deceased Donor Kidney Transplant Patients. Int J Organ Transplant Med 5(1):7–14

Dueland S, Syversveen T, Solheim JM et al (2020) Survival Following Liver Transplantation for Patients With Nonresectable Liver-only colorectal metastases. Ann Surg 271(2):212–218

Erim Y, Beckmann M, Valentin-Gamazo C et al (2006) Quality of life and psychiatric complications after adult living donor liver transplantation. Liver Transpl 12(12):1782–1790

Erim Y, Senf and W, Heitfeld M, (2003) Psychosocial impact of living donation. Transplant Proc 35(3):911–912

Ethun CG, Lopez-Aguiar AG, Anderson DJ et al (2018) Transplantation versus resection for Hilar Cholangiocarcinoma: an argument for shifting treatment paradigms for resectable disease. Ann Surg 267(5):797–805

Fujita M, Akabayashi A, Slingsby BT et al (2006) A model of donors' decision-making in adult-to-adult living donor liver transplantation in Japan: having no choice. Liver Transpl 12(5):768–774

Fukunishi I, Sugawara Y, Takayama T et al (2002) Psychiatric problems in living-related transplantation (II): the association between paradoxical psychiatric syndrome and guilt feelings in adult recipients after living donor liver transplantation. Transplant Proc 34(7):2632–2633

Fukunishi I, Sugawara Y, Takayama T et al (2002) Association between pretransplant psychological assessments and posttransplant psychiatric disorders in living-related transplantation. Psychosomatics 43(1):49–54

Galle PR, Forner A, Llovet JM et al (2018) EASL clinical practice guidelines: management of hepatocellular carcinoma European Association for the Study of the Liver. J Hepatol 69:182–236

Gordon EJ (2012) Informed consent for living donation: a review of key empirical studies, ethical challenges and future research. Am J Transplant 12(9):2273–2280

Gordon EJ, Rodde J, Skaro A et al (2015) Informed consent for live liver donors: a qualitative, prospective study. J Hepatol 63(4):838–847

Hagness M, Foss A, Line PD et al (2013) Liver transplantation for nonresectable liver metastases from colorectal cancer. Ann Surg 257(5):800–806s

Hameed B, Mehta N, Sapisochin G et al (2014) Alpha-fetoprotein level > 1000 ng/mL as an exclusion criterion for liver transplantation in patients with hepatocellular carcinoma meeting the Milan criteria. Liver Transpl 20(8):945–951

Hays RE, Rudow DL, Dew MA et al (2015) The independent living donor advocate: a guidance document from the American Society of Transplantation's Living Donor Community of Practice (AST LDCOP). Am J Transplant 15(2):518–525

Hibi T, Itano O, Shinoda M et al (2017) Liver transplantation for hepatobiliary malignancies: a new era of "Transplant Oncology" has begun. Surg Today 47(4):403–415

Hibi T, Sapisochin G (2019) What is transplant oncology? Surgery 165(2):281–285

Hsu CC, Chen CL, Wang CC et al (2016) Combination of FDG-PET and UCSF Criteria for Predicting HCC Recurrence After Living Donor Liver Transplantation. Transplantation 100(9):1925–1932

Humar A, Carolan E, Ibrahim H et al (2005) A comparison of surgical outcomes and quality of life surveys in right lobe vs. left lateral segment liver donors. Am J Transplant 5(4 Pt 1):805–809

Hwang S, Lee SG, Lee YL et al (2006) Lessons learned from 1,000 living donor liver transplantations in a single center: how to make living donations safe. Liver Transpl 12(6): 920–927

ILTS (2019) ILTS Consensus Conference. ILTS, (2019) Consensus Conference: Transplant Oncology—the Future of Multidisciplinary Management. International Liver Transplantation Society, Rotterdam, The Netherlands

Jennings T, Grauer D, Rudow DL (2013) The role of the independent donor advocacy team in the case of a declined living donor candidate. Prog Transplant 23(2):132–136

Karliova M, Malagó M, Valentin-Gamazo C et al (2002) Living-related liver transplantation from the view of the donor: a 1-year follow-up survey. Transplantation 73(11):1799–1804

Kim SH, Moon DB, Kim WJ et al (2016) Preoperative prognostic values of α-fetoprotein (AFP) and protein induced by vitamin K absence or antagonist-II (PIVKA-II) in patients with hepatocellular carcinoma for living donor liver transplantation. Hepatobiliary Surg Nutr 5(6): 461–469

Kim-Schluger L, Florman SS (2002) Quality of life after lobectomy for adult liver transplantation. Transplantation 73(10):1593–1597

Knibbe ME, Maeckelberghe EL, Verkerk MA (2007) Confounders in voluntary consent about living parental liver donation: no choice and emotions. Med Health Care Philos 10(4):433–440

Königsrainer A, Templin S, Capobianco I et al (2019) Paradigm Shift in the Management of Irresectable Colorectal Liver Metastases: Living Donor Auxiliary Partial Orthotopic Liver Transplantation in Combination With Two-stage Hepatectomy (LD-RAPID). Ann Surg 270(2): 327–332

Kornberg A, Schernhammer M, Friess H (2017) (18)F-FDG-PET for assessing biological viability and prognosis in liver transplant patients with Hepatocellular Carcinoma. J Clin Transl Hepatol 5(3):224–234

Lai Q, Nicolini D, Inostroza Nunez M et al (2016) A Novel Prognostic Index in Patients With Hepatocellular Cancer Waiting for Liver Transplantation: Time-Radiological-response-Alpha-fetoprotein-INflammation (TRAIN) Score. Ann Surg 264(5):787–796

Lai Q, Feys E, Karam V et al (2017a) Hepatic Epithelioid Hemangioendothelioma and Adult Liver transplantation: proposal for a prognostic score based on the analysis of the ELTR-ELITA Registry. Transplantation 101(3):555–564

Lai Q, Vitale A, Iesari S et al (2017b) Intention-to-treat survival benefit of liver transplantation in patients with hepatocellular cancer. Hepatology 66(6):1910–1919

Lee HW, Song GW, Lee SG et al (2018) Patient Selection by Tumor Markers in Liver Transplantation for Advanced Hepatocellular Carcinoma. Liver Transpl 24(9):1243–1251

Lee JG, Lee KW, Kwon CHD et al (2017) Donor safety in living donor liver transplantation: the Korean organ transplantation registry study. Liver Transpl 23(8):999–1006

Liang W, Wu L, Ling X et al (2012) Living donor liver transplantation versus deceased donor liver transplantation for hepatocellular carcinoma: a meta-analysis. Liver Transpl 18(10):1226–1236

Lieber SR, Schiano TD, Rhodes R (2018) Should living donor liver transplantation be an option when deceased donation is not? J Hepatol 68(5):1076–1082

Line PD, Hagness M, Berstad AE et al (2015) A novel concept for partial liver transplantation in nonresectable colorectal liver metastases: the RAPID concept. Ann Surg 262(1):e5-9

Line PD, Hagness M, Dueland S (2018) The potential role of liver transplantation as a treatment option in colorectal liver metastases. Can J Gastroenterol Hepatol 2018:8547940

Mazzaferro V, Sposito C, Coppa J et al (2016) The long-term benefit of liver transplantation for hepatic metastases from neuroendocrine tumors. Am J Transplant 16(10):2892–2902

Mazzaferro V, Sposito C, Zhou J et al (2018) Metroticket 2.0 model for analysis of competing risks of death after liver transplantation for hepatocellular carcinoma. Gastroenterology 154(1): 128–139

Merani S, Majno P, Kneteman NM et al (2011) The impact of waiting list alpha-fetoprotein changes on the outcome of liver transplant for hepatocellular carcinoma. J Hepatol 55(4): 814–819

Middleton PF, Duffield M, Lynch SV et al (2006) Living donor liver transplantation–adult donor outcomes: a systematic review. Liver Transpl 12(1):24–30

Miller C (2014) Preparing for the inevitable: the death of a living liver donor. Liver Transpl 20(Suppl 2):S47–S51

Miller CM (2008) Ethical dimensions of living donation: experience with living liver donation. Transplant Rev (Orlando) 22(3):206–209

Miyagi S, Kawagishi N, Fujimori K et al (2005) Risks of donation and quality of donors' life after living donor liver transplantation. Transpl Int 18(1):47–51

Nadalin S, Capobianco I, Konigsrainer I et al (2015) Living liver donor: indications and technical aspects. Chirurg 86(6):609–621;quiz 622

Nadalin S, Malagó M, Broelsch CE (2006) Historical Notes, Liver Transplantation. Pediatric Solid Organ Transplantation. R. N. Fine, A. K. Deirdre, S. A. Webber, E. H. William and K. M. Olthoff. Blackwell Publishing 2:193–198

Nadalin S, Malago M, Radtke A et al (2007) Current trends in live liver donation. Transpl Int 20(4):312–330

Otto G (2013) Liver transplantation: an appraisal of the present situation. Dig Dis 31(1):164–169

Panocchia N, Bossola M, Silvestri P et al (2013) Ethical evaluation of risks related to living donor transplantation programs. Transplant Proc 45(7):2601–2603

Parikh ND, Waljee AK, Singal AG (2015) Downstaging hepatocellular carcinoma: A systematic review and pooled analysis. Liver Transpl 21(9):1142–1152

Pascher A, Neuhaus P (2003) Ethical considerations regarding living donation for patients with malignant liver tumors. Transplant Proc 35(3):1169–1171

Patel S, Orloff M, Tsoulfas G et al (2007) Living-donor liver transplantation in the United States: identifying donors at risk for perioperative complications. Am J Transplant 7(10):2344–2349

Petrini C (2010) Ethical issues with informed consent from potential living kidney donors. Transplant Proc 42(4):1040–1042

Pomfret EA, Lodge JP, Villamil FG et al (2011) Should we use living donor grafts for patients with hepatocellular carcinoma? Ethical Considerations. Liver Transpl 17(Suppl 2):S128–S132

Post SG (2005) Altruism, happiness, and health: it's good to be good. Int J Behav Med 12(2): 66–77

Samoylova ML, Dodge JL, Yao FY et al (2014) Time to transplantation as a predictor of hepatocellular carcinoma recurrence after liver transplantation. Liver Transpl 20(8):937–944

Schiano TD, Rhodes R (2015) The Ethics of living related liver transplantation when deceased donation is not an option. Clin Liver Dis (Hoboken) 6(5):112–116

Shimamura T, Akamatsu N, Fujiyoshi M et al (2019) Expanded living-donor liver transplantation criteria for patients with hepatocellular carcinoma based on the Japanese nationwide survey: the 5-5-500 rule - a retrospective study. Transpl Int 32(4):356–368

Siegler J, Siegler M, Cronin DC (2004) Recipient death during a live donor liver transplantation: who gets the "orphan" graft? Transplantation 78(9):1241–1244

Strong RW, Lynch SV (1996) Ethical issues in living related donor liver transplantation. Transplant Proc 28(4):2366–2369

Sugarman J, Lavori PW, Boeger M et al (2005) Evaluating the quality of informed consent. Clin Trials 2(1):34–41

Suh KS, Suh SW, Lee JM et al (2015) Recent advancements in and views on the donor operation in living donor liver transplantation: a single-center study of 886 patients over 13 years. Liver Transpl 21(3):329–338

Trevisani F, Garuti F, Neri A (2019) Alpha-fetoprotein for diagnosis, prognosis, and transplant selection. Semin Liver Dis 39(2):163–177

Trotter JF, Talamantes M, McClure M et al (2001) Right hepatic lobe donation for living donor liver transplantation: impact on donor quality of life. Liver Transpl 7(6):485–493

Venkat KK, Eshelman AK (2014) The evolving approach to ethical issues in living donor kidney transplantation: a review based on illustrative case vignettes. Transplant Rev (Orlando) 28(3): 134–139

Verbesey JE, Simpson MA, Pomposelli JJ et al (2005) Living donor adult liver transplantation: a longitudinal study of the donor's quality of life. Am J Transplant 5(11):2770–2777

Vibert E, Azoulay D, Hoti E et al (2010) Progression of alphafetoprotein before liver transplantation for hepatocellular carcinoma in cirrhotic patients: a critical factor. Am J Transplant 10(1):129–137

Volk ML, Marrero JA, Lok AS et al (2006) Who decides? Living donor liver transplantation for advanced hepatocellular carcinoma. Transplantation 82(9):1136–1139

Walter M, Bronner E, Pascher A et al (2002) Psychosocial outcome of living donors after living donor liver transplantation: a pilot study. Clin Transplant 16(5):339–344

Walter M, Dammann G, Küchenhoff J et al (2005) Psychosocial situation of living donors: moods, complaints, and self-image before and after liver transplantation. Med Sci Monit 11(11): Cr503–509

Walter M, Pascher A, Jonas S et al (2005) Living donor liver transplantation from the perspective of the donor: results of a psychosomatic investigation. Z Psychosom Med Psychother 51(4): 331–345

Xia W, Ke Q, Guo H et al (2017) Expansion of the Milan criteria without any sacrifice: combination of the Hangzhou criteria with the pre-transplant platelet-to-lymphocyte ratio. BMC Cancer 17(1):14

Yao FY, Mehta N, Flemming J et al (2015) Downstaging of hepatocellular cancer before liver transplant: long-term outcome compared to tumors within Milan criteria. Hepatology 61(6): 1968–1977

Yaprak O, Acar S, Ertugrul G et al (2018) Role of pre-transplant 18F-FDG PET/CT in predicting hepatocellular carcinoma recurrence after liver transplantation. World J Gastrointest Oncol 10(10):336–343

Ethical Challenges in Pediatric Oncology Care and Clinical Trials

11

Daniel J. Benedetti and Jonathan M. Marron

11.1 Introduction—Why is Pediatric Ethics Different?

Clinically, the care of pediatric cancer patients is a vast departure from cancer care of adults. While the available treatment modalities—chemotherapy, radiation, and surgery—are the same, the diseases, care-delivery, and outcomes differ greatly. And just as 'children are not just little adults,' pediatric bioethics occupies a distinct place within the broader field of bioethics. In this chapter, we highlight the framework for understanding ethical issues in pediatrics and explore common ethical dilemmas pediatric oncologists encounter.

We must begin with a caveat that is important for readers of this text. We are pediatricians and pediatric hematologists/oncologists in the USA (US), where we were both born, raised, and professionally trained. The US medical and legal systems are different from those in other countries (Blake et al. 2011) and reflect unique American social and cultural values. Because ethics and law are inextricably linked, and profoundly influenced by societal and personal values, the frameworks we discuss will reflect our US-centric background and may not be completely applicable in other settings. We will denote where US laws are a major factor in our ethical analysis. But to appropriately think through ethical dilemmas in pediatric

D. J. Benedetti (✉)
Division of Hematology-Oncology, Department of Pediatrics,
Vanderbilt University Medical Center, 2220 Pierce Avenue 397 PRB,
Nashville, TN 37232-6310, USA
e-mail: daniel.benedetti@vumc.org

J. M. Marron
Division of Pediatric Hematology/Oncology, Harvard Medical School,
Center for Bioethics, Dana-Farber/Boston Children's Cancer and Blood Disorders Center,
Boston, MA 02215, USA
e-mail: jonathan_marron@dfci.harvard.edu

© Springer Nature Switzerland AG 2021
A. W. Bauer et al. (eds.), *Ethical Challenges in Cancer Diagnosis and Therapy*,
Recent Results in Cancer Research 218,
https://doi.org/10.1007/978-3-030-63749-1_11

149

oncology, the reader must have a firm understanding of the value-system and legal standing in their country of practice.

Why are ethical issues in pediatrics different? Most clinical encounters for the adult patient are dyadic, involving a patient and physician jointly making decisions for the patient. But because (most) children are unable to make decisions for themselves, decisions about their medical care are made by others, usually their parents. Therefore, pediatrics involves a triadic relationship, with the child-patient and parents as independent parties in the relationship. The child's healthcare is thus subject to the views and values of both the parent and physician, and yet the child experiences the effects of decisions they had little-to-no part in making. The parent is a fiduciary of the child, with an obligation to protect and promote the health and non-health-related interests of the child. The physician is a fiduciary of the child-patient, with an obligation to protect and promote the health-related interests of their patient (McCullough 2010). At its core, 'pediatric ethics explores how to make the best choices for children [...] seeks to define parental and clinician obligations to children and [...] attempts to protect the interests of children' (Fleischman 2016).

Another critical layer of pediatric ethics is the concept of emerging and future autonomy. While children generally lack the ability to make decisions for themselves at the time a decision must be made, most will eventually acquire the ability to make such decisions. Most develop their own values and become autonomous adults, capable of making choices that reflect these values and preferences. Therefore, the parents and physicians, as co-fiduciaries of the child, have a duty to promote and protect the emerging and future autonomy of the child. They should promote the child's emerging autonomy by allowing the child to participate in decision-making to the extent she is developmentally capable at that time. And they should promote the child's future autonomy by making choices that optimize the chance that the child will become an autonomous adult. Often described as the child's 'right to an open future' (Feinberg 1980), this concept comes to the forefront in such decisions as performing germline sequencing in children, which we will explore further later in this chapter.

It is in this background that ethical dilemmas occur in pediatrics and pediatric cancer care. In this chapter, we will describe ethical challenges commonly encountered by pediatric oncologists, examining issues involving (a) informed consent; (b) research involving children; (c) end of life; and (d) genetic and genomic testing.

11.2   Informed Consent, Assent, and Developing Autonomy in Pediatric Cancer

11.2.1   Parental Decision-Making for Children as Incompetent Patients

Central to the discussion of informed consent especially for children is an understanding of the concepts of competence and informed consent for patients who lack capacity. While *capacity* is a medical determination, and *competence* is a legal judgment, many argue that this difference is inconsequential in practice (Appel-baum 2007; Beauchamp and Childress 2013). For our purposes, we will use them interchangeably to indicate a person's ability to cognitively, psychologically, and legally complete the necessary tasks to make a decision. And because by law in the USA—where the age of majority is 18 years—children lack capacity, we will briefly examine informed consent for the incompetent adult prior to explicating the framework for informed consent in children. An adult who becomes incapacitated (temporarily or permanently) must have a surrogate decision-maker appointed to make decisions on her behalf. Identifying the appropriate surrogate for a patient depends on many factors, and while all 50 US states have statutes that address surrogate decision-making, there is wide variability (DeMartino et al. 2017). Accordingly, physicians should be familiar with relevant laws in their jurisdiction or should consult with ethics or legal teams at their institution.

There are two main frameworks a surrogate can use to make decisions for the patient, the *substituted judgment standard* and the *best interests standard*. Substi-tuted judgment is the preferred framework, asking a surrogate to make the decision that the patient would if she were not incapacitated. This decision can be informed by personal conversations about specific circumstances, by knowledge of the patient's general values, or by written preferences documented in an advanced directive. While this framework strives to preserve patient autonomy by encour-aging decisions that approximate the choice the incapacitated patient would make, surrogates often lack sufficient knowledge to make choices just as the patient would. When this occurs, the *best interests standard* is the more appropriate framework to use. One definition of this standard is 'acting so as to promote maximally the good of the individual' (Buchanan and Brock 1989). More simply stated, this standard asks surrogates to make the decision they believe to be in the patient's best interest.

Minor children are by definition incompetent and therefore require a surrogate to make health decisions on their behalf. The surrogate is almost always the child's parent, and with a strong moral and legal justification. Society allows parents wide leeway to make decisions for their children, including value-based decisions such as what they eat, what school they attend, and whether they practice a religion. Deference to parental choices is justified in most situations, because parents are uniquely positioned to know and understand the child's interests. Parents instill values in the child, meaning the child will share many if-not most of the parents' values. Accordingly, most of a parents' decisions are likely to reflect the decisions the child would make once they become competent. Additionally, parents almost always have the best interest of the child in mind. Lastly, parents—more than anyone else—will bear the consequences of choices that impact the child. For all of these reasons, parents are the appropriate surrogate decision-makers for children for most health decisions. At times, parents must weigh familial interests, such as the interests of other children, the parents themselves, and the family unit itself. But because familial interests usually align with the child's interests, and the child's interests often depend on the familial interests, it remains appropriate for parents to balance these interests.

There is a subtle but important distinction to make between parental autonomy and parental authority. 'Autonomy is the right of a rational person to make his or her own decisions, and provides a moral justification for … informed consent' (Unguru 2011). When parents make health decisions on behalf of someone else (the child), they do not exercise autonomy. It is more accurate to describe what they do as exercising parental authority. A corollary is that parents do not provide informed consent for medical interventions for the child, and they provide informed permission. This distinction highlights the fact that parents are surrogate decision-makers and do not have carte blanche to make whatever decision they want. Rather, they are morally obligated to use the established frameworks for surrogate decision-making outlined above.

It is inappropriate to use substituted judgment to make decisions for children. Substituted judgment is ideal for the adult who has become incompetent but at one time had the capacity to develop and express autonomous values and wishes. Because children lack capacity, application of the best interests standard is appropriate for pediatric decision-making (Kopelman 1997).

11.2.2 Participation of Children in Medical Decision-Making

Children at all stages of development will develop and express opinions relevant to their care, and children should be given choices about aspects of their care that they are developmentally capable of making. In most situations, it is appropriate to use a sliding-scale, with more weight given to a younger child's opinion about lower-stakes decisions (e.g., which arm to place an IV), but with higher-stakes decisions typically restricted to older and more mature children (Katz et al. 2016). Parents may choose to incorporate the child's values or opinion into the parents' decisions, but until a child reaches adulthood their values should rarely override parental choices, particularly about major medical decisions. In many circumstances it is appropriate to solicit the assent of the child. *Assent* refers to a child's agreement or approval to participate in the care agreed upon by the parent (Committee on Bioethics 2016). It is a way to give children a voice, respect their dignity, and promote and protect their interests (Unguru et al. 2008). There is no consensus about the age at which a child can provide assent; however, some suggest that most children are developmentally capable of giving assent at 7 years of age (Diekema 2006). Despite this ideal, it remains controversial how the minor's voice should be included in medical decisions, particularly in the setting of decisional conflict.

In the USA, there are two circumstances in which we allow minors to make autonomous healthcare decisions; that of emancipated minors and mature minors. An *emancipated minor* is granted legal status as an adult to make decisions on her behalf. A minor may become emancipated permanently if she lives independently of her parents, usually living on her own, being married, and being financially independent from her parents. A minor may also be emancipated based on predetermined health conditions, including pregnancy, sexually transmitted infections, mental health disorders, or substance use disorders. A child emancipated under these conditions may independently consent for care only as it relates to these conditions. The rationale for these exceptions is not based on the child having capacity for these decisions. Historically, adolescents have not sought care for these conditions when parental permission was required, and society's public health interests—that adolescents seek and secure treatment for these conditions—generally outweigh concerns over minors' incomplete capacity to make these decisions (Katz et al. 2016). A *mature minor* is a child who is determined by a judge to have sufficient capacity to give informed consent or refusal for a particular medical decision. Not all US states have mature minor statutes (Coleman and Rosoff 2013). Furthermore, when a child successfully petitions for status as a mature minor, her decision-making authority is limited to the specific decision approved by the court.

11.2.3 Ethical Dilemmas Involving Informed Consent

11.2.3.1 Parental Refusal of Cancer Treatment

While most parents agree to recommended cancer treatment, some families resist or refuse curative cancer therapy, and the oncologist must decide whether to support the refusal, or attempt to persuade the parents. In general, when the prognosis is extremely poor, or the morbidity of treatment extremely high, it may be appropriate to allow parental refusal. In contrast, when the prognosis is good, or the morbidity of treatment is low, persuasion should be attempted. These deliberations can be contentious, can lead to significant distress for the oncologist (Rosenberg 2015), and some even draw widespread media attention (Goldschmidt 2015). If attempts to persuade a family are unsuccessful, the oncologist may request court-ordered treatment, claiming that failure to treat would constitute medical neglect. There is no consensus about how to decide when to request court-ordered treatment. Some believe the best interests standard should guide this decision (Pope 2011), while others have proposed alternative ethical frameworks for these decisions, including the *Harm Principle* (Diekema 2004), *Constrained Parental Autonomy* (Ross 1998), and the *Zone of Parental Discretion* (Gillam 2016). Requests for compelled treatment are not always granted, as some judges defer to parents' wishes or find the child to be a 'mature minor' (In re EG 1989). Other judges may compel chemotherapy, even for children just under the age of majority (In re Cassandra C 2015).

Pediatric oncologists should be familiar with the relevant medical neglect laws in their jurisdiction, as well as their obligations as mandated reporters of abuse and neglect. Most agree that legal involvement should be a last resort. To avoid this, it may be appropriate for oncologists to consider alternative treatment options, compromises or making alterations to the treatment that would be acceptable to the family without significantly reducing the chances of cure and/or risk of toxicity. Consultation with experts in other disciplines may help navigate these cases, including social work, psychology, child life, chaplaincy, ethics, palliative care, legal or risk management, and child abuse. Despite persuasion or legal involvement, some patients abscond to avoid treatment (Caruso Brown and Slutzky 2017).

11.2.3.2 Child Refusal of Treatment

Children, particularly adolescents, may object to aspects of their cancer care when they experience or worry about side effects. In some circumstances, this may be easily overcome by good communication from the child's parents and the oncology team. Psychosocial team members (e.g., child life specialists, psychologists, social workers, etc.) may be helpful, particularly if there are concerns about depression, or when refusal occurs shortly after a child's diagnosis, such as a teenager refusing chemotherapy due to not wanting to lose her hair. In other situations, a child's refusal can pose significant challenges, as adolescents can be difficult to convince to do something against their will, and may even run away to avoid being forced to comply with treatment (Ross 2009).

11.2.3.3 Parental Requests for Non-recommended Treatments

When a child develops refractory and progressive cancer, parents may ask oncologists for treatment options that have no meaningful chance of benefiting the child. Sometimes these options include early-phase clinic trials, which despite a low likelihood of clinical benefit (explored in greater detail below), advance scientific knowledge and may provide psychological benefits from hope and from making a contribution to science. At other times, however, parents may request treatment without evidence of efficacy, and not available through a clinical trial. Physicians are not obligated to provide care they believe to be inappropriate (Bosslet et al. 2015). Historically such requests were labeled as 'futile'; however, the term 'futility' is controversial, and its use is falling out of favor (Burns and Truog 2007). Most scholarly attention to this problem centers around requests for care in intensive care unit settings and has resulted in a series of policies—e.g., the Texas Advance Directives Act of 1999 (Texas Health and Safety Code 1999)—or procedural approaches for resolving conflicts (Truog 2009). Some criticize the approach of 'exclusively leaning on policy, [as it] underplays the ethical significance of the decision and insufficiently recognizes the singular role of the parent' (Marron 2018). Because technological and scientific advances continue to expand the range of treatment options available to pediatric cancer patients, future work is needed to develop an ethical framework for how to best consider and navigate these requests.

11.2.3.4 Minors as Hematopoietic Stem Cell Donors

Some children with aggressive or refractory cancers require allogeneic stem cell transplants to maximize their chance of being cured. HLA-matched, biologically related donors are preferred due to lower risks of transplant-related complications, and siblings are the most likely family members to be an HLA match. Because siblings are often children—and therefore unable to provide autonomous consent to the procedure—there are unique ethical issues and arguments to consider (Kesselheim et al. 2009). Most agree that minors may ethically serve as donors, however due to rare cases of significant psychological harms to donors (Opel and Diekema 2006), the American Academy of Pediatrics recommends a risk/benefit calculation that takes into account both the physical and psychological well-being of the donor, including how this relates to the recipient's survival (Committee on Bioethics 2010).

11.3 Research Involving Children

Around the world, the efforts of cooperative groups dedicated to pediatric cancer research receive significant funding and have resulted in an increase in cure rates from approximately 10% in 1950 to greater than 80% today (O'Leary et al. 2008). Despite the overwhelming success of this research model, there are numerous ethical issues that must be considered and addressed when conducting research involving children.

11.3.1 Children as a Vulnerable Population

Children have long been recognized as a vulnerable population that could be subjected to unethical research (Grodin and Glantz 1994), and stringent protections exist to minimize their exposure to harm, yet also to ensure they aren't excluded from the benefits of research (Office for Protection from Research Risks 1983). Because children require surrogate decision-makers, parental permission is required for a child's participation in research. This process of permission should be identical to informed consent for an adult research participant (Diekema 2006). Assent may be required depending on a child's age, maturity, psychological state, and the determination of the research ethics board [e.g. Institutional Review Board (IRB)]. Assent holds more weight in research deliberations than in routine clinical care, and a child's dissent (i.e., refusal to assent) ought to be respected for nearly all research, except where research participation offers prospect of direct benefit, and is unavailable outside of the research context (Office for Protection from Research Risks 1983).

11.3.2 Therapeutic Misconception

The *therapeutic misconception* is 'the belief that the purpose of a clinical trial is to benefit the individual patient rather than to gather data for the purpose of contributing to scientific knowledge' (National Bioethics Advisory Commission 2001). This misconception occurs 'when individuals do not understand that the defining purpose of clinical research is to produce generalizable knowledge, regardless of whether the subjects enrolled… may potentially benefit from the intervention under study or other aspects of the clinical trial' (Henderson et al. 2007). This belief is problematic for the conduct of clinical research, as it calls into question and undermines the validity of subjects' informed consent. Other types of misunderstandings can similarly undercut and compromise research consent, including *therapeutic misestimation, therapeutic optimism* (Horng and Grady 2003), and *unrealistic optimism* (Crites and Kodish 2013), and these misunderstandings may sit on a continuum (Sisk and Kodish 2018). Evidence of these misunderstandings has prompted calls for new approaches to clinical trial enrollment. While some have suggested that clinicians ought not present study details or offer enrollment (Flory and Emanuel 2004; Eder et al. 2007), this would be a significant challenge in pediatric oncology, where most physicians also serve as investigators on clinical trials.

The two best-studied examples of misunderstandings during clinic trial consent revolve around understanding of randomization, and consent to phase I clinical trials.

11.3.2.1 Randomization

In audiotaping informed consent conferences (ICCs) between pediatric oncologists and parents of children with Acute Lymphoblastic Leukemia, Kodish et al. found that a significant percentage of parents offered enrollment on a randomized controlled trial mistakenly believed that enrolled children would receive the treatment arm that the clinician felt was the best fit for the child (Kodish et al. 2004). Many of these children (84%) were ultimately enrolled on the trial, and while not statistically significant, parents who did not understand randomization were more likely to consent to the study than those who understood it. This raises the question of whether parents, were they to understand randomization, would not enroll their children in randomized clinical trials.

11.3.2.2 Phase I Research Consent

Phase I trials are a critical part of clinical research, particularly in the emerging era of 'targeted therapies.' The goal of a phase I trial is to explore the safety of a new drug, by determining the dose-limiting toxicities and maximum tolerated dose of the agent, with hopes of finding a safe dose for subsequent trials to examine efficacy. These early-phase trials are limited to small numbers of subjects, and while the hope is that novel agents will prove to be safe and efficacious, there is no therapeutic intent to the phase I trial. This lack of therapeutic intent is a source of confusion for parents. Daugherty et al. found that barely one third of adults enrolling in phase I trials understood the purpose of the trial to include 'dose/toxicity determination.' The vast majority reported 'seeking anticancer response' such as remission or cure as the main reason for participation (Daugherty et al. 2000). Cousino et al. found that parents of children with cancer who participated in ICCs had poor understanding of the safety and dose-finding purposes of phase I trials (Cousino et al. 2012). While the cause of misunderstandings is unclear, efforts are underway to improve pediatric oncologists' communication skills for ICCs (Cousino et al. 2011, Johnson et al. 2015).

11.3.3   Is There a Prospect of Direct Benefit in Phase I Clinical Trials?

Whether phase I trials offer the prospect of direct benefit to subjects is a critical question to decide whether it is permissible to enroll children with cancer on these studies (Kodish 2003; Ross 2006; Weber et al. 2015; Kimmelman 2017). A recent meta-analysis of phase I pediatric oncology trials from 2004 to 2015 found that 10% of participants had an objective response (Waligora et al. 2018). In addition to citing tumor response rates as direct benefits, others insist that participants benefit from maintaining hope, and making scientific contributions that benefit future children with cancer (Kodish et al. 1992). An added layer of complexity is that parents, who are not the research subjects and yet provide informed permission, may derive these benefits (e.g., hope) from the child's trial enrollment.

11.3.4   Randomized Clinical Trials and the Challenge of Equipoise

Randomized controlled trials (RCTs) compare the efficacy of two treatments by randomly assigning participants to the treatment arms. It would not be ethically justifiable to subject study participants to less efficacious treatment if one of the options were known to be superior. *Equipoise*—the 'state of professional uncertainty about [the] relative therapeutic merits' of the two treatments being studied—is an important justification for the conduct of RCTs (Miller and Joffe 2011); however, there are many criticisms and challenges to the concept.

First, while this theoretic 'state of uncertainty' is conceptually appealing, oncologists may have a preference for a novel treatment, given the level of evidence of efficacy required for an investigational therapy to make it to a RCT. Promising preliminary data may be sufficient to move expert opinion even before validation in a RCT. Secondly, most patients expect their physician to recommend the best therapeutic option based on their experience, knowledge of existing data, and of the patient. Equipoise requires that patients accept having their treatment chosen randomly, without their physician's input. Thirdly, equipoise ignores the fact that patients may have preferences between treatment arms, even if the oncology community does not. Lastly, even if equipoise exists at the onset of a study, there may reach a point when study data favors one treatment over the other. At this point, equipoise is disturbed, and continuing the trial—if justified by equipoise alone—would be considered unethical. This last concern led to the formation of Data Safety Monitoring Committees, whose role is to evaluate interim data and determine whether to halt a trial. When interim data are equivocal, equipoise remains intact, and a trial continues until completion or until another interim analysis triggers early stopping rules.

11.3.5   Timely Access to Novel Therapies

The clinical research pathway to drug approval is a formal and highly regulated path to enabling access to new medical therapies that are safe and efficacious. Testing new therapies for children with cancer takes far longer than for adults, delaying approval and access to potentially efficacious treatments (Neel et al. 2019). Of the 126 drugs approved by the FDA for oncology indications from 1997 to 2017, only 6 had a pediatric indication with the approval. The fact that childhood cancer is rare, combined with the additional regulations on pediatric research, prompted the passage of laws to promote the development and approval of drugs for children, including the Best Pharmaceuticals for Children Act (US Food and Drug Administration 2002), Pediatric Research Equity Act (United States Congress 2003), and Research to Accelerate Cures and Equity for Children Act (Schmidt 2017). Many hope these measures, along with age-agnostic development of targeted drugs (Drilon et al. 2018), will help expedite the delivery of new therapies to children with cancer (Shulman and DuBois 2019).

11.3.6   'Right to Try' and Compassionate Access

Historically, access to unapproved and unproven therapies has been restricted to 'compassionate use' or 'expanded access' programs, which are intended to provide the rare patient who cannot participate in a clinical trial with a mechanism to seek a novel therapy that *may* benefit her (US Food and Drug Administration (FDA)). In 2018, the US congress passed a controversial 'right-to-try' law that attempts to expand and streamline access to non-FDA-approved therapies (United States Congress 2018). Supporters argue that patients' right to self-determination and self-preservation means they ought to be able to choose to accept the unknown side effects of investigational drugs for the chance the drug will benefit them. But in the USA, physicians are not required to give patients anything they want, and courts have found that 'there is no fundamental right… to experimental drugs for the terminally ill' (Abigail Alliance For Better Access v Von Eschenbach 2007).

Right-to-try opponents worry that terminally ill patients' desperation makes them vulnerable and in need protection, a fact recognized by the US Congress when drafting the Pure Food and Drug Act (Piel 2016). Children with incurable cancer are particularly vulnerable, as there is little parents wouldn't do for any perceived chance to save their child's life. And yet harms may occur from untested drugs, or from the consequences of such laws. Some state right-to-try laws prevent patients from obtaining hospice care or home health care for a period of time after receiving the experimental treatment (Kearns and Bateman-House 2017). For children with progressive cancer, these services are critical to alleviate suffering, and help achieve high-quality end-of-life care. A final concern is that expansion of right-to-try laws may undermine the existing research enterprise and impede approval of medications. At the time of this writing, it is too soon to know what consequences, intended or otherwise, right-to-try legislation will have on pediatric cancer patients.

11.4   Additional Ethical Issues in Pediatric Oncology Care

11.4.1   Drug Shortages

There are between 170 and 200 drug shortages each year in the USA, and these shortages are becoming more frequent and lasting longer (Council on Science and Public Health 2018). Over the past decade, there have been severe shortages in vasopressors, intravenous fluids, neurologic agents, chemotherapeutics, among others. Unfortunately, children with cancer are not immune to the effects of such shortages. One study found that 50% of pediatric patient-subjects enrolled on a clinical trial were impacted by drug shortages, and two-thirds had their clinical care impacted by shortages (Salazar et al. 2015). In recent years, the USA has experienced shortages in chemotherapeutics commonly used in pediatric oncology, including vincristine, methotrexate, etoposide, daunorubicin, and asparaginase. While an equivalent alternative drug may be available, replacing medications of proven efficacy with alternatives can have dire consequences. When the shortage of mechlorethamine necessitated its replacement with cyclophosphamide for children with Hodgkin lymphoma, this substitution resulted in a significant decrement in event-free survival for children with this otherwise highly curable cancer (Metzger et al. 2012).

Drug shortages are not unique to pediatric oncology, but they are particularly impactful in this field given the central role of generic injectable medications (those most commonly affected by drug shortages) in the treatment of children with cancer. It is best to avoid making rationing/allocation decisions being made by the treating clinician at the patient bedside, as this presents a conflict of interest for the clinician, who must both consider how to allocate the drug in scarce supply and simultaneously vouch for the best interests of their patient. It is advisable to have procedures in place for managing drug shortages and to minimize conflicts of interest and maintain public trust, and the allocation strategies should be transparent to physicians, patients/families and to the general public and should involve just application of allocation principles (Decamp et al. 2014; Drug Shortages Task Force 2019).

11.4.2   Requests to Withhold a Cancer Diagnosis

Parents occasionally ask that the oncology team hide a cancer diagnosis from a child. Clinicians who encounter this request should explore the parents' motivation for the request. Some families come from cultures that believe in withholding cancer diagnoses from all patients, including autonomous adults. More commonly, however, parents want to protect their child, and worry about causing additional distress or anxiety at a time when they are already sick and undergoing medical procedures and treatments. Despite this natural parental desire to protect their child, it is important to be transparent with the child about their diagnosis. Disclosing this information exemplifies respect for the child's emerging autonomy, so that she understands why she is sick and the nature of the tests and treatments she will undergo. Often it is appropriate to disclose a cancer diagnosis to the parents and child at the same time, particular when the patient is an adolescent. Other times, the cancer diagnosis may be disclosed to the parents separately, and the oncologist should seek the parents' input into the best way to inform the child. Soliciting this information recognizes and respects parents' unique understanding of their child's psychological needs (Mack and Grier 2004) and ensures that disclosure is done in age and developmentally appropriate language, and with appropriate social and psychological support surrounding the child. Most children take the news of a cancer diagnosis better than parents fear, as the word 'cancer' is less likely to trigger the same negative stigma that it does for adults.

The second, practical reason not to honor parents' request for non-disclosure is that it will be impossible to hide this information from a child who is likely to visit a 'cancer center' for appointments, interact with providers whose badges or clothing refer to cancer, receive chemotherapy, and meet or see other children with alopecia due to chemotherapy. An observant child is likely to put the pieces together and deduce that she has cancer. Additionally, even if an oncologist agreed to withhold this information from a child, the child will interact with dozens of healthcare providers each hospital day or visit to the clinic. It would be impractical to expect everyone else not to use the word 'cancer,' and accidental disclosure is inevitable. Withholding this information may have negative consequences for a child, including fear or anxiety knowing that their parents and doctor are keeping a secret from them. Some may interpret this to mean that the situation is worse than it really is; for example, a child may think she is dying when in fact she has a highly curable cancer. Other children will have difficulty trusting their parents and physicians, with negative consequences on their cancer treatment experience or adherence (Mack et al. 2018; Lin et al. 2019).

11.5 Ethical Issues at or Near the End of Life

Many ethical challenges arising in the care of children with cancer at or near the end of life are similar to those encountered in the care of adults; however given the unique nature of pediatric bioethics, some features of pediatric end-of-life (EOL) care are particularly noteworthy.

11.5.1 Requests not to Tell a Child They Are Dying

When a child is not expected to survive, parents may wish to not tell their child that they are dying. This is challenging for all involved, and similar principles and considerations apply as above, when a parent wishes to not tell a child about their cancer diagnosis. In this case, however, the stakes are even greater and most would agree that the telling the truth to the child is imperative. Doing so can support the dying child's burgeoning autonomy, allowing them to participate in their EOL care plans and express what they would like to do with their remaining time. The level of involvement will depend on the child's age, developmental status, and clinical scenario, but most minors express a strong desire to be told of their prognosis and expected treatment course (Mack et al. 2018).

Openly speaking about prognosis and death in both children and adults with cancer is a relatively recent phenomenon. As recently as 1961, 90% of physicians reported not telling patients that they had cancer (Oken 1961). Today, nearly all oncologists believe they have an 'ethical imperative' to disclose a cancer diagnosis (Daugherty and Hlubocky 2008), yet it is not universal. Complicating these prognostic discussions are cultural differences in how this truth-telling about prognosis is perceived (Rosenberg et al. 2017). Whether to tell a child about their prognosis when a parent requests to withhold this information, represents a unique conflict between the rights of the child and the authority of the parent. With limited data on how to navigate this dilemma, oncologists should explore and thoughtfully address parents' reasons for wishing to withhold this information and explore ways to deliver the truth that are acceptable to all involved.

11.5.2 Refusal of Life-Sustaining Therapies

While typically the goal of treatment is to prolong the child's life and/or enhance their quality of life, sometimes the decision is made to forgo life-sustaining therapies (LST) when a child appears to be nearing the end of their life. Adults have the legal and ethical right to refuse medical treatment, and in most circumstances, parents have the authority to refuse treatment on behalf of their minor children, including all types of EOL care, be it palliative chemotherapy, mechanical ventilatory support, or other therapies (Katz et al. 2016). In 1983, the President's Commission for the Study of Ethical Problems in Medicine and Biomedical and Behavioral Research developed a framework for considering both the perspectives of the medical team and the preferences of the parents when faced with a decision whether to continue or forgo a particular LST for a child (President's Commission 1983). Communication and collaboration among clinicians, parents, and the patient are of particular importance in such scenarios, and legal and/or ethics support may be advisable, particularly if there is disagreement about the decision (Weise et al. 2017).

Pediatric oncologists occasionally encounter the challenging question: can parents refuse all therapies in all scenarios for their children at or near the end of life? Factors such as the child's prognosis, risks and benefits of treatment, quality of life, and patient/family preferences should be considered. Decisional frameworks discussed above—such as the *Best Interest Standard, Harm Principle, Zone of Parental Discretion*, and *Constrained Parental Autonomy*—can aid clinicians in deciding whether to attempt to override refusal of EOL therapies, or to respect the refusal. The clinical and ethical considerations for a minor child at the end of life are quite different than those at other points in the care continuum. For example, while a child with incurable cancer may derive some measurable benefit from palliative, oral chemotherapy, the harms from legal involvement and conflict would almost certainly exceed those benefits if the child's parents did not wish to provide such therapy. As a result, parents should generally be given wide discretion regarding EOL treatment decisions, with attempts to override these decisions made only in unique (and rare) circumstances.

11.5.3 Withholding and Withdrawing Life-Sustaining Therapies

Although withholding and withdrawing medical interventions are generally considered to be ethically equivalent, many clinicians report these to be psychologically quite distinct. It is often stated that it feels more difficult to withdraw a LST (e.g., mechanical ventilation) than to choose not to initiate such a therapy. There are further differences in how it feels to withdraw different types of medical therapies. For example, it is less controversial to withdraw intensive, invasive, or burdensome interventions (e.g., surgery, chemotherapy, mechanical ventilation), sometimes referred to as 'extraordinary' measures. But the same cannot always be said for more 'ordinary' measures such as artificial nutrition and hydration (via intravenous fluids, nasogastric feeds, etc.). While most agree that it is ethically permissible to withdraw life-sustaining artificial hydration and/or fluids for a child at the end of life, many experts recommend consultation with local experts from ethics, legal, and/or other support services given the complexity of and emotional response to such withdrawals (Diekema and Botkin 2009).

11.5.4 Palliative Care and Palliative Sedation

The field of pediatric palliative care has grown substantially since early work identified that children who die of cancer often experience significant symptom burden as they approach the end of life (Wolfe et al. 2000). Some also experience existential distress about their pending death. Given the great improvements in supportive care and palliative care in the inpatient and outpatient settings, most symptoms can be controlled for children dying of cancer. Rarely, symptoms cannot be adequately controlled despite maximal supportive therapies, and palliative sedation is an important consideration for such uncommon scenarios. The purpose of palliative sedation is to alleviate the dying child's symptoms, while acknowledging that doing so may unintentionally hasten the child's death (American Academy of Pediatrics 2000). The doctrine of double effect (DDE), a guiding principle first developed by Catholic clerics in the Middle Ages, provides justification for palliative sedation in children and adults (Quill et al. 1997; McIntyre 2018). According to the DDE, a given intervention is ethically permissible as long as it meets each of four conditions:

1 The act itself is morally neutral or good. In the case of palliative sedation, the act is the administration of a medication such as morphine.

2 The provider intends for the 'good' effect of this intervention but not for a possible 'bad' effect (though the bad effect may be foreseen). In this case, the good (intended) effect is relief of the child's pain/suffering and the bad (unintended) effect is hastening of the child's death.

3 The bad effect cannot be the means by which the good affect is achieved. In palliative sedation, pain relief is due to the primary effect of the morphine, not to death itself (contrast this with administration of a very large dose of intravenous potassium chloride: Potassium has no pain-relieving properties, the child's pain relief would result solely from her death).

4 Finally, the benefits of the good effect must outweigh the harms of the bad effect. While this assessment is subjective and may be debated, given the degree of uncontrollable pain that would warrant consideration of palliative sedation, relief of pain and suffering outweighs even the possibility of hastened death.

In addition to the ethical support the DDE provides for the practice of palliative sedation, this practice also has legal support. In 1997, the US Supreme Court invoked the DDE in stating that it is legal to provide medication to alleviate suffering to a dying patient 'even to the point of causing unconsciousness and hastening death' (Vacco v Quill 1997). There are ethical and legal distinctions, however, between palliative sedation, physician aid in dying (sometimes referred to as medical aid in dying, physician-assisted suicide, etc.) and euthanasia. A full review of these practices is outside of the scope of this chapter, but at the time of writing, neither are legal for minor children in the USA, though they are legal for children in Switzerland, the Netherlands (for children over age 12) and Belgium (for children with terminal illnesses). These legal standards may change, so clinicians should consult with both ethics and legal consultants regarding such practices in their home country.

11.6 Ethical Issues in Genetics, Genomics, and Precision Cancer Medicine

Recent advances in genetics, genomics, and personalized medicine have ushered in a new era in medical and pediatric oncology. Paradigm-shifting success with imatinib first highlighted the potential for the use of genomically targeted therapies in cancer. In pediatric oncology, molecular profiling of tumors demonstrates great promise (Mody et al. 2015; Harris et al. 2016; Parsons et al. 2016) and genomically-targeted therapies are rapidly moving from the laboratory to the pediatric oncology clinic (Laetsch et al. 2018; Donadieu et al. 2019). Ongoing worldwide efforts are underway to better understand the genomic landscape of pediatric cancers and identify how to harness genomics to improve care of children with cancer.

With the hope brought by these advances come new ethical considerations. How can pediatric oncologists balance the hope (or, possibly, hype) surrounding genomic technologies with the limitations of the current state of clinical pediatric cancer genomics? How should clinicians communicate with patients and parents about the subtleties in this growing field? It can be difficult to explain nuances like differences between clinical sequencing and research sequencing, differences between germline and somatic alterations, and the uncertainty inherent in much of clinical cancer genomics.

11.6.1 Somatic (Tumor) Sequencing

A great amount of research aims to identify actionable mutations in pediatric cancers, particularly driver mutations. The hope is that identification of a driver mutation will lead to development of a targeted drug, and that this drug might prove more efficacious and less toxic than the non-specific cytotoxic agents presently used to treat pediatric cancers. Numerous studies have performed widescale sequencing of pediatric tumors, including iCat, the GAIN Consortium, BASIC3, Genomes4Kids, MOSCATO-01, the LEAP Consortium, and Pediatric MATCH. Despite significant hope behind these efforts, under 20% of pediatric patients appear to experience direct benefit from receiving targeted therapy, and even fewer demonstrate an improvement in overall survival (Mody et al. 2015; Chang et al. 2016; Harris et al. 2016; Parsons et al. 2016; Harttrampf et al. 2017).

The hopes of young adults and parents of children with cancer outpace the present state of this technology, as most hope genomic sequencing will provide more treatment options and/or a greater chance of cure (Marron et al. 2016). As the lines between clinical and research testing become blurred—tumor sequencing initially performed only through a research study is now often sent as a clinical test (Marron et al. 2019)—pediatric oncologists face the challenge of communicating these nuances, and managing patient/parent hopes for tumor sequencing with the realities of what it can provide. This communication is particularly challenging given that genomics depends on statistical probabilities, heritability, and other complex concepts. At present, these complexities mean that many pediatric oncologists lack confidence in their ability to incorporate tumor genomic findings into their practice and/or counsel patients and parents about genomic findings (Cohen et al. 2016).

11.6.2 Germline Sequencing

Approximately 10–15% of children diagnosed with cancer have an underlying cancer predisposition syndrome (Zhang et al. 2015; Chang et al. 2016; Harris et al. 2016). Most patients and parents in the pediatric oncology setting want this information, even if no screening or prevention is available (Marron et al. 2016). These findings mirror data from outside of pediatric oncology (Gray et al. 2012).

Despite the importance of identifying such syndromes, and desire for this information, there are numerous ethical challenges inherent in germline sequencing of children with cancer.

Notably, not all patients and families want data about cancer risk (Gray et al. 2012; Marron et al. 2016), and anecdotally, some report this information adds worry and stress at a time when they want to focus their energy on the patient with cancer. It remains controversial whether learning information about an underlying cancer predisposition should be mandated as part of tumor genomic sequencing. Further, some have raised the question of whether the minor child should have a say in whether or not to learn about their risk of cancer and/or other disorders. This so-called right to not know is closely related to arguments made regarding a child's right to an open future (Feinberg 1980). In this line of thinking, children's future prospects should not be limited whenever possible, so that they can make informed choices for themselves at a future date, once they have the capacity to do so. Applied to this type of testing, the debate is whether cancer predisposition testing should be delayed until children reach the age of majority (age 18 in the USA) so that they can make the decision to undergo the testing for themselves. The argument in favor of delaying testing is stronger if it is expected that the child will not benefit from the testing until they are an adult. Testing for *BRCA1* is one example of such an ethical quandary, since cancers linked to *BRCA1* mutations do not present in most patients until adulthood. Many adults who are known to be at risk of inheriting BRCA1 mutations choose not to undergo diagnostic testing, raising the concern that some children who undergo testing without a say in the decision may grow to regret the knowledge.

11.6.3   Incidental Findings

Incidental findings are results discovered as part of a genomic test but not the intended or expected result of that test. While incidental findings are not unique to genomics—'incidentalomas' are sometimes found on imaging studies such as MRI or CT—they are more frequent, more controversial, and potentially more ethically treacherous in genomic medicine. In 2016, the American College of Medical Genetics and Genomics (ACMG) published a list of 56 germline genomic alterations it felt should always be reported when found through clinical genomic sequencing, regardless of the clinical indication (Green et al. 2013). The ACMG argued that the value of knowledge about these alterations outweighs any potential drawbacks, even if the individual tested is a child and/or the patient does not desire these results. Many took issue with these recommendations, particularly regarding genomic testing for children (Burke et al. 2013), leading the ACMG to slightly change its recommendations (ACMG Board of Directors 2015). Because many tumor sequencing methodologies include germline sequencing, this controversy is of great relevance to pediatric oncology.

Incidental findings also raise concerns about genetic discrimination. Legal protections against such discrimination vary greatly by jurisdiction, though in the

USA, the Genetic Information Nondiscrimination Act of 2008 provides protection against discrimination for health insurance and employment based on genetic findings (United States Congress 2008). This bill does not, however, prevent discrimination in other forms of insurance (e.g., life, disability, long-term care) or for some subgroups (e.g., government employees). Though negative effects on insurance and employment are a common concern about genetic testing among the public (Gollust et al. 2012), these concerns appear to be less prevalent in the pediatric oncology population (Marron et al. 2016). To date, it is reassuring that few reports of such discrimination have been uncovered (Hall and Rich 2000).

11.6.4 Additional Ethical Challenges in Pediatric Cancer Genomics

Because genomics is rapidly being integrated into standard clinical practice in pediatric oncology, the consequences of this paradigm shift are only beginning to be fully understood, and other areas of ethical complexity are emerging.

11.6.4.1 Big Data in Cancer Genomics

Because of the vast amounts and specificity of genomic data, there are concerns about privacy and confidentiality regarding collection and publication of this so-called big data. When a patient's laboratory results or clinical data are gathered in clinical or research contexts, there is a reasonable assurance that these data will remain de-identified, and the patient's or subject's identity will remain confidential. Because genomic data are more detailed and more identifiable, confidentiality is less certain. Studies of the genetic basis of diabetes in Havasupai Native Americans demonstrate the hazard of big data, when, given the small population studied and specificity of genomic data, it was discovered that published genomic data could be linked to particular individuals (Drabiak-Syed 2010). Without adequate protections, similar problems could arise with genomic data in pediatric oncology. That said, these concerns must be balanced with the importance of sharing these data to maximize its utility and the efficiency of clinical investigation. There is growing recognition of the importance of collaborative research and open access to genomic repositories, with efforts underway through the National Cancer Institute's Genomic Data Commons, CBioPortal, and other similar resources, to pool data and optimize investments of patient-subjects and society at large.

11.6.4.2 Direct-To-Consumer Genetic Testing

Developments in genomic technologies have been commercialized through direct-to-consumer (DTC) genetic testing, and numerous companies offer and advertise such testing. Many of the ethical challenges described above are augmented in their magnitude due to the absence of clinician involvement with such testing. If a child with cancer has a cancer predisposition syndrome identified on a sequencing panel performed at their oncologist's office, the physician, genetic counselor, and other trained professional are available to help interpret the results and discuss their clinical implications. This is not available with DTC testing, and many worry about misinterpretation of results and inadequate support for patients and families. Further, while most companies report not allowing minor children to get sequenced, enforcement of such policies is difficult. There are additional concerns about the accuracy/reliability of this testing (Covolo et al. 2015; Gill et al. 2018) and the growing recognition that data from such testing are sold to large tech conglomerates, pharmaceutical companies, governments, and law enforcement agencies (Martin 2018). Despite concerns, supporters of DTC argue that there is a 'right to know,' and that testing enables patients and families to take ownership over their health. Because DTC genetic testing will continue to be part of the clinical landscape for the foreseeable future, further work is needed to understand the ethical challenges it presents to pediatric oncology and more broadly.

11.6.4.3 Future Advances

Just thirty years after the Human Genome Project began, genomic science has become a core feature of pediatric oncology practice. Progress in this area continues at a rapid pace, and gene therapy, CRISPR-Cas9, proteomics, epigenomics, and immunotherapy represent but a small portion of the genetic/genomic advances likely to impact the care of children with cancer in coming years. While it is exciting to consider the role of future advances in pediatric oncology, it is paramount that we consider the potential ethical hazards and unintended consequences of these technologies. Discussions about germline gene editing in the wake of the CCR5 scandal can serve as a guide for how scientific advancement can be balanced with conscientious discourse (Regalado 2018), with the goal of ensuring the safe and effective application of these advances to patients.

References

Abigail Alliance For Better Access v Von Eschenbach (2007) Abigail alliance for better access v. Von Eschenbach. F. 3d, vol 495, pp 695. Court of Appeals, Dist. of Columbia Circuit

Administration, U. F. a. D (2002) Best pharmaceuticals for children act. Public Law: 107–109

American Academy of Pediatrics (2000) American academy of pediatrics. committee on bioethics and committee on hospital care. Palliative care for children. Pediatrics 106(2 Pt 1):351–357

Appelbaum PS (2007) Clinical practice. Assessment of patients' competence to consent to treatment. N Engl J Med 357(18):1834–1840

Beauchamp TL, Childress JF (2013) Principles of biomedical ethics. Oxford University Press, New York

Blake V, Joffe S, Kodish E (2011) Harmonization of ethics policies in pediatric research. J Law Med Ethics 39(1):70–78

Bosslet GT, Pope TM, Rubenfeld GD, Lo B, Truog RD, Rushton CH, Curtis JR, Ford DW, Osborne M, Misak C, Au DH, Azoulay E, Brody B, Fahy BG, Hall JB, Kesecioglu J, Kon AA, Lindell KO, White DB (2015) An Official ATS/AACN/ACCP/ESICM/SCCM policy statement: responding to requests for potentially inappropriate treatments in intensive care units. Am J Respir Crit Care Med 191(11):1318

Buchanan AE, Brock DW (1989) Deciding for others: the ethics of surrogate decision making. Cambridge University Press, Cambridge England; New York

Burke W, Antommaria AH, Bennett R, Botkin J, Clayton EW, Henderson GE, Holm IA, Jarvik GP, Khoury MJ, Knoppers BM, Press NA, Ross LF, Rothstein MA, Saal H, Uhlmann WR, Wilfond B, Wolf SM, Zimmern R (2013) Recommendations for returning genomic incidental findings? We need to talk! Genet Med 15(11):854–859

Burns JP, Truog RD (2007) Futility: a concept in evolution. Chest 132(6):1987–1993

Caruso Brown AE, Slutzky AR (2017) Refusal of treatment of childhood cancer: a systematic review. Pediatrics 140(6)

Chang W, Brohl AS, Patidar R, Sindiri S, Shern JF, Wei JS, Song YK, Yohe ME, Gryder B, Zhang S, Calzone KA, Shivaprasad N, Wen X, Badgett TC, Miettinen M, Hartman KR, League-Pascual JC, Trahair TN, Widemann BC, Merchant MS, Kaplan RN, Lin JC, Khan J (2016) Multi dimensional clinomics for precision therapy of children and adolescent young adults with relapsed and refractory cancer: a report from the Center for Cancer Research. Clin Cancer Res 22(15):3810–3820

Cohen B, Roth M, Marron JM, Gray SW, Geller DS, Hoang B, Gorlick R, Janeway KA, Gill J (2016) Pediatric oncology provider views on performing a biopsy of solid tumors in children with relapsed or refractory disease for the purpose of genomic profiling. Ann Surg Oncol 23 (Suppl 5):990–997

Coleman DL, Rosoff PM (2013) The legal authority of mature minors to consent to general medical treatment. Pediatrics 131(4):786–793

Committee On B (2016) Informed consent in decision-making in pediatric practice. Pediatrics 138(2)

Committee on Bioethics, American Academy of Pediatrics. (2010) Children as hematopoietic stem cell donors. Pediatrics 125(2):392–404

Congress U (2003) Pediatric research equity act of 2003. Public Law 108(155):117

Cousino, M., R. Hazen, A. Yamokoski, V. Miller, S. Zyzanski, D. Drotar, E. Kodish and T. Multi-site Intervention Study to Improve Consent Research, 2011. Cousino M, Hazen R, Yamokoski A, Miller V, Zyzanski S, Drotar D, Kodish E (2011) Multi-site intervention study to improve consent research. Parent participation and physician-parent communication during informed consent in child leukemia. Pediatrics 128(6):e1544–1551

Cousino MK, Zyzanski SJ, Yamokoski AD, Hazen RA, Baker JN, Noll RB, Rheingold SR, Geyer JR, Alexander SC, Drotar D, Kodish ED (2012) Communicating and understanding the purpose of pediatric phase I cancer trials. J Clin Oncol 30(35):4367–4372

Covolo L, Rubinelli S, Ceretti E, Gelatti U (2015) Internet-based direct-to-consumer genetic testing: a systematic review. J Med Internet Res 17(12):e279

Crites J, Kodish E (2013) Unrealistic optimism and the ethics of phase I cancer research. J Med Ethics 39(6):403–406

Daugherty CK, Banik DM, Janish L, Ratain MJ (2000) Quantitative analysis of ethical issues in phase I trials: a survey interview of 144 advanced cancer patients. IRB 22(3):6–14

Daugherty CK, Hlubocky FJ (2008) What are terminally ill cancer patients told about their expected deaths? A study of cancer physicians' self-reports of prognosis disclosure. J Clin Oncol 26(36):5988–5993

Decamp, M., S. Joffe, C. V. Fernandez, R. R. Faden, Y. Unguru and O. Working Group on Chemotherapy Drug Shortages in Pediatric, 2014. Decamp M, Joffe S, Fernandez CV, Faden RR, Unguru Y, Working Group on Chemotherapy Drug Shortages in Pediatric (2014) Chemotherapy drug shortages in pediatric oncology: a consensus statement. Pediatrics 133(3): e716–724

DeMartino ES, Dudzinski DM, Doyle CK, Sperry BP, Gregory SE, Siegler M, Sulmasy DP, Mueller PS, Kramer DB (2017) Who Decides when a patient can't? Statutes on alternate decision makers. N Engl J Med 376(15):1478–1482

Diekema DS (2004) Parental refusals of medical treatment: the harm principle as threshold for state intervention. Theoret Med 25:243–264

Diekema DS (2006) Conducting ethical research in pediatrics: a brief historical overview and review of pediatric regulations. J Pediat 149(1 Suppl):S3-11

Diekema DS, Botkin JR (2009) Clinical report–Forgoing medically provided nutrition and hydration in children. Pediatrics 124(2):813–822

Directors, A. B. o. (2015)ACMG policy statement: updated recommendations regarding analysis and reporting of secondary findings in clinical genome-scale sequencing. Genet Med 17(1):68–69

Donadieu J, Larabi IA, Tardieu M, Visser J, Hutter C, Sieni E, Kabbara N, Barkaoui M, Miron J, Chalard F, Milne P, Haroche J, Cohen F, Helias-Rodzewicz Z, Simon N, Jehanne M, Kolenova A, Pagnier A, Aladjidi N, Schneider P, Plat G, Lutun A, Sonntagbauer A, Lehrnbecher T, Ferster A, Efremova V, Ahlmann M, Blanc L, Nicholson J, Lambilliote A, Boudiaf H, Lissat A, Svojgr K, Bernard F, Elitzur S, Golan M, Evseev D, Maschan M, Idbaih A, Slater O, Minkov M, Taly V, Collin M, Alvarez JC, Emile JF, Heritier S (2019) Vemurafenib for refractory multisystem langerhans cell histiocytosis in children: an international observational study. J Clin Oncol 37(31):2857–2865

Drabiak-Syed K (2010) Lessons from Havasupai tribe v. Arizona state university board of regents: recognizing group, cultural, and dignity harms as legitimate risks warranting integration into research practice. J. Health Biomed L. 6:175

Drilon A, Laetsch TW, Kummar S, DuBois SG, Lassen UN, Demetri GD, Nathenson M, Doebele RC, Farago AF, Pappo AS, Turpin B, Dowlati A, Brose MS, Mascarenhas L, Federman N, Berlin J, El-Deiry WS, Baik C, Deeken J, Boni V, Nagasubramanian R, Taylor M, Rudzinski ER, Meric-Bernstam F, Sohal DPS, Ma PC, Raez LE, Hechtman JF, Benayed R, Ladanyi M, Tuch BB, Ebata K, Cruickshank S, Ku NC, Cox MC, Hawkins DS, Hong DS, Hyman DM (2018) Efficacy of Larotrectinib in TRK fusion-positive cancers in adults and children. N Engl J Med 378(8):731–739

Eder ML, Yamokoski AD, Wittmann PW, Kodish ED (2007) Improving informed consent: suggestions from parents of children with leukemia. Pediatrics 119(4):e849-859

Feinberg J (1980) The child's right to an open future. In: Aiken W, Lafollette H (eds) Whose child? Children's rights, parental authority, and state power. Littlefield Adams, pp 124–153

Fleischman AR (2016) Pediatric ethics: protecting the interests of children. Oxford University Press, New YorK, NY

Flory J, Emanuel E (2004) Interventions to improve research participants' understanding in informed consent for research: a systematic review. JAMA 292(13):1593–1601

Force DST (2019) Drug shortages: root causes and potential solutions. United States Food and Drug Administration

Gill J, Obley AJ, Prasad V (2018) Direct-to-Consumer genetic testing: the implications of the US FDA's first marketing authorization for BRCA mutation testing. JAMA 319(23):2377–2378

Gillam L (2016) The zone of parental discretion: an ethical tool for dealing with disagreement between parents and doctors about medical treatment for a child. Clin Ethics 11(1):1–8

Goldschmidt D (2015) Teen's forced chemo may continue. Connecticut court rules

Gollust SE, Gordon ES, Zayac C, Griffin G, Christman MF, Pyeritz RE, Wawak L, Bernhardt BA (2012) Motivations and perceptions of early adopters of personalized genomics: perspectives from research participants. Public Health Genom 15(1):22–30

Gray SW, Hicks-Courant K, Lathan CS, Garraway L, Park ER, Weeks JC (2012) Attitudes of patients with cancer about personalized medicine and somatic genetic testing. J Oncol Pract 8 (6):329–335, 322 p following 335

Green RC, Berg JS, Grody WW, Kalia SS, Korf BR, Martin CL, McGuire AL, Nussbaum RL, O'Daniel JM, Ormond KE, Rehm HL, Watson MS, Williams MS, Biesecker LG, American College of Medical and Genomics G (2013) ACMG recommendations for reporting of incidental findings in clinical exome and genome sequencing. Genet Med 15(7):565–574

Grodin MA, Glantz LH (1994) Children as research subjects: science, ethics, and law. Oxford University Press, New York

Hall MA, Rich SS (2000) Laws restricting health insurers' use of genetic information: impact on genetic discrimination. Am J Hum Genet 66(1):293–307

Harris MH, DuBois SG, Glade Bender JL, Kim A, Crompton BD, Parker E, Dumont IP, Hong AL, Guo D, Church A, Stegmaier K, Roberts CWM, Shusterman S, London WB, MacConaill LE,

Lindeman NI, Diller L, Rodriguez-Galindo C, Janeway KA (2016) Multicenter feasibility study of tumor molecular profiling to inform therapeutic decisions in advanced pediatric solid tumors: the individualized cancer therapy (iCat) study. JAMA Oncol 2(5):608–615

Harttrampf AC, Lacroix L, Deloger M, Deschamps F, Puget S, Auger N, Vielh P, Varlet P, Balogh Z, Abbou S, Allorant A, Valteau-Couanet D, Sarnacki S, Gamiche-Rolland L, Meurice G, Minard-Colin V, Grill J, Brugieres L, Dufour C, Gaspar N, Michiels S, Vassal G, Soria JC, Geoerger B (2017) Molecular screening for cancer treatment optimization (MOSCATO-01) in pediatric patients: a single-institutional prospective molecular stratification trial. Clin Cancer Res 23(20):6101–6112

Health, C. o. S. a. P. (2018) Drug shortages: update. American Medical Association

Henderson GE, Churchill LR, Davis AM, Easter MM, Grady C, Joffe S, Kass N, King NM, Lidz CW, Miller FG, Nelson DK, Peppercorn J, Rothschild BB, Sankar P, Wilfond BS, Zimmer CR (2007) Clinical trials and medical care: defining the therapeutic misconception. PLoS Med 4(11):e324

Horng S, Grady C (2003) Misunderstanding in clinical research: distinguishing therapeutic misconception, therapeutic misestimation, and therapeutic optimism. Irb 25(1):11–16

In re Cassandra (2015) In re Cassandra C. A. 3d, vol 112, pp 158. Supreme Court, Conn

In re EG (1989) In re EG. NE 2d, vol 549, pp 322. Supreme Court, Ill

Johnson LM, Leek AC, Drotar D, Noll RB, Rheingold SR, Kodish ED, Baker JN (2015) Practical communication guidance to improve phase 1 informed consent conversations and decision-making in pediatric oncology. Cancer 121(14):2439–2448

Katz AL, Webb SA, Committee On B (2016) Informed consent in decision-making in pediatric practice. Pediatrics 138(2)

Kearns L, Bateman-House A (2017) Who stands to benefit? Right to try law provisions and implications. Therap Innov Regul Sci 51(2):170–176

Kesselheim JC, Lehmann LE, Styron NF, Joffe S (2009) Is blood thicker than water? Ethics of hematopoietic stem cell donation by biological siblings of adopted children. Arch Pediatr Adolesc Med 163(5):413–416

Kimmelman J (2017) Is participation in cancer phase I trials really therapeutic? J Clin Oncol 35 (2):135–138

Kodish E (2003) Pediatric ethics and early-phase childhood cancer research: conflicted goals and the prospect of benefit. Account Res 10(1):17–25

Kodish E, Eder M, Noll RB, Ruccione K, Lange B, Angiolillo A, Pentz R, Zyzanski S, Siminoff LA, Drotar D (2004) Communication of randomization in childhood leukemia trials. JAMA 291(4):470–475

Kodish E, Stocking C, Ratain MJ, Kohrman A, Siegler M (1992) Ethical issues in phase I oncology research: a comparison of investigators and institutional review board chairpersons. J Clin Oncol 10(11):1810–1816

Kopelman LM (1997) The best-interests standard as threshold, ideal, and standard of reasonableness. J Med Philos 22(3):271–289

Laetsch TW, DuBois SG, Mascarenhas L, Turpin B, Federman N, Albert CM, Nagasubrama-nian R, Davis JL, Rudzinski E, Feraco AM, Tuch BB, Ebata KT, Reynolds M, Smith S, Cruickshank S, Cox MC, Pappo AS, Hawkins DS (2018) Larotrectinib for paediatric solid tumours harbouring NTRK gene fusions: phase 1 results from a multicentre, open-label, phase 1/2 study. Lancet Oncol 19(5):705–714

Lin B, Gutman T, Hanson CS, Ju A, Manera K, Butow P, Cohn RJ, Dalla-Pozza L, Greenzang KA, Mack J, Wakefield CE, Craig JC, Tong A (2019) Communication during childhood cancer: systematic review of patient perspectives. Cancer

Mack JW, Fasciano KM, Block SD (2018) Communication about prognosis with adolescent and young adult patients with cancer: information needs, prognostic awareness, and outcomes of disclosure. J Clin Oncol 36(18):1861–1867

Mack JW, Grier HE (2004) The day one talk. J Clin Oncol 22(3):563–566

Marron JM (2018) Not all disagreements are treatment refusals: the need for new paradigms for considering parental treatment requests. Am J Bioeth 18(8):56–58

Marron JM, Cronin AM, DuBois SG, Glade-Bender J, Kim A, Crompton BD, Meyer SC, Janeway KA, Mack JW (2019) Duality of purpose: participant and parent understanding of the purpose of genomic tumor profiling research among children and young adults with solid tumors. JCO Precis Oncol 3

Marron JM, DuBois SG, Glade Bender J, Kim A, Crompton BD, Meyer SC, Janeway KA, Mack JW (2016) Patient/parent perspectives on genomic tumor profiling of pediatric solid tumors: the Individualized Cancer Therapy (iCat) experience. Pediatr Blood Cancer 63 (11):1974–1982

Martin N (2018) How DNA companies like Ancestry and 23AndMe are using your genetic data. Retrieved December 10, 2019, from https://www.forbes.com/sites/nicolemartin1/2018/12/05/how-dna-companies-like-ancestry-and-23andme-are-using-your-genetic-data/#3806fdca6189

McCullough LB (2010) Contributions of ethical theory to pediatric ethics: pediatricians and parents as co-fiduciaries of pediatric patients. In: Miller G (ed) Pediatric bioethics. Cambridge University Press, New York, pp 11–21

McIntyre A (2018) Doctrine of double effect. In: Zalta EN (ed) The stanford encyclopedia of philosophy

Metzger ML, Billett A, Link MP (2012) The impact of drug shortages on children with cancer–the example of mechlorethamine. N Engl J Med 367(26):2461–2463

Miller FG, Joffe S (2011) Equipoise and the dilemma of randomized clinical trials. N Engl J Med 364(5):476–480

Mody RJ, Wu YM, Lonigro RJ, Cao X, Roychowdhury S, Vats P, Frank KM, Prensner JR, Asangani I, Palanisamy N, Dillman JR, Rabah RM, Kunju LP, Everett J, Raymond VM, Ning Y, Su F, Wang R, Stoffel EM, Innis JW, Roberts JS, Robertson PL, Yanik G, Chamdin A, Connelly JA, Choi S, Harris AC, Kitko C, Rao RJ, Levine JE, Castle VP, Hutchinson RJ, Talpaz M, Robinson DR, Chinnaiyan AM (2015) Integrative clinical sequencing in the management of refractory or relapsed cancer in youth. JAMA 314(9):913–925

National Bioethics Advisory Commission (2001) Ethical and policy issues in international research: clinical trials in developing countries, vol 1. https://bioethics.georgetown.edu/nbac/clinical/Vol1.pdf

Neel DV, Shulman DS, DuBois SG (2019) Timing of first-in-child trials of FDA-approved oncology drugs. Eur J Cancer 112:49–56

O'Leary M, Krailo M, Anderson JR, Reaman GH (2008) Progress in childhood cancer: 50 years of research collaboration, a report from the Children's Oncology Group. Semin Oncol 35(5):484–493

Office for Protection from Research Risks (1983) Protection of human subjects. Bethesda, Md., National Institutes of Health (U.S.)

Oken D (1961) What to tell cancer patients. A study of medical attitudes. JAMA 175:1120–1128

Opel DJ, Diekema DS (2006) The case of A.R.: the ethics of sibling donor bone marrow transplantation revisited. J Clin Ethics 17(3):207–219

Parsons DW, Roy A, Yang Y, Wang T, Scollon S, Bergstrom K, Kerstein RA, Gutierrez S, Petersen AK, Bavle A, Lin FY, Lopez-Terrada DH, Monzon FA, Hicks MJ, Eldin KW, Quintanilla NM, Adesina AM, Mohila CA, Whitehead W, Jea A, Vasudevan SA, Nuchtern JG, Ramamurthy U, McGuire AL, Hilsenbeck SG, Reid JG, Muzny DM, Wheeler DA, Berg SL, Chintagumpala MM, Eng CM, Gibbs RA, Plon SE (2016) Diagnostic yield of clinical tumor and germline whole-exome sequencing for children with solid tumors. JAMA Oncol 2(5):616–624

Piel J (2016) Informed consent in right-to-try cases. J Am Acad Psychiatry Law 44(3):290–296

Pope TM (2011) The best interest standard: both guide and limit to medical decision making on behalf of incapacitated patients. J Clin Ethics 22(2):134–138

President's Commission for the Study of Ethical Problems in Medicine and Biomedical and Behavioral Research (1983) Deciding to forego life-sustaining treatment: a report on the ethical, medical, and legal issues in treatment decisions. United States, Government Printing Office, Washington, DC

Quill TE, Dresser R, Brock DW (1997) The rule of double effect–a critique of its role in end-of-life decision making. N Engl J Med 337(24):1768–1771

Regalado A (2018) Exclusive: Chinese scientists are creating CRISPR babies—a daring effort is under way to create the first children whose DNA has been tailored using gene editing. MIT Technol Rev

Rosenberg AR (2015) Poison. J Clin Oncol

Rosenberg AR, Starks H, Unguru Y, Feudtner C, Diekema D (2017) Truth telling in the setting of cultural differences and incurable pediatric illness: a review. JAMA Pediatr 171(11):1113–1119

Ross L (2006) Phase I research and the meaning of direct benefit. J Pediatr 149(1 Suppl):S20-24

Ross LF (1998) Children, families, and health care decision making. Clarendon Press, Oxford; New York

Ross LF (2009) Against the tide: arguments against respecting a minor's refusal of efficacious life-saving treatment. Camb Q Healthc Ethics 18(3):302–315; discussion 315–322

Salazar EG, Bernhardt MB, Li Y, Aplenc R, Adamson PC (2015) The impact of chemotherapy shortages on COG and local clinical trials: a report from the Children's Oncology Group. Pediatr Blood Cancer 62(6):940–944

Schmidt C (2017) Children with cancer get more access to experimental drugs. Science 357 (6351):540

Shulman DS, DuBois SG (2019) Winning the RACE: Expanding pediatric cancer drug approvals. Pediatr Blood Cancer 66(8):e27705

Sisk BA, Kodish E (2018) Therapeutic misperceptions in early-phase cancer trials: from categorical to continuous. IRB 40(4):13–20

Texas Health and Safety Code (1999) Texas Advance Directives Act of 1999. Texas Health and Safety Code

Truog RD (2009) Counterpoint: the Texas advance directives act is ethically flawed: medical futility disputes must be resolved by a fair process. Chest 136(4):968–971

Unguru Y (2011) Pediatric decision-making: informed consent, parental permission, and child assent. In: Diekema DS, Mercurio MR, Adam MB (eds) Clinical ethics in pediatrics: a case-based textbook. Cambridge University Press, Cambridge, pp 1–6

Unguru Y, Coppes MJ, Kamani N (2008) Rethinking pediatric assent: from requirement to ideal. Pediatr Clin North Am 55(1):211–222, xii

United States Congress (2008) Genetic Information Nondiscrimination Act of 2008 (GINA). HR 493. United States of America

United States Congress (2018) Trickett Wendler, Frank Mongiello, Jordan McLinn, and Matthew Bellina Right to Try Act. United States of America, 115th Congress

US Food and Drug Administration (FDA). Expanded access (Compassionate Use). Retrieved 1 Aug 2017, from https://www.fda.gov/NewsEvents/PublicHealthFocus/ExpandedAccessCompassionateUse/default.htm

Vacco v. Quill (1997) Vacco v. Quill, vol 521, pp 793. Supreme Court, US

Waligora M, Bala MM, Koperny M, Wasylewski MT, Strzebonska K, Jaeschke RR, Wozniak A, Piasecki J, Sliwka A, Mitus JW, Polak M, Nowis D, Fergusson D, Kimmelman J (2018) Risk and surrogate benefit for pediatric Phase I trials in oncology: a systematic review with meta-analysis. PLoS Med 15(2):e1002505

Weber JS, Levit LA, Adamson PC, Bruinooge S, Burris HAT, Carducci MA, Dicker AP, Gonen M, Keefe SM, Postow MA, Thompson MA, Waterhouse DM, Weiner SL, Schuchter LM (2015)American society of clinical oncology policy statement update: the critical role of phase I trials in cancer research and treatment. J Clin Oncol 33(3):278–284

Weise KL, Okun AL, Carter BS, Christian CW, Committee On B, Section On H, Palliative M, Committee On Child and Neglect A (2017) Guidance on forgoing life-sustaining medical treatment. Pediatrics 140(3)

Wolfe J, Grier HE, Klar N, Levin SB, Ellenbogen JM, Salem-Schatz S, Emanuel EJ, Weeks JC (2000) Symptoms and suffering at the end of life in children with cancer. N Engl J Med 342 (5):326–333

Zhang J, Walsh MF, Wu G, Edmonson MN, Gruber TA, Easton J, Hedges D, Ma X, Zhou X, Yergeau DA, Wilkinson MR, Vadodaria B, Chen X, McGee RB, Hines-Dowell S, Nuccio R, Quinn E, Shurtleff SA, Rusch M, Patel A, Becksfort JB, Wang S, Weaver MS, Ding L, Mardis ER, Wilson RK, Gajjar A, Ellison DW, Pappo AS, Pui CH, Nichols KE, Downing JR (2015) Germline mutations in predisposition genes in pediatric cancer. N Engl J Med 373 (24):2336–2346

Ethical Pain and Terminal Chaperonage

12

Robert E. Feldmann Jr. and Justus Benrath

12.1 Introduction

Principles of palliative care and pain relief, based on a widely accepted integrated approach to humane medicine, resonate with human reasoning, and with emotional and spiritual needs. In recent decades, they have undergone significant developments and advances. Most of all, palliative care, including access to pain and symptom control, are seen as part of a fundamental human right, the right to health (WHO 2019a). Palliative pain relief has also been declared an imperative of universal health coverage (Knaul et al. 2018). In practice, the World Health Organization (WHO) defines it as an essential objective of primary health care and integrated people-centred health services (WHO 2019a). The 2014 World Health Assembly Resolution Number 67.19 recognized that "palliative care, when indicated, is fundamental to improving the quality of life, well-being, comfort, and human dignity for individuals, being an effective person-centred health service that values patients' need to receive adequate, personally and culturally sensitive information on their health status, and their central role in making decisions about the treatment received" (WHO 2014). Guidelines for planners, implementers and managers on integrating palliative needs into health care have been issued (WHO

R. E. Feldmann Jr. (✉) · J. Benrath
Department of Anesthesiology, Pain Center, Medical Faculty Mannheim,
Heidelberg University, Theodor-Kutzer-Ufer 1-3, 68167 Mannheim, Germany
e-mail: robert_feldmann@gmx.li

J. Benrath
e-mail: justus.benrath@umm.de

R. E. Feldmann Jr.
Swiss Red Cross, Canton St. Gallen, Center for Psychotraumatology - Gravita SRK,
Bahnhofplatz 5, 9000 St. Gallen, Switzerland

© Springer Nature Switzerland AG 2021
A. W. Bauer et al. (eds.), *Ethical Challenges in Cancer Diagnosis and Therapy*,
Recent Results in Cancer Research 218,
https://doi.org/10.1007/978-3-030-63749-1_12

2019a) and palliative care and pain management have now been established in many health systems worldwide.

The philanthropic concepts of palliative care and pain control are well embedded in the World Medical Association's Declaration of Geneva (WMA 2017), which irrevocably interweaves medical agency with the well-being of clients and respect for their autonomy and dignity. While implementation of palliative care and pain control in medicine is not only clearly advocated by societies and legislators internationally and is also actively demanded by almost all affected parties, their sensitive translation into practice demands reflection on the often unseen ethical challenges that lie more deeply below the surface of ordinary, honest benevolence.

This chapter addresses important ethical aspects arising in terminal pain and palliative chaperonage and highlights the importance of affect and thought homeostasis.

12.2 Tumour Pain and Palliative Symptom Management

Included in the International Association for the Study of Pain's definition of pain is "unpleasant sensory and emotional experience" (Merskey et al. 1979). Alterations of or amendments to this definition are currently being discussed (Treede 2018). The immediate causal relationship between such an (acute) experience and the intensity of subjective suffering links pain perception with involuntary reaction to evade a potentially life-threatening condition (somato-psychic interface). This signalling effect is phylogenetically conserved across vertebrates and non-vertebrates, and has become detached from its evolutionary role in chronic pain, reflecting maladaptation to sub-threshold menace. Acute and chronic pain may occur together and increase the burden of suffering. Ethically, subjectively unpleasant sensory experiences, including but not limited to pain, nausea, vomiting, or dyspnoea associated with neoplasia qualify for immediate alleviation by virtue of the Declaration of Geneva in that they (in most cases) directly compromise the well-being of clients and their quality of life. It is generally agreed that informed consent is obligatory for pain and other symptom control, as it is for any treatment. However, pain in the mammalian brain shares network structures with emotional processing, causing the discomfort of the sensory pain experience to become intertwined with emotional suffering. A stimulus that somatically hurts in the tissue in a severe and prolonged fashion may equally hurt the mind, predisposing to emotional expression of restlessness, moaning, anger, dysphoria, agitation, aggression, depression, angst and other affects which may themselves entail consequences for the body. All of this together adds to the subjective sense of intolerability. Thus, the evolutionary meaning of pain and the burden of its suffering has led modern medicine to assume an implicit consent to pain control in (most) cases where it cannot be directly obtained (e.g., impaired consciousness), unless otherwise specified. It is commonly considered unethical to allow a client to experience (intense) pain and subsequent suffering. In practice, this means that analgesic treatment is regarded as acceptable, even imperative, even in the absence of informed consent, where subjective discomfort and suffering are likely to occur without the remedy. This implies that the client will not be informed of the potential risks, adverse reactions, unwanted side effects or other consequences of the treatment prior to its administration. It also implies that consent would most likely have been given if appraisal of the detriments and communication had been possible, assuming that the burden of discomfort and suffering of untreated pain or other symptoms would not have been a viable alternative for most clients.

While these considerations are probably not false, (opioid-based) pain and palliative symptom control has a number of implications that are less frequently and sometimes not openly and critically discussed within the framework of an informational conversation. But their ethical overtones necessitate fundamental and careful consideration of the moral rights of the client, in that they may directly impact (cancer) treatment choices, perhaps even those laid out in an advance directive. They necessarily demand critical consideration and reasoning.

For palliative pain management in oncology, especially in advanced terminal disease, Dame Cicely Saunders' (1918–2005) multidimensional concept of 'total pain' (Saunders 1986) and the related bio-psycho-social model of pain (Blanchard et al. 1984) have become the gold standard. On the therapeutic side, modern multimodal pain management reflects this well, its principles (Khatami and Rush 1982) addressing the target areas of body, mind, spirit and social needs. Functional categories of multimodal pain management include pharmacotherapy, invasive/interventional therapy including radiotherapy, psychotherapy including psycho-oncology and psychosocial support, manual, physical and physiotherapy, as well as complementary therapy. The comprehensive two-fold conceptual partnership of total pain and multimodal management factoring in both causes and effects, if honestly implemented, must be considered best clinical practice in (cancer) pain therapy. Hence, identification of the sources of the pain and the options of appropriate responses render notions about (1) what kind of pain (type, origin, correct medical diagnosis) requires treatment, (2) what kind of treatment should be considered, and (3) what kind of delivery should be chosen and why. As pain and many other components of palliative suffering are critical determinants of well-being and quality of life, it is obligatory to address them therapeutically. By modern standards, insufficient pain management or none at all must be considered unethical. Several ethical imperatives surface when the details are examined:

First and foremost, effective comprehensive pain management depends on the correct underlying diagnosis, hence the correct identification of the cause(s) and type(s) of pain. This is contingent on the overall professional qualifications and experience of the team as well as the diagnostic tools available in the health facility. As specialists and well-trained personnel incur higher labour costs and technical upgrades involve financial investment, austerity measures in a medical clinic are associated with stress for clients from (possibly total) pain. For this reason, balanced economic policies that observe the nature of the palliative mandate and make sufficient allowances for adequately meeting its demands must be considered an ethical imperative.

Second and linked to the above, effective tumour pain and palliative symptom management is associated with the availability of specialist provider resources. The widespread global unavailability and other limitations of these spark an ethical dilemma. For example, when pain therapy is performed, not in a multimodal but solely in a medication-based fashion (most often seen), or if multimodal is offered, but not all its aspects are included, or if all disciplines are involved, but are not provided by specialists in their field (who are more expensive), it is less likely to be effective, leading to more suffering and reduced quality of life, which is in conflict with the palliative mandate and the ethical imperative. It is a misunderstanding that pain and palliative symptom management around terminal chaperonage, existential psychology and palliative psychiatry can be performed by self-caring, unencumbered, compassionate and healthy personnel as a matter of routine, during their regular work shifts and without physical or mental health emergencies. Still less does medical training to become an excellent physician predispose one to competence in high-quality supervision of a complex multimodal therapeutic mission for a client on the verge of death in a situation of financial austerity. In the end, each existentially threatened sufferer presents with their own individual combination of total pain constituents and requires a highly individually tailored selection from the multimodal treatment tray. It is a complex undertaking, but an ethically compelling one that calls for adequate qualified human resources.

Third, people with severe acute and chronic pain used to suffer worldwide, among other reasons because of a lack of standardized scientific approaches to therapy. With recognition of this came the development of guidelines by WHO, member states and cooperating professional organizations (WHO 2007). Prior to 2019, the last set of WHO guidelines on cancer pain management had been published in 1996. In light of the new scientific evidence that has emerged since then regarding the risks associated with the use of medication in the management of pain, WHO discontinued and revised former versions of its clinical guidelines, and in January 2019 issued the latest *WHO Guidelines for the pharmacological and radiotherapeutic management of cancer pain in adults and adolescents 2019* (WHO 2019c). As basic and applied research and development in the field of pain management continues, regular updates of the guidelines translating these findings into clinical practice will be mandatory. Consequently, the current needs-driven increase in state-of-the-art pain and palliative management availability to prevent a pain and suffering pandemic worldwide represents a moral challenge in terms of consolidation and harmonization of expertise, resources for its evaluation and translation, as well as adherence to the guidelines.

Fourth, more than 200 years after its first isolation from opium by the pharmaceutical assistant Friedrich Wilhelm Sertürner (1783–1841) in the Westphalian prince-bishopric Paderborn in 1805, the alkaloid morphine and some of its (later synthetic) derivatives have today become available in different pharmaceutical forms (opiates and opioids). Their application was based initially on the battlefield expertise of military doctors, but later on the growing experience in anaesthesiology, perioperative medicine and intensive care. Moreover, the pharmacotherapy of pain associated with neoplasia in the first half of the twentieth century, regarded as part and parcel of the emerging diverse medical cancer services (which became oncology), at the time was not (yet) profoundly scientifically evidence based, but was, rather, linked to subjective experience, or the 'style' of the supervising medical director. Today's scientific evidence suggests that comprehensive medication-based treatment of tumour pain and control of several palliative symptoms necessitates the differential use of opioids, non-opioids and adjuvants. WHO's three-step pain ladder has become the standard tool for cancer pain relief in adults (WHO 2019b). However, after decades of experience with opioid application, the WHO

> …recognized that the need for access to pain relief must be balanced with concerns about the harm arising from the misuse of medications prescribed for the management of pain, including opioids. Scientific evidence indicates there are risks associated with the use of these medications - such as the development of dependence [including iatrogenic origin], overdose and accidental death. Even when prescribed according to established clinical guidelines and clients' needs, and used as directed, certain factors may increase these risks … (WHO 2019d).

The lessons learned here imply the need for ethical considerations. While opioid application is indispensable and is justified under the moral imperative, given its ability to reduce suffering and increase quality of life in tumour disease, it must be guaranteed before initiation (1) that the prescriber is a trained specialist pain management consultant well-versed in pharmacology of narcotics, adjuvants and psychotropic compounds in general, and (2) that the prescriber comprehensively informs and educates clients, families or legal guardians, enabling them to become informed participants in the healthcare decision processes. Topics must include the rationale for a pharmacotherapy with opioids and psychotropic adjuvants, their properties and pharmacodynamics, benefits, side effects (often well treatable), drug interactions, risks and uncertainties associated with their use. Also, multimodal and medication alternatives to opioid and/or adjuvant treatment for pain management must be compared, including relevant benefits and risks. Finally, client under-standing must be evaluated, followed by the necessary approval of the pharma-cotherapy by the client. Naturally, all of the above applies when employing opioids to palliate anxiety and existential suffering in terminal dyspnoea.

Given the broad spectrum of physiological and pathophysiological effects of opioids and psychotropic adjuvants, the usual informational routines are often inadequate, and caution is advised. Specifically, parties must be empowered to clearly comprehend the consequences of their informed consent, or waiver, with particular reference to those rare, but not unseen and sometimes difficult to control, adverse effects. These include impairment of consciousness and mental capacity, possibly rendering clients confused, anxious, delirious, somnolent, comatose, even leading to death, as well as intoxication (overdose), dependence (including iatro-genic in origin)/withdrawal symptoms, opioid-induced hyperalgesia (Fletcher and Martinez 2014) and accidental death.

Overdosing can happen anywhere in pharmacotherapy but may have severe consequences if narcotics, including opioids or psychotropic adjuvants, are used in (cancer) pain management and palliative care. These compounds are to be distinguished from other analgetic agents. While non-steroid anti-inflammatory drug-induced nephropathy and acetaminophen-related hepatotoxicity may primarily lead to somatic sequelae (other than renal or hepatic encephalopathy), opioids and psychotropic adjuvants can directly compromise cerebral networking. This can impair or even completely override mental capabilities, including those for generating consciousness, orientation, apperception, thought processes, reasoning, appraisal and decision making, and for experiencing emotions, as well as the concept of self (integrity) or social connectivity - all faculties that have maximum relevance at the end of life. Hence, changes in mental status have direct implications for a client's ability to interact and experience their environment, the world, and their subjective quality of life, one of the cornerstones of palliative care. Ultimately, this affects the way the client will die.

A state of painlessness under sedation, substance craving, psycho-vegetative excitation, or possibly an incipient opioid-induced sudden death - impairing, unexpected and approved by neither client or kin - cannot be appreciated in the context of fostering quality of life and may be in conflict with both the palliative intention and the moral mandate (assuming here that they are separable). Further, is a prescriber morally justified in imposing such a particularly unexpected or unapproved, potentially difficult to control and significant harm (e.g., sedative amputation from reality) on the terminal client without infringing the *primum nihil nocere*? And, specifically, how much detachment from reality would be acceptable and how can the client decide on that? Who decides which of *these* demons to choose, if not the client?

Yet, pain relief in the absence of (or with impaired) conscious awareness of the world *might* be morally acceptable if the party has been well informed, has been given the opportunity to consider and proactively decide to approve or not, and has been able to anticipate the changes in mental status beforehand. Knowledge of the risk of such changes, the conditions under which they may take place, and the variability of their clinical manifestations can make a major difference to the affected individual. Although those changes presumably occur, from a physiological point of view, independently of their anticipation, awareness beforehand can abate their traumatic impact and help to lessen the perceived helplessness and loss of control, thereby restoring conformity with the palliative notion and the moral imperative.

Importantly, mental status fluctuations influence appraisal of quality of life, as do subjective well-being, expectations, preconceptions or bias, all of which themselves depend on the mental status. In addition, a subjective lack of quality of life or related concerns will not be communicated directly by a confused, sedated or delirious client, which requires the client's relevant bearings, mindsets and appraisals to be proactively explored and addressed by the provider, ideally beforehand. Moral integrity beyond the imperative to do no harm clearly demands that client information and comprehension, including differential balancing of pros and cons, are obligatory constituents of informed consent. If this cannot be accomplished, the ethical framework of opioid-based cancer pain management has not been adequately taken into account. Of course, this does not render invalid a client's moral right to receive only selected pieces of information, or to receive information in a dosed manner, or to obtain no information at all. Where necessary, the extent of information desired or the minimum that is acceptable to the client may have to be defined with the help of the provider. Ethically, the right not to know is tantamount to the right to know.

It is crucial to realize that clients who have full mental capacity when they give informed consent for opioid and/or psychotropic adjuvant use will agree to accept the risk of losing that capacity in the course of the therapy, temporarily or for a longer time. This is not always taken fully into account in clinical settings, when clients are informed about the risk of sedation or other mental status changes but their mental capacity is often not reassessed in the course of the therapy, not even when signs of overdose are evident. In part, this may be because clinical capacity assessments are mostly performed not by pain management specialists but by liaison psychiatrists, rarely or not at all available, depending on the medical institution. It also emphasizes the importance of advance directives dealing with this particular aspect. If no legal guardian has been appointed by the client, then in most Western countries medical staff are obliged to request that a court appoints a guardian, which can be undesirable and stressful for client and family in a palliative situation. All of the above facets imply considerable consequences for the quality of our care as providers. Limitations in mental capacity are also observed in palliative care outside opioid therapy. Among others, clouded consciousness can occur in renal and hepatic encephalopathy, cerebral metastases, addiction or near the end of life.

Last but not least, (deep) sedation and psycho-vegetative decoupling can sometimes be actively requested by clients if severe and uncontrollable pain causes intensive subjective distress and its downstream sequelae. This may indicate electively induced palliative sedation (Ciancio et al. 2020). Other clients may seek sedation in advance of death as a shield against anxiety and/or the outside world as the biological demise approaches. In contrast, an opposite trend towards explicit preservation, or acquisition, of full mental alertness has been increasingly noticed in the Western world. The objective, based on dedicated spiritual beliefs, is to facilitate selective sensual perception and thought control at the very moment of death.

Many adverse effects associated with opioid and other psychotropic drug use must in fact be considered iatrogenic in origin. While medication management has not been consigned to machine-learned artificial intelligence, and a productive human error culture is on the rise in the Western hemisphere, iatrogenic drug dependence or overdose-based intoxication are problematic if caused by insufficient prescriber experience, lack of specialist training, inappropriate attempts to meet client expectations, pressure to succeed or economic motives. An increasing number of recent examples of iatrogenic opioid addiction necessitating regulatory action includes the oxycodone epidemic in the United States (Okie 2010). It also includes, in Germany, the soaring off-label use of the synthetic μ-agonist methadone outside the FDA-approved detoxification treatment of opioid addiction as an adjuvant in the management of cancer, even in the absence of clinically relevant cancer pain. Claims of an antiproliferative effect on certain tumour cells in-vitro in a disease model were taken up and generalized by the lay press in 2017, leading to an increase in client requests for (co)prescription as an adjuvant cancer treatment. Astonishingly, the absence of scientific evidence has not prevented physicians outside specialized pain management exposing oncology outpatient clients without opioid addiction and even without pain-related indication for opioid intake to the severe risks associated with methadone's long half-life, lipophilic properties and cardiac toxicity. From an ethical standpoint, these examples re-emphasize the importance of the global debate about how much training psychiatrists and physicians withdrawing narcotics, benzodiazepines and other dopaminergic compounds in addiction medicine should receive in evidence-based prescription of these substances in the context of (multimodal) pain management and about how the relevant psychiatry skills should be acquired by anaesthesiologists, pain specialists and family doctors handling psychotropic drugs. After all, pain, dying and the psyche are deeply and inextricably interwoven. The fourth ethical imperative calls for specialty-trained narcotics prescribers cooperating with pharmacologists, who take mental status assessment and follow-up into account, and who accentuate the processes of obtaining informed consent, detailing on opioid application.

12.3   In Pursuit of a *Decent* Death - Palliative Imperatives for Terminal Chaperonage

Palliative care does not imply failure, or termination of medical agency. Likewise, a palliative, i.e., non-curative, concept is not incompatible with a medical mandate. Rather, it has become part of the latter, voicing the desire for self-determination in the face of finiteness and irreversibility. In recent years, the idea of informed consenting and its objectives - the facilitation of client understanding and decision making - have led ethicists to foster the completion of advance directives in which clients advise, for example, under which circumstances (further) treatment is to be withheld or withdrawn and what clinicians *should not do* when that occurs. However, clinicians are rarely advised what they *should do*. The following section recaps fundamental moral imperatives for palliative providers during terminal chaperonage en route to a *decent* client death, one, which might ideally be anticipated by the client with greater peace of mind.

Many societies share a historically and culturally formed conception of death and its potential meanings, its wider context and its implications for the life that precedes it. This also involves the longstanding notion of death being merely the end of *this* life but not the end overall. Imaginations are often associated with a guiding ethos and with certain often ritualized behaviours of society members reflecting their goal of living a (personally and socially) desired life and dying a (personally and socially) desired death. These precepts, in turn, are most often embedded in a framework of psychological or spiritual beliefs which itself may culminate in the image of an ideal death and how it can be achieved. While the physical, mental and social needs and (perhaps unconscious, explicit and implicit) expectations of a client at any given time on the palliative road are aligned with these often 'monomorphic', rather static convictions, they frequently vary according to the circumstances. Meeting them with the help of end-of-life care may provide the client with the comfort of believing that certain aspects of this ideal, if not all, can be targeted and approached, possibly closely, and ultimately realized. Facilitation of that experience may alleviate the client's journey to the edge. Conversely, diffuse and unprocessed, unaccomplished hopes and expectations can lead to the opposite and impede preparations for a serene transition to the Shangri-La. The high therapeutic relevance of cultivating belief and building faith, imagining and visualizing them and drawing hope from them, is addressed later in this chapter.

Individual understanding of death shapes preferences with respect to its approach. Clinical terminal chaperonage teaches that questioning clients about their personal understanding of (life and) death, its meaning, ideal form and favoured approaches in a sincere, compassionate and non-judgemental fashion can create trust and nourish the therapeutic relationship. Further, helping the client to not only verbalize but eventually (believe they will be able to) realize some of those predilections may become anxiolytic. These processes may allow denial and resistance to be diluted and possibly pave the way for unlocking and modifying forms of abyssal existential (terminal) angst. And they may alter painful emotions and cognitions linked to deep regret. In this regard, a non-scientific assemblage of regrets voiced by clients prior to their passing is indicative of the profound nature of human sentiment. Clients report regretting not having had the courage to live a life true to themselves instead of the life others expected of them, not having worked less, not having had the courage to express their feelings, not having stayed in touch with their friends, and not having let themselves be happier (Ware 2012). Aspects of overcoming terminal angst and terminal regret will be considered later in this chapter.

Other client preferences and requests conducive to a *decent* death have been experientially observed in the context of palliative situations in a university medical centre. Regarding somatic experiencing, all clients emphasize their request for effective pain and other symptom control (anxiety, shortness of breath, nausea). With respect to social communication and awareness, many confess to longing for a humane and compassionate team showing emotional honesty and sincerity. To be able to die in the preferred state of consciousness (alert and conscious or in elective sedation), to have the dying process attended by loved ones and possibly not to have to die alone, is important to many. Likewise, an affirmation of love and being able to say farewell to important people can make a difference. Many, but not all, would like to be sure that they have received sufficient information and gained enough understanding of their medical condition, including the underlying oncological or other terminal disease. Regarding sense of control, many clients indicate that it is essential for them to maintain autonomy while approaching death, or for their personal decision making and understanding to be taken account of in the palliative chaperone process. Almost all terminally ill clients express a wish to be able to die in accordance with their spiritual beliefs and customs. Medically, many seek reassurance that their last wishes as expressed in an advance directive are being adhered to, specifically, that no stressful interventions are conducted which would not impact the onward decision-making process of the team, and that 'do not resuscitate/do not intubate' (DNR/DNI) instructions are respected and not considered at the last minute. Clients also deem it important to know before they die that their personal wishes (estate, inheritance, etc.) will be fulfilled post mortem. Many seek to complete final worldly personal commitments and tasks.

Scientifically analyzed attributes, rated by end-of-life clients as *very important,* comprise (in descending order): be kept clean, name a decision maker, have a nurse with whom one feels comfortable, know what to expect about one's physical condition, have someone who will listen, maintain one's dignity, trust one's doctor, have financial affairs in order, be free of pain, maintain a sense of humour, say goodbye to important people, be free of shortness of breath, be free of anxiety, have a doctor with whom one can discuss fears, have a doctor who knows one as a whole person, resolve unfinished business with family or friends, have physical touch, know that one's doctor is comfortable talking about death and dying, share time with close friends, believe family is prepared for one's death, feel prepared to die, experience presence of family, have treatment preferences in writing, not die alone, remember personal accomplishments, and receive care from their own doctor (Steinhauser et al. 2000).

It should be kept in mind that end-of-life preferences differ according to role (clients, families, providers) and by individual. However, while they are empiric collections of subjective mindsets (not all of which can be realized), bedside experience in the Western world appears to confirm their high relevance for dying clients. They may provide an important lead for setting priorities in palliative care and terminal chaperonage.

12.4   Savour the Thought, Appreciate the Feeling: The Holy Grail of Humane Terminal Chaperonage

The mental state of the dying client - well beyond subjective predilections (reflecting explicit and implicit views) - requires special attention during terminal chaperonage. A distressing, painful or prolonged advance towards death, possibly involving unwanted invasive or intensive care, for example, may elicit profound physical and emotional suffering.

Emotions, the affect appraised by our counterpart, fluctuations of the mental energy field, rule the kingdom of subjectivity and its cohesion and broadly unfold the mental space between dopamine delight and aversion, approach and repulsion, between wanting and avoiding. Along its scaffold, myriad choices spring up, each associated with unique challenges and - more importantly - consequences, stealthily navigating the evolution of our individual life path between birth and death as it attempts to increase lust and deflect sorrow. Emotions enable us to sense that we are alive, they serve as an informational authority to validate or dismiss our perception of the momentary world, they are communication and they drive our actions.

Bereavement theories postulate sequences of (potentially alternating and variable) emotions to precede death. They share an initial rejection, negation or denial phase, to all intents and purposes an emotional resource, after which resistance or anger may be followed by a catharsis based on qualities such as lethargy or despair. A bargaining phase may then predate a final continuum between the two ultimate poles of integration and acceptance of the irrevocable changes and - at worst - resignation, depression and deep crisis. Angst is often perceived underneath throughout.

Natural primary affects of high relevance in palliative care are angst (which includes fear and anxiety), grief, anger, joy and shame, all of which are widely recognized transculturally. It is thought that the human mind–body system seeks to discharge them to effectuate transmission of their implicit meaning to the outside world. Prevention of that clearing, for whatever reason, may disrupt congruence between affect (emotion), body perception and cognitive appraisal, and individuals may discover a subtle disunity between their reason and intuition, leaving them with insecurity and possibly amplification of the angst. Furthermore, regret, guilt and lack of acceptance are believed to play a dominant role during contemplation of impending death with the potential to exhaust the dying.

The appearance of these emotions in the context of death is not detrimental as such. In fact, they may be an essential component of individual healing and psycho-spiritual development and its associated choice-based learning tasks during adaptation, all of which can reflect post-traumatic growth. However, their particular expression, their subjective appraisal, degree of entanglement, indissolubility and unsuccessful closure can suggest intense psychological discomfort in a dying client. Together with thoughts and other cognitions, emotions represent complex intertwined states of mind that are embedded in or related to deeply rooted existential processes, and hence may reflect painful maladaptive coping before or during the threat of death and death itself. Ancient wisdom and traditions suggest that an essential preparation for death embraces the wholehearted, sincere, authentic recognition - disclosure, as it were - of all subjective perceptions, emotions and sentiments. The client should be given the freedom to express *anything* rising to the surface of the mind at any time, unfiltered and devoid of negative appraisal and this inner transformation should resonate with unconditional love, free of expectations and reflecting the qualities of the heart (*anahata*). Interactions like this imply certain requirements in the mindset and behaviour of the attender, who should engage with loving kindness, empathy, equanimity and joy to serve - the hallmarks of compassion. The dying often see through insincerity, their profound sensitivity in the face of the irrevocability of their worldly demise compelling them to discard protective disguise and superficiality. They are about to lose their entire world, unavoidably, permanently and without limitations. This leads to greatly increased vulnerability and immense subjective suffering often precipitated, among others, by depressive mood swings, deep regrets, guilt or angst. There may actually be a situation worse than dying: dying in suffering - physically, mentally or both. Dying is tough!

Being humans, we tend to choose our bearings according to how we have once been conditioned and how familiar they are. To master life's complexity, we efficiently construct patterns in which our habits and customs of thought, emotions and behaviour are internally buffered in our mind to be retrieved on demand under certain circumstances. This is no different when we die. Cultural wisdom indicates that the mindset just immediately prior to death is of paramount importance. Our ethos, our conscious thoughts and our sentiments during that moment exert a powerful influence on death itself and on the proceedings afterwards. However, their quality, quantity and subjective internal impact can become excessively amplified and possibly preoccupy the dying, flooding their entire perception. Specifically, aversive and unchangeable threats often melt into a learned helplessness-like perception and behaviour, with negative appraisals and global attribution, liberating previously formed emotional patterns and, eventually, their dysfunctional regulation. This may occupy, cloud or sidetrack the mind from the actual goals of death preparation, namely unintentional affirmation of positive emotions, love and compassion. Negative appraisals and their associated homopolar emotions, however, *can* be repelled and neutralized prior to death because they were likewise once acquired by experience and learning and are not considered to be a congenital entourage. Small children, for example, have generally not yet heard or gathered a lot of them. In addition to the terminal composure of our mind, the quality and intention of our past deeds, reflected by their formerly underlying emotions, cognitions, words, decisions and actions, are thought to become decisive entities as death is contemplated. What we think, feel and how we act is critical - at all times!

To support alleviation and facilitate liberation from attachment to longing and grasping, the dying client should ideally be at ease, free of pain and other suffering, as well as awake and fully conscious. The fact that ideal pharmacological options for treating angst and anxiety without simultaneously impairing wakefulness, consciousness and cognition are not available challenges common clinical concepts of chemical anxiolysis and emotion attenuation by induction (including palliative sedation) or the side effects of opioid application (including overmedication). It favours communicative, supportive psychological and spiritual approaches, toge-ther with client autoregulation of mental homeostasis via meditation, mindfulness and practices such as praying or reciting mantras prior to death.

Lastly, the qualities of the setting - location, social and sensory environment - play a crucial role and should be thoughtfully controlled both by the providers of palliative chaperonage and by the next of kin.

12.5   The Art of Mindful Dying *or* the Essentials of Terminal Thought Plasticity and Affect Catharsis

How does one approach the client's emotional realm supportively and address the mindset prior to death appropriately? It should be recalled that all emotional expe-riences, without exception, comprise projections of the human mind (*Geist*). As such, emotions should be identified as what they really are, namely nothing but the natural radiance of the mind. Clients should be guided to recognize this and to become conscious of its significance, and to practise the ultimate goal of composing themselves in this nature of their mind. Success in this contest often requires the exploration, work-up and abandonment of habitually accumulated emotional and cognitive patterns. This is the time to give up the quantified ego and cease self-tracking. The very moment of death can become a mighty opportunity for clearing.

Clinically, paradigms of thought and emotion are rarely discarded in vain, but the process can be very arduous and challenging. While individual differences based on psychological strain and the associated subjective degree of suffering exist, certain mental concepts appear highly relevant for most dying adults across different societies and cultural backgrounds. Bedside terminal chaperone practice shows that these include angst and anxiety, valediction and grief, anger, joy, hope and faith, regret, forgiveness and reconciliation, shame and guilt, as well as acceptance. None reigns supreme, and each can be equally important and valuable. Addressing them is paramount and often paves the way towards the goal.

The following sections identify and advocate eight most fundamental affective, respectively cognitive fields of the human mind, termed the "*Ensemble of the essential eight iridescent fields of relinquishment*", whose sincere, mindful conceptual reframing can be of immense psychological benefit for dying clients. Adaptable and culturally sensitive facilitation of client development in this area must be regarded as an indispensable duty, possibly even the core imperative in terminal chaperonage.

12.5.1 Support Relief of Terminal Angst, Fear and Anxiety

Angst, fear and anxiety project into the future, as opposed to grief reflecting on the past and anger responding to the present. They declare that something is frightening in response to a perceived threat or danger. Phylogenetically conserved in mammals and other species to secure essential safety and survival through fight-or-flight responses to danger, no other sentiments directly control human behaviour in a similar fashion. Codetermining almost everything we do, they help to govern our behaviour, guarding against failure and ultimately death. Inevitably, they are an integral part of our lives. If the intensity mounts and angst or fear prevail, excessive fear may arise and take over. Possible responses, besides 'fear of the fear', may include psycho-vegetative hyperarousal with the potential to entirely debilitate perceptive faculties, mental access to reason, emotion regulation and action control, which in turn may lead to incapacitation, even paralysis-like or dissociative states, possibly lacking coherent association with the here and now. Frequently, secondary emotions such as anger, shame, aversion and powerlessness may arise from angst and fear and disable the mind further. The existential nature of having to face the unknown at the end of life, which itself gives rise to angst, complicates this. After all, a dying client is, often involuntarily, about to surrender to this unknown and leave their entire world behind, completely, and without any conscious control.

Consequently, the spearhead of terminal anxiolysis, ideally long before affective overflow sets in, requires ways of helping the dying to comprehend and to vanquish, to surmount, really to *over*come and honestly leave behind the angst and its causes instead of *under*mining them by suppression. This may require an individual view of the unknown to be built and the central senses of ultimate helplessness and lack of control to be contextually reframed, complemented by mindfulness- and meditation-based (body-mind) control of psycho-vegetative arousal, including breathing exercises (*pranayama*). Imaginative ties with the concepts of *inner safe space*, *inner helper* and *inner healer* can help to further suppress restlessness. Over time, affective strain along the existential fringe can ease and attune to the equanimity and calmness conducive to a *decent* death. In addition to sincere humane compassion, only genuine human succour, providence, presence, sharing, holding and other qualities of true human encounter can empower this reframing.

Over the decades, the authors personally have had the honour of working with a multitude of fully mentally alert dying clients in both Western and Eastern hemispheres, and have experienced that interactive measures reflecting deeply humane social qualities, including, but not limited to, desired and appropriate nearness, non-judgemental empathy, respect, attentive kindness, reassurance, sometimes in tranquil wordlessness, together with sensibly and mindfully offered gentle touch (ideally holding the hand or the arm and not the head or the face unless requested by the client), with or without eye contact, jointly contribute to mitigating their otherwise unbearable abyssal angst. As much as it is possible to say in *this* world, these and other visceral hallmarks of a truly humane poise, sacred and magical, not measurable or quantifiable, neither to be operationalized nor standardizable, perhaps connecting with the intuitive practice of the heart (*anahata*), appear to reflect the very essence of the shared meaning of life and being: love. And, finally, transcending human interaction, true faith and hope, constructive mental fields and visionary convictions together can become powerful attenuators of angst in view of the current reality and that which is to come. Further considerations on that are discussed below in this chapter.

In contrast, pharmacological anxiolysis via sedation, especially in cases of accumulation or overdose, may deepen affective and contextual dissociation, interfering with mental agency and reducing the human ability to sense, experience and to share just that. If angst remains unaddressed, panic may result whose consequences are likely to be detrimental to a *decent* death, obstructing awareness and the view of the natural radiance of the mind.

12.5.2 Comfort Allowing Farewell, Embracing Grief and Gently Letting Go

Grief indicates that something is missing or sad. Reflecting the past, it appears in response to imminent or acute loss. Just as sadness serves to close with adverse conditions that we cannot change, so grief assists resolution of an unalterable loss within the tribe. It rarely reveals itself in a uniform fashion, often quickly altering its appearance. Often preceded by diffuse anguish and associated with distress, it may initially be accompanied by subjective (secondary) sensations of despair, horror, sadness, inner conflict and sometimes fierce anger, vengeance, rebellion or (self)-loathing. Emptiness, senselessness or numbness may build up later until the emotional momentum eventually flows more smoothly (again).

Normal grief, allowing for adjustment to the novel situation, usually declines gradually over time. But for the terminal client, active commitment to releasing grief and achieving true farewell prior to the biological end can be a quintessential emotional preparation for what is to come. Individual disposition or circumstances, however, may perpetuate despair or anger before changing worlds, impeding clearance of the affective field, and leaving the dying client with a potentially heavy load of undesired affective tension and consequently a diminished palliative quality of life. Intense attachment and grief of loved ones immediately before death occurs can also be a burden for the dying client whose consciousness is vulnerable and unprotected. Dimming these feelings may be important for preventing transferred emotional suffering, compromising the ability to let go in peace of mind.

Ideally, grief, the farewell to loved ones, and the abandonment of longing, grasping and attachment to ego qualities should have been achieved and completed before the final dying commences. In some circumstances, loved ones themselves may risk transferring the sorrow into their own lives, giving rise to prolonged and often tremendous suffering and functional impairment. In extreme cases, persistent complex bereavement may occur, conflicting the meaning and function of grief within the tribe. Endlessly responding to a loss with desperation will not lead to healing. Unfinished grief and failed integration of the loss may in the long run encumber individual psycho-social and psycho-spiritual growth.

Despite the required formal distinction in clinical psychiatry between *normal* (adequate) and *pathological* (complicated, traumatic, prolonged, etc.) grief and its traits, the concept behind *normal*(ized) grief may necessitate second thoughts in (acute) terminal chaperonage. This is because the features of any internal emotional debate of this kind are highly individual and strongly influenced by education, experience, personality and socialization, as well as by cultural and anthropological variables, despite several common manifestations. Thus, the bereavement of loved ones (and clients) at any given moment pre and post mortem, but especially in the time window immediately before death, may differ quite significantly from what the 'Gaussian bell' indicates, with clinical consequences. A cardinal assertion is that the unexpected must be expected.

Authentic bereavement is crucial for being able to return to content and brio. Attending appropriately to grief, and integrating the loss into our earthly life to come and its conclusion will foster humane growth in all of us over time. It may even represent an important individual learning assignment in the lives of the survivors. It is vital for the continuing and for those who are left behind to mourn together on the basis of their true individual needs, reflecting the power of shared experience. Shared bereavement in palliative practice, carried by the fine qualities of human bonding, can increase peace of mind for the terminal client, and for the survivors often outweighs the desperation of having to face life without the deceased in the long run. Although painful, saying farewell is deeply anchored within our human longing to be recognized, appreciated and loved. One of the most compelling contributions to an emotionally *decent* death may be personally attending to the dying, being present, thanking, dignifying, forgiving and reconciling where necessary, and - most of all - (perhaps temporarily) saying farewell. Culturally specific or individual rituals and ceremonies, all of which can take place by the palliative bedside, can help to facilitate this and sufficient resources should be offered. Furthermore, bedside interventions targeting transformational changes towards an individually 'effective' and beneficial bereavement to be completed before death may become necessary.

In practical terminal chaperonage, experience indicates that mindfulness, meaning-oriented interventions, retrospection, cognitive reframing, and relaxation and meditation approaches, or a combination of these, are helpful in practice. Mindfulness, ideally, brings profound acceptance that as humans, we all face life and - sooner or later - its losses, pains and ultimately its end - death - and, if nothing else, ourselves. While this is neither good nor bad, it may have relevance within a much higher context unknown to us. It demands that we acquire our own skills and devise our own ways of handling these remarkable features of our humanity. We take our inner balance with us wherever we go, including towards cessation of our biological existence. Helpful cognitive reframing often includes reminders: first, that the time and experience one had in life and with loved ones may have been and possibly still may be given to us as a gift for which gratitude is worthwhile; second, that all living beings have to walk the same road one day, the client now, followed by their kin at a later time; third, that an enduring yet incomprehensible spiritual connectivity may one day reconnect loved ones; and finally, that our past and present development may reflect a deeper meaning that for now is hidden. The aim of meaning-oriented interventions is to induce meaningful appraisal by promoting the dignifying and appreciation of past and current experiences, achievements and social interactions. Here, retrospection methods (such as narration-based ones) can help bereave roles, realized and unrealized goals, and dreams.

Assisted bereaving should also include relaxation and meditation methods fostering mental and physical catharsis and stress relief to help master the exceptional mental challenges. Obstacles interfering with rewarding bereavement, including physical and medical factors, must not be neglected. Clouded consciousness or treatment at an intensive care ward, for example, may partly or completely compromise the terminal client's ability to grieve.

12.5.3 Help Unmasking and Dissolving Anger

Anger occurs in response to a perceived threat. Its purpose is to mobilize defences and evoke changes required to meet our needs in response to something which we do not feel is right for us and consequently do not want. If anger is "justified" and our responsive behaviour proves successful, relief may occur; otherwise, anger may be converted into guilt, shame, fear, self-contempt or grief - all seen in terminal disease - or be amplified or prolonged by them. Wrath and grudges can be forms of anger. Anger can flare up as a secondary response to a negative, dissatisfying, frustrating or threatening appraisal of a situation or its outcome. Subjective help-lessness and lack of control, which may either give rise to it or amplify it, are found in almost all palliative situations (inevitably leading to the threat of death), although not all dying clients express anger in their behaviour. Formally, anger is thought to comprise one potential reactive affect in the abovementioned models of phasic bereavement experienced by terminal clients prior to death. (Unresolved) anger and its sequelae may induce or intensify psycho-vegetative arousal with all its physical (including cardiovascular and neurologic) and mental consequences, particularly detrimental in pre-terminal and terminal processes. It has been observed that clients who die in unresolved anger allow a large amount of their mental energy to be absorbed by non-constructive and degradative processes of both mind and matter (body). This may obstruct the gentle closure of life and compromise access to a *decent* death.

Supportive unburdening of anger in terminal chaperonage is of paramount importance. First and foremost, anger must be identified before it can be con-sciously addressed. This should be followed by reflection on whether transforma-tion should originate from the client occupied by the anger, or whether evoking changes by the outside world is necessary and adequate and is in keeping with the individual's internal values. Essential techniques for aiding anger resolution before demise include practising non-appraisal, overcoming helplessness and lack of control, radical acceptance of full personal accountability for absolutely all personal cognitions, affects, decisions and deeds, and finally, disengagement and letting go of all negative emotions, and fostering their dyadic partners, affirmative and friendly ones, at the other end of the spectrum of choices. Truthful and forgiving gentle smiles accompanied by mindful breathing, the common denominator of any detoning relaxation, may signify successful closure of the task.

12.5.4   Encourage Invigorating Joy

Joy indicates that something is right. Being a reverberation of success, it represents one end of the affective valence spectrum and might be seen as the antagonist of angst. Being conscious creatures, we obey the pattern of seeking (dopamine-mediated) pleasure by experiencing joy (represented by wanting, desire, attachment, attraction) and avoiding pain propagated by angst (represented by aversion, repulsion). Life outside the ethereal world has taught us that superficial joy is more readily available and less cumbersome to obtain, which often deter-mines the behavioural strategies we adopt to meet most of our fundamental needs. Higher-order needs, however, are not always addressed and are often even less successfully fulfilled, despite our honest desire to do so. As our matter corrodes, losing its affinity towards dopamine zest, we realize that joy's superficial sisters vanish into thin air and that true and substantial satisfaction renders a call for depth.

Having rarely or perhaps never thought about the underlying meaning and the essence of our sub-lunar existence, terminal clients often share the realization that their past life has been full of once indispensable gains and preoccupation with the satisfaction of shallow needs; but once the surface has been ransacked sufficiently, such as now when they face their biological end, they sense a desire to dig deeper. Higher-order needs often demand attention almost automatically as we approach death.

Superficial joy depends on external triggers; in their absence it dulls as our biological options irrevocably narrow. Once we realize that, we are challenged with accepting the gift of joy over ontological entities and their deeper conscious meaning in our life. The process of actually letting go of the triggers, their attributions and their intrinsic vacuity and meaninglessness may then lead towards the experience and radiation of pure and authentic joy. Due to our learned helplessness while attempting to prioritize the innumerable developmental choices of daily life, many of us have lost connection with this powerful intrinsic and tangible property of our conscious being. This joy, genuinely independent from external stimuli, consists in delight over what really lies *behind* or can be discovered *within* all worldly entities, not their momentary and contingent yield, or in bliss over the essentiality and connectedness of all things, and not their limitation to our functional gains. This natural, we might say true and fundamental form of joy arises out of the moment as each and every one of them fills us with awe and wonder. Humans are capable of rejoicing in the pervasive simplicity of things independently of the sadness, grief, attachment and greed that constantly demand fulfilment of our material desires and needs - desires that easily metabolize to woes if unaddressed. It is this joy over our being, together with humbleness and thankfulness, which is to be uncovered. Naturally, these ideas do not imply a recommendation to en*joy* the advent of death. But while physical death may be regarded as a relief in certain situations, they remind us that these omnipresent forms of joy may balance affects and strengthen self-composure and equanimity to serve the higher needs that are critical prerequisites for a *decent* death. As the biological evolution of a conscious life sooner or later requires us to cope with its end or even an imminent unexpected threat of death, experiencing joy can become more than an antidote against angst and should not only not be compromised, but actually practised - in humbleness and gratitude.

12.5.5 Guide to Defy the Illusion of Objectivity, Building Faith and Drawing Hope

Everything we have ever learned about death has been taught by the living. Thus, a dying client must surrender to the unknown, must forfeit everything they ever loved and cared for, including meaning and purpose, unasked, helpless, lacking control and without the option of ever turning back. Awareness of this presents an unprecedented challenge to the human mind and may provoke subjectively strong (aversive) affects, even more so if entirely unprepared. Since neither matter-based perspectives nor scientifically proven knowledge are available and death itself and the afterworld are hidden, there are no certain adjustments but at most vague and uncertain ones. In an attempt to overcome this lack of control and helplessness, different minds turn to different heuristic beliefs. Some turn to the hard sciences, some approach the humanities and the arts, while others choose metaphysics or spirituality or combinations of concepts on which there is consensus. What all of them, all of us, share is that we believe in, have faith in, stand for something, some *thing*, based on our personal conviction, which is subject to many variables including our education, socialization and biology. Importantly, this also comprises ideas about the meaning and purpose of our lives.

Yet, everything, including that *thing*, whether scientifically proven (within a defined reference system) or not, is inevitably based on assumptions, conjectures and predefined axioms, as well as on personal predilections and antipathies, all of which reflect varying degrees of subjectivity. In the absence of an absolute absoluteness, *this* finite world, the world as *we* (in a body), and *each one of us individually,* perceive it and everything in it, phenomenologically *appears* to be a mere construct with subjective validity predetermined and maintained on the basis of our biological properties. Human ideas and concepts in the intellectual domain are not free of appraisal, and they are not nonjudgmental, yielding perception, awareness and knowledge (*Erkenntnis*) to be observer variables. In the physical domain, energy and matter obey the laws of quantum physics in quantized spacetime, and the (human or machine) observer is a no less decisive constituent of the reality generated. Variations in observation provoke variations in reality (see below), thus true objective knowledge is unattainable. In the Gottfried Wilhelm Leibniz`s (1646–1716) theory of possible worlds, modal realism suggested different worlds whose knowledge and beliefs are given by their epistemic and doxastic access, that is, worlds that we realize and believe to live in (Lewis 1986). All possible worlds are real in the same way. Hence, the actual world and its reality is not this or that, it is this *and* that. Logically, this is also true for the life and the death within it. We are invited to choose what we believe and have faith in and what conclusions we draw from that. Choices include anything between 'proven' science, which quickly imposes its characteristic limitations, and - opening up to a diffuse but intuitive mindset - the unproven, heterodox, ever hypothetical realm. If we choose for our mind to believe hard science, even become convinced of its attractive results and alleged proofs, we will still not know for sure. All we know is that our experiments can probe our theories, which again may or may not confirm our observations. Yet, how do we know that it was the appropriate experiment, indeed that the underlying theory is appropriate? Life itself unravels as a series of experimental choices, but where is the source of the options, where is *their* dao (*Urgrund*)? Can we ever awaken to it, being as we are among the living? And what are the right questions to lead to that knowledge? To make it more complicated, the human predisposition to accept a scientific proof is itself highly modulated by volatile affective energy, besides reason working underneath. Knowledge and experience mutually bias one another, although they do not necessarily presuppose each other - strictly speaking, knowledge cannot only be experienced and experience cannot only be known. Even the most scientific science is emotional, in that it is driven by subtle survival-promoting ego forces conclusively acting within all of us. The Janus-headed requisition of acceptance demands consensus consulting both reason *and* affect. But what if our intrinsic framework associated with their corresponding field ensembles does not endorse certain observations? Can a brain comprehensively understand *itself* at all? Paving the way for enlightenment, Leibniz may have had some central premonition suggesting that the cause of thoughts, sentiments and perceptions ("*Gedanken, Empfindungen, Perceptionen*") should be sought *outside* the "machine" or the "composito" from which they emerge (Leibniz 1714). We are bound by the applicability of the laws of nature to within *our* degrees of freedom and reference system. Any expansion necessitates its translation to coordinates *outside* the box.

What is more, energy is also condensed in *this* world, which is why we are hurt falling off a bicycle. Every material entity - the stars, earth, every carbon atom, pyrophosphate, protein, cell, tissue and organ, every living and non-living being - consists of, actually *is*, condensed energy. But the matter-based state of energy is not its unique feature. It is just one of many states into which energy has been translated to yield biology and the organic substrate of human consciousness and intelligence in *this* uni(que)-verse. This renders all of our perceptions projections of the illusion of our current material energetic form, i.e., our biological being, as assessed by our equally matter-based cognitive faculties. With respect to death and the afterworld, this implies that we will not know as long as we are biologically alive and still *inside* the box. We are tied to the hypothetical as per our systems properties. "*Die Wahrheit* [dass das so ist] *ist dem Menschen zumutbar!*" (freely adapted from Ingeborg Bachmann (1926–1973)).

Something that cannot be known with absolute certainty, however, challenges the initially unprejudiced and later biased human mind to be believed, even more so if the mind of the believer has become emotionally attached to it. In contrast to absolute certainty, belief, Bayesian in nature, or faith, entails uncertainty and parallels reductionism to probability, which is noetically reminiscent of the stochastic nature of quantum mechanics, particularly featured by probability amplitudes of quantum states and by the uncertainty of an observation beyond $\hbar/2$. The latter was formulated in 1927 by Werner Heisenberg (1901–1976) and most elegantly derived five years later by John von Neumann (1903–1957) (Neumann 1968). With reference to the former, Max Born (1883–1970) suggested that wave functions describe a probabilistic, but not an absolute distribution of microcosmic particles in space upon observation. Fascinatingly, the process of observation itself alters the quantum state and modifies the system: if we measure something, we change it. Observation changes reality in that is shifts an undetermined, multivalent state into a distinct, ostensibly unambiguous and univalent condition by making a choice. Should that perhaps be the very same in our empirical, macroscopic world? (For an outstanding original introductory lecture on probability amplitudes by Richard Feynman (1918–1988), see Feynman et al. (1989). Rae (2004) provides excellent additional and more comprehensive reading.) Belief and faith are non-deterministic and involve our cultural socialization, including religious and spiritual propensity and conditioning. And that has important implications for how humans live and die, because we are endowed with thinking and imagination, the mental power to create any-*think*, any-*thing*, in our psyche, for the time being, and devoid of any material correlate, in addition to belief, respectively faith. Despite the matterlessness of an image, there is no reason why the subtle neural electrical and magnetic field (energy) pattern that intricately represents its composition and meaning within the brain, the facilitator of our consciousness, is not specifically interactive with the rest of the biological and non-biological matter, i.e., condensed energy, over short and long distance, bringing about diverse changes in its character, and amenable to the (mathematical and physical) laws of nature. Macroscopically, imagination causes priming of neuronal catenation, well known to professional athletes. Also, imagined and real matters of apperception exhibit measurable similarity in their underlying neural processes. Moreover, belief, faith, imagination and affectively derived expectations are powerful in that they may simulate pharmacological and mental interventions. Placebo research has fascinatingly shown that mental fields (beliefs, faith, composure, imaginations, expectations) carry modulating powers in both the physical (i.e., biological) and the mental world, and can, bilaterally, significantly influence medical variables. Just like observing, thinking itself changes, creates, reality. Looking deeper, thinking *is* observing and observing *is* choosing – *this one* and *not that one* – from the multeity. Concerning the above concepts of reality, the mind overcomes the constraints of two (or more) preliminary, ever changing worlds, *this* world, the (alleged objective) external frame around us and all of its appearances, and our internal (subjective) selves in it, by means of thinking and choosing, thereby creating. The creative mind is becoming a creating one.

Belief and faith (in something) comprise an attitude, a bearing, in the sense of trust and confidence. Across most cultures, this involves spirituality or religion and should always be actively explored and addressed in terminal chaperonage, if the desire has been voiced. It is not about what is right or wrong, it is about assisting the terminal client to benefit from or not suffer from their individual interpretation of relevant spiritual topics, including about the life lived and the contemplation of death. Given the nature of the human mind, even in severe depression, conscious terminal clients incapable of believing, having faith, imagining and holding expectations, are rare. Because of the transformative power of the mindset, it is not only socially acceptable to believe, to have faith, and to imagine and visualize, it is essential in order to unlock the unknown space of prospects. Conversely, having nothing to believe and have faith in may lead to a lack of meaning, which may imply other painful consequences. These processes can be assisted by offering encouragement and guidance to the imagination and by building faith in the agency of intention, ethos, thought, wishing and dedication, together with supportive sensory facilitation using, for example, music, prayer and mantras. And this should include hope, a conceptual mental field that can be seen as an affective representation of the reassuring conviction that what we have faith in will become true (for us). Hope renders possibility from reality. And that is limitless.

Providing the dying with assistance to cultivate the purity of their individual beliefs and thoughts, build faith and finally draw hope seems an indispensable element of comprehensive terminal chaperonage.

12.5.6 Advocate Overcoming Regret

Regret is a sentiment that almost always involves an existential dimension if it occurs in the context of the end of life. Accordingly, its underlying catalysts need to be particularly addressed in terminal chaperonage. In the balance of a life, retrospection may yield affirmative and reassuring recollections, a pleasing earthly afterglow, as well as disappointing or otherwise displeasing and wearing imagery. Unfulfilled or unrealized dreams, wishes, plans or opportunities that were perhaps once emotionally intense and important, as well as subjectively false decisions in the past, can often not be made up for or corrected in later stages of life, even less so when facing its end. These missed opportunities usually concern personal development in social areas including choice of partner, offspring and family, as well as educational or professional domains. If any related intense discontent has not previously been alleviated and closure achieved, regret may occur. While regret as a cognitive emotion may naturally arise in the context of any decision making in life, and while it does train personality development and coping skills for the individual, it may become extremely painful under the heavy threat of a biological end. The terminal client faces the challenge of having to accept that neither former decisions nor their consequences can be reversed ex post. Because of that, forgiveness and acceptance (both further discussed below in this chapter) are among the most potent mental manoeuvres to forego and close painful regret and associated secondary affective fields. The confident (subjective) conception that one's life had a true and possibly higher-ordered meaning and purpose given these past decisions and consequences, together with one's choices of coping, or precisely *because of them*, opens another often most helpful, yet inevitable space of relief. Since modifications to the past will remain inaccessible, open-mindedness for what is to come while wholeheartedly embracing the past become imperative, closing the loop with regard to death preparation, as outlined above. Working with regret should be an important focus of bedside terminal guidance.

12.5.7 Facilitate Mitigation of Guilt and Shame and Practising Forgiveness

Critical end-of-life topics include coping with the cognitive emotions guilt and shame, two culturally deeply preserved emotional appraisals associated with codes of socially desired versus undesired conduct that regulate social behaviour within the tribe through operant learning. Guilt and shame are often encountered in terminal chaperonage and their unsuccessful or ineffective relief are major obstacles when working towards a *decent* death. Ancient cultural lore of the emotional and existential needs of the human psyche, body and spirit teaches us that sincere forgiveness of others and of oneself can be instrumental in the process of their healing. Sincere forgiveness, especially of oneself, can sometimes be arduous and often turns out to be a most painful and challenging mental manoeuvre that demands a great deal from the dying client. The sense of not being able to afford to forgive oneself and of not deserving forgiveness at all regularly causes emotional suffering in terminal chaperonage. Frequently, this plays a potent inhibitory role during affect regulation aimed at achieving equanimity and calmness while facing death. Therapeutically, the acknowledgement that this idea exists exclusively in the client's mind and not elsewhere, may become a relieving lead. Terminal clients should aspire to unconditionally reconcile with relatives, friends and foes, leaving no traces of resentment and grudges for having been hurt and made to suffer. Truly rewarding human relationships allowing for forgiveness may become a powerful personal resource prior to the end of life.

12.5.8   Strengthen the Building and Mastering of Acceptance

Clinically, one of the most challenging psychological barriers to a *decent* death can be lack of acceptance - acceptance of the current situation, ultimately acceptance of the loss of participation and the imminent end of the biological life. The very demanding mental faculty of an unreserved radical acceptance may require the ability to overcome a strong sense of helplessness and lack of control. Relieving end-of-life chaperonage often requires addressing these latter two.

True acceptance consists in the willingness to allow and let be what irrevocably is and cannot be altered, in contrast to expending mental energy on unsuccessfully attempting to drive impossible changes. Repeated disappointments due to the emotionally exhausting rejection of the unwanted, together with depletion of internal resources trying to reverse the process, can be halted by the conviction that some things are unchangeable, come rain or shine, however deep the desire. Death is one such thing. The more the impossible is enforced, the more the mind will become imprisoned by the repetitive failure. By adopting radical acceptance, the tension between wanting and never achieving may recede and possibly help to make the client's mindset more placid. Hidden affective powers of despair and anger over the subjective conclusion of having no choice may be repolarized and redirected from frustrating change behaviour towards other terminal emotional needs, helping to improve the current condition. Acceptance of the situation, its evolution and consequences, is a most powerful manoeuvre. Acceptance means gently letting go. It is not an escape but a coming home. Honouring and coming to terms with life and death in deep faith will become liberating in that very moment and in what is to come. This is true for all of mankind. There is no other way!

Therapeutically, approaches to emotion regulation based on millennia-old Eastern concepts of mindfulness have been refined and advanced in the third wave of psychotherapy in the last 30 years or so, building on the assumption that there is ultimately no alternative to developing acceptance. Similar to efforts to overcome regret, experience from bedside chaperonage suggests that the initially unacceptable and traumatic sense of threat to one's life (in terminal disease) is ameliorated by personal beliefs about the meaning of life and death, a shared meaning, possibly in a higher-order sense, including past or present individual earthly tasks. Aside from that, adherence to the cognitive modes of non-appraisal and abandonment of attachment and aversion described above may help to expedite acceptance in mental pre-terminal preparation.

12.6   Vista – quid nunc?

We are slowly beginning to achieve a better understanding of the importance of the mind and specifically of thought and affect processes surrounding both life and death. Based on what we assume today, it appears possible for each and every conscious and unconscious terminal client to die with peace of mind, if the right and individually appropriate choices are made on both sides (client/kin and providers) at the right time. Absence or displacement of consciousness does not exclude this, rather it serves as a re-*mind*-er of the importance of becoming intellectually and emotionally concerned with the end of our biological life while still among the conscious living. Despite some of the latest trends, globally this is currently not often seen. Death has meaning only in life. Yet, every day we live is a day we die, inevitably!

There is no alternative to a philanthropic understanding in palliative and terminal chaperonage (and elsewhere in medicine). It renders compassion one of the characteristic attributes of *humanitas*. Hence, adequate and sufficient state-of-the-art 'somatic' pain therapy and palliative symptom control *pari passu* with culturally and individually sensitive psychological and spiritual guidance are not only desirable but must be considered non-negotiable moral imperatives. The ultimate goal is to aid the dying in the process of discovering and utilizing their personal assets and power and to facilitate the transition pursuant to their individual needs. Clearly, the ethical implications of philanthropy should surmount evidence-based probability and cost-effective rationalization and call for advocacy to permit just that.

Terminal chaperonage involves observing boundaries, edges and constraints, and demanding equality of intuitive approaches with evidence-based ones. Ultimately, there is the age-old and cross-culturally held fundamental conviction that death is transitory and becomes solely mental once the physical boundaries of condensed matter have been completely left behind, perhaps opening the door for continuation of the psycho-spiritual development assigned to us. Thoroughly attending to thoughts and emotions prior to our biological death is, then, only logically consistent. They make up what we humans are and account for our true identity. Bearing that in mind - mind over matter - is evidence of candour, impartiality and humility, which themselves are mental dispositions, since we will not know for sure during this life.

References

Blanchard EB, Andrasik F, Arena JG, Neff DF, Jurish SE, Teders SJ, Saunders NL, Pallmeyer TP, Dudek TB, Rodichok LD (1984) A bio-psycho-social investigation of headache activity in a chronic headache population. Headache 24(2):79–87

Ciancio AL, Mirza RM, Cinacio AA, Klinger CA (2020) The use of palliative sedation to treat existential suffering: a scoping review on practices, ethical considerations, and guidelines. J Palliat Care 35(1):13–20

Feynman RP, Leighton RB, Sands M (1989) Probability Amplitudes. In: The Feynman lectures on physics, vol 3. Addison-Wesley, Redwood City. https://www.feynmanlectures.caltech.edu/ Accessed 13 Mar 2020

Fletcher D, Martinez V (2014) Opioid-induced hyperalgesia in patients after surgery: a systematic review and a meta-analysis. Br J Anaesth 112(6):991–1004

Khatami M, Rush A-J (1982) A One Year Follow-Up of the Multimodal Treatment for Chronic Pain. Pain 14(1):45–52

Knaul FM et al (2018) Lancet commission on palliative care and pain relief study group. alleviating the access abyss in palliative care and pain relief—an imperative of universal health coverage. The Lancet Commission report. The Lancet 391 (10128):1391–1454

Leibniz GW (1714) Monadologie §17. German translation from the French original in 1720 by Heinrich Koehler. Projekt Gutenberg-DE. https://www.projekt-gutenberg.org/leibniz/monaden/monaden.html Accessed 13 Mar 2020

Lewis DK (1986) On the plurality of worlds. Blackwell, Oxford

Merskey H, Albe Fessard D, Bonica JJ, Carmon A, Dubner R, Kerr FWL, Lindblom U, Mumford JM, Nathan PW, Noordenbos W, Pagni CA, Renaer MJ, Sternbach RA, Sunderland S (1979) Pain terms: a list with definitions and notes on usage. Recommended by the IASP subcommittee on taxonomy. Pain 6(3):249–252

Neumann J (1968) Mathematische Grundlagen der Quantenmechanik. Unveränderter Nachdruck der 1. Auflage von 1932, in der Reihe Grundlehren der mathematischen Wissenschaften, Band 38. Kapitel III Die quantenmechanische Statistik, Abschnitt 12.4 Unbestimmtheitsrelationen. Erste Auflage. S. 123–124. Springer, Berlin. English translation: Mathematical Foundations of Quantum Mechanics. Princeton University Press, Princeton, 1955

Okie S (2010) A flood of opioids, a rising tide of deaths. N Engl J Med 363(31):1981–1985

Rae AIM (2004) Quantum physics: illusion or reality?, 2nd edn. Cambridge University Press, New York

Saunders C (1986) The nature and nurture of pain control. J Pain Symptom Mange 1(4):199–201

Steinhauser KE, Christakis NA, Clipp EC, McNeilly M, McIntyre L, Tulsky JA (2000) Factors considered important at the end of life by patients, family, physicians, and other care providers. JAMA 284(19):2476–2482

Treede R-D (2018) The International Association for the Study of Pain definition of pain: as valid in 2018 as in 1979, but in need of regularly updated footnotes. Pain Rep 3(2):e643

Ware B (2012) Top five regrets of the dying: a life transformed by the dearly departing. Hay House UK, London

WHO (2007) World Health Organization Normative guidelines on pain management. Report of a Delphi Study to determine the need for guidelines and to identify the number and topics of guidelines that should be developed by WHO. https://www.who.int/medicines/areas/quality_safety/delphi_study_pain_guidelines.pdf. Accessed 28 Dec 2020

WHO (2014) World Health Assembly Resolution # 67.19 "Strengthening of palliative care as a component of comprehensive care throughout the life course". https://apps.who.int/gb/ebwha/pdf_files/WHA67/A67_R19-en.pdf. Accessed 28 Dec 2020

WHO (2019a) World Health Organization Palliative care. https://www.who.int/health-topics/palliative-care. Accessed 28 Dec 2020

WHO (2019b) World Health Organization Cancer pain ladder for adults. Annex 1 in https://www.who.int/ncds/management/palliative-care/cancer-pain-guidelines/en/. Accessed 28 Dec 2020

WHO (2019c) World Health Organization Guidelines for the pharmacological and radiothera-
    peutic management of cancer pain in adults and adolescents. World Health Organization,
    Geneva. Licence: CC BY-NC-SA 3.0 IGO. https://www.who.int/ncds/management/palliative-
    care/cancer-pain-guidelines/en/. Accessed 28 Dec 2020
WHO (2019d) World Health Organization Web statement on pain management guidance. https://
    www.who.int/medicines/areas/quality_safety/guide_on_pain/en/. Accessed 28 Dec 2020
WMA (2017) World Medical Association, Declaration of Geneva, as amended by the 68th WMA
    General Assembly, Chicago, United States, Oct 2017. https://www.wma.net/policies-post/
    wma-declaration-of-geneva/. Accessed 28 Dec 2020

Advance Directives for Medical Decisions

13

R. Beckmann

13.1 Introduction

Just a few decades ago, patients were happy if the doctor did 'everything' in his power, because often, that was not too much. There was no reason to fear overtreatment. The patient generally agreed with what the doctor suggested. Nowadays, the medical possibilities have expanded to such an extent that there are often several options for treatment, some of them going way beyond what the patient is willing to accept. In legal terms, too, there has been a change. While the doctor can determine an indication for treatment, it is ultimately up to the patient to decide whether to accept a particular treatment or not. Patient autonomy has become the guiding principle of medical treatment.

Many patients want to influence their future treatment even if they are no longer able to make decisions on their own. Advance directives, in particular living wills and powers of attorney, serve as a means to this end. These legal institutions will be discussed in this chapter on the basis of the German legal context with particular reference to cancer patients. (For useful information on living wills and advance directives in the US health care system see Mayo Clinic Staff 2018.)

R. Beckmann (✉)
History, Philosophy, and Ethics in Medicine, Medical Faculty Mannheim,
Heidelberg University, Ludolf-Krehl-Strasse 13-17, 68167 Mannheim, Germany
e-mail: mail@rainerbeckmann.de

© Springer Nature Switzerland AG 2021
A. W. Bauer et al. (eds.), *Ethical Challenges in Cancer Diagnosis and Therapy*,
Recent Results in Cancer Research 218,
https://doi.org/10.1007/978-3-030-63749-1_13

13.2 Basics: Defining the Areas of Competence

Every medical treatment rests on two pillars: the medical indication and the informed consent of the patient. The two aspects cannot always be clearly separated from each other. In particular, an unduly broad understanding of the concept of 'indication' can affect patients' rights.

In medical statements, great weight is given to shared decision making between doctor and patient (or their legal representative). For example, the principles of the German Medical Association on terminal care state: "The decision on the initiation, further implementation or termination of a medical measure is taken in a *shared decision-making process* by doctor and patient or patient representative" (Bundesärztekammer 2011, 347). This attempt to find a consensus is reasonable, since without trust and cooperation between doctor and patient it will scarcely be possible to achieve successful treatment. This is also taken into account by the legal provisions of Sec. 630c (1) BGB (German Civil Code), according to which the treating person should "cooperate" in carrying out the medical treatment. Regardless of this, however, the legal competences for each treatment decision have to be distinguished clearly from each other.

13.2.1 The Correlation Between Indication and Informed Consent

Even if every medical treatment is initially based on two pillars, the existence of a medical indication and the patient's consent, the indication is of particular importance. It has a kind of filter function. There is no room for the consent of a patient (or their representative) to treatment if the doctor does not offer such treatment because there is no medical indication for it (Bundesgerichtshof 2003, Sec. 63). It is therefore of great importance that the limits of the physician's decision-making competence are not drawn too wide, in order to leave the patient enough room for their own independent decision making.

This danger arises in particular if, with regard to decision-making competence, one does not focus on the individual treatment measure, but rather considers the medical procedures and the general living conditions of the patient as a unit. The physician would then have to assess the overall situation and, if they judged it to be unsatisfactory, could deny the indication for an individual measure, although it would in itself be medically indicated. For example, if an appendicitis occurs in a patient who already has severe cognitive impairment and whose life the physician perceives only as 'vegetative', then the physician must not deny the medical indication for the removal of the appendix, just because they think that the quality of life will remain low and the patient's 'suffering' will be extended as a result of the intervention. The same applies to permanent medication or life-sustaining substitution treatment if additional acute illnesses occur. Even in such situations, the physician cannot end the original treatment, which continues to fulfil its purpose, by arguing that the medical indication has ceased because the overall situation of the patient is not improving.

Whether a particular medical intervention should be continued or discontinued due to additional medical symptoms and/or the deterioration of the patient's overall quality of life—which is often the case with terminal cancer—is not a question of determining a specific medical indication. It must be left to the patient (or their representative) to decide, in view of their changing life situation, whether to revoke consent to an indicated and ongoing medico-technical procedure or to refuse to consent to further treatment that could be stressful. An over-extension of the physician's competence in the area of determining the medical indication would undermine the patient's right of self-determination.

13.2.2   Area of Competence of the Physician

The physician is responsible for determining the indication (see also Sec. 1901b (1) BGB). There are three essential aspects to this (cf. Beckmann 2018, 556):

1. A reason for medical treatment, that is, an illness or functional impairment or disability of the affected person.
2. A therapeutic goal towards which a treatment can be described as useful. This goal may be the healing of an illness, the alleviation of symptoms or compensation for a missing/disordered bodily function.
3. A medical procedure that has the potential to achieve the therapeutic goal (with a specific probability).

The initiative for treatment initially comes from the patient, because he has 'complaints' that make him seek medical help. It is part of the doctor's competence to determine whether these complaints actually give cause for medical action because of a disease or functional impairment. The diagnosis is made by the physician, the only one with the necessary expertise to recognize pathological conditions or functional limitations and their causes.

The possible therapeutic goals can also only be described and presented appropriately by the physician. The patient can express their wishes. If these cannot be fulfilled, they will not be considered therapeutic goals. However, it is important to recognize that the physician does not 'determine' or set the treatment goal(s). The physician is only able to present and describe which goals could realistically be aimed at with professional medical skills. First and foremost, a causal cure will be the goal, but if this is not possible, at least an alleviation of symptoms might be aimed at. In some cases, symptomatic and curative procedures are available alternatively or cumulatively. While all these options with their specific advantages and disadvantages are to be offered to the patient by the physician, it is the patient who decides whether one of the therapeutic goals offered should actually be pursued.

The medical procedure by which the therapeutic goal may be achieved is again up to the professional assessment of the physician. If several methods can lead to the goal (e.g., medical intervention or drug treatment), these must be explained to the patient as part of the information given to enable them to make an informed decision.

13.2.3 Area of Competence of the Patient

In exercising their right of self-determination, it falls within the patient's competence to decide whether and how they want to be treated. If there are several ways of approaching the therapeutic goal, they decide the aim of the treatment (e.g. curative or symptomatic) as well as the method of treatment. This is not an 'intervention' in the competence of the medical profession, but the exercise of the patient's 'autonomy', expressed in German law as the patient's "body-related right of self-determination" according to Article 2 (2) GG (German Basic Law). By refusing to consent to certain forms of treatment, the patient can exclude all options that do not correspond to their own personal preferences. "Clinicians (not patients) provide indications, patients (not clinicians) decide on their realisation" (Raspe 2015, 98).

The division of responsibilities between doctor and patient does not change if the patient is no longer able to give consent. The patient is then replaced by their legal representative, an authorized proxy, or the guardian (see below). They must enforce the patient's wishes (Sec. 1901a (1) BGB) or, if these are not known, determine the patient's preferences for treatment and ultimately their presumed wishes (Sec. 1901a (2) and (6) BGB). If the presumed wishes of the patient cannot be determined on the basis of concrete evidence, their well-being remains the final criterion for the decision-making process (see Sec. 1901 (2) BGB; Deutscher Bundestag 2008a, 16). It is the responsibility of the patient's representative to make a decision on whether to consent to or refuse the indicated medical measures, taking the patient's well-being into account.

13.3 The Legal Framework for Living Wills in Germany

Since 2009, medical advance directives have been legally regulated in Germany under the term *Patientenverfügung* (see Deutscher Bundestag 2008a), which corresponds to 'living will' in Anglo-American usage.

13.3.1 Legal Definition

According to Sec. 1901a (1) BGB, the basic statement of the law on living wills is:

> If a person of full age who is able to consent has determined in writing, in the event of his becoming unable to consent, whether he consents to or prohibits specific tests of his state of health, treatment or medical interventions not yet directly immanent at the time of

determination (living will), the guardian must examine whether these determinations correspond to the current living and treatment situation. If this is the case, the guardian must see to it that the wish of the person under guardianship is carried out.

Although this provision is located in the 'guardianship' section of the BGB, it defines in a general way—whether guardianship exists or not—what is meant by a living will under the law (legal definition). Thus, the legislator has recognized advance directives intended to give consent to or to refuse diagnostic, therapeutic or other medical procedures as legally binding in the field of health care.

The patient's decisions are primarily to be observed and enforced by the patient's legal representative. Corresponding references in the law specify that representatives (authorized person, legal proxy) appointed by the patient themselves with power of attorney have the same rights and duties with regard to living wills as guardians appointed by the court (see Sec. 1901a (5), 1901b (3), 1904 (5) BGB).

Of particular practical importance are decisions by the patient to refuse certain treatments in the future. In Austria, a living will is defined a priori as a document "by which a patient refuses medical treatment" (Sec. 2 (2) *Österreichisches Patientenverfügungsgesetz* - öPatVG). Declarations denying further treatment often refer to life-prolonging procedures such as artificial nutrition and hydration, ventilation, resuscitation, etc. This practical context links to the topic of euthanasia. The cessation of treatment at the request of the patient is also described as 'passive euthanasia'. The following considerations take particular account of the situation of such a refusal of treatment.

13.3.2 General Aspects

With regard to the preparation and practical application of living wills, German law requires the following aspects to be observed.

13.3.2.1 Distinction from the Actual Wishes of the Patient

A living will must first be distinguished from the actual wishes of the patient. If a patient has been informed about the intended course of treatment or discontinuation of treatment at the same time, or nearly the same time, as a treatment or discontinuation of treatment and has given their decision to the physician, then this actual decision is binding on the physician (and also on any third party). The patient's decision must be observed. This also applies if the patient loses their ability to give consent within a short time. A living will in the technical sense is not necessary for this purpose because the patient has made a decision about an imminent medical treatment. Only decisions which are intended to have an effect on "not immediately" imminent tests of the state of health, treatment or medical intervention must be made in the form of a living will (see Sec. 1901 (1) BGB).

13.3.2.2 Field of Application

Prior to the legal regulation of living wills, there had been discussion in Germany about whether a patient should only be allowed to refuse treatment if they are suffering from an "irreversibly fatal disease" (Enquetekommission des Deutschen Bundestages 2004, 38). The legislature decided against this and explicitly made clear that treatment decisions in a living will are permitted "irrespective of the nature and stage of the illness" of the person concerned (Sec. 1901a (3) BGB). It therefore makes no difference whether the patient's condition is hopeless and they will die in a short time anyway, or whether they could be saved by a simple and harmless intervention or the administration of inexpensive drugs with minimal side effects. If the patient has refused to give their consent to the specifically indicated treatment in their living will, the decision to refrain from treatment must be respected.

13.3.2.3 Information and Counselling

The legal regulations on living wills do not contain any provisions on 'information' or counselling—unlike those in the Austrian Patient Living Will Act (see Sec. 5 and 6 öPatVG). Although medical advice prior to the drafting of a living will is generally considered useful and is recommended (Deutscher Bundestag 2008a, 19), the legislator has not made it a general precondition for the validity of living wills. Refusal of medical interventions can be declared without prior consultation. In such cases, the patient is personally responsible for ensuring that they are sufficiently informed about the consequences of their decisions and must bear the risk of informational deficit.

13.3.2.4 Revocation

A living will can be revoked informally at any time (see Sec. 1901a (1) s. 3 BGB). The only criterion is that the change of will "is expressed with sufficient clarity" (Deutscher Bundestag 2008a, 13). As long as the patient is capable of giving consent, revocation is no problem. The patient can either destroy the document to be revoked altogether and replace it with a new one, or make changes to the original document. A verbal revocation before witnesses can also be sufficiently clear.

However, the situation is problematic if the patient is only able to communicate with limitations or if they are no longer fully able to give consent. A reduced ability to express one's own wishes in itself results in considerable difficulties of interpretation, especially if non-verbal expressions—such as gestures or signs—have to be evaluated. If a revocation cannot be clearly identified, the advance directive continues to apply.

13.3.2.5 Duration of Validity

The validity of expressions of intent documented in writing is unlimited. All provisions are valid for an indefinite period of time. A regular review and confirmation of the living will, as provided, for example, in the Austrian Patient Living Will Act (see Sec. 7 öPatVG), is not required under German law.

However, it can still be useful to re-evaluate a living will if, for example, the therapeutic options for a particular disease have changed. If a patient confirms their wishes in such a case, it is clear that the new medical developments have not changed their attitude. However, the patient's wishes could be unclear if, due to the age of the decision, it must be assumed that they were not aware of newer therapeutic alternatives at the time of writing the living will. In Austria, Sec. 10 (1) no. 3 öPatVG declares living wills to be invalid if "the state of medical science has changed significantly with regard to the content of the living will since its establishment".

13.3.2.6   Filing, Registration and Disclosure

Under German law, it is not necessary to file or register the living will. Here, too, the principle of personal responsibility ultimately applies: the patient has to ensure that their living will is known to their legal representative or the attending physician, or that it will become known as soon as possible in the cases described in the living will. It is advisable to inform at least near relatives and close friends about the existence of a living will and where it is kept, so that it can be taken into account without delay.

Special precautions should be taken in the event of an emergency. The purpose of the emergency medical service is to apply life-saving measures as quickly as possible. Therefore, it is not the task of an emergency physician to obtain information about the patient's wishes before providing initial aid. In most cases the physician must act immediately. Hence the patient is responsible for making it clear to the doctor that they do not want any treatment. For example, an essential instruction (e.g., "Do not resuscitate") can be placed, clearly visible, above the nursing bed or on the bedside table. It makes even more sense to disclose instructions to reject medical treatment to relatives and, if necessary, to the nursing staff. This is the best way of guaranteeing that in the situations described in the living will the emergency doctor is not called in at all.

13.3.3   General Requirements for Validity

In Germany, the legislator has laid down only a few formal and personal prerequisites for the validity of living wills.

13.3.3.1   Written Form

The only formal prerequisite for validity is that the living will must be in writing (see Sec. 1901a (1) BGB). The written form is intended to protect against haste and misinterpretation and guarantees a minimum of authenticity, clarity and verifiability. Certification or even recording by a solicitor is not required.

In German law, 'in writing' means that the author must sign the living will. A ready-made pro forma can be used. However, it must be signed. If the author of the living will is not (or is no longer) in a position to sign it, a mark can replace a signature—individual letters or, if necessary, "three crosses", provided the procedure is legally validated (see Sec. 126 (1) BGB). In such cases, particular care must be taken to ensure that there is no doubt as to the signatory's ability to give consent.

13.3.3.2 Capacity to Give Consent

At the time the living will is drafted, the patient must have been "able to give consent". The capacity to give consent is the patient's natural ability to understand and control the nature, significance, scope and risks of a therapeutic treatment measure and to determine their wishes accordingly (see Deutscher Bundestag 2008a, 9). In principle, therefore, persons who are not of full age may already be able to give consent. Equally, however, the capacity to give consent can be lost in adults due to disease-related limitations, such as degenerative processes or cancer metastases in the brain. If such diseases are imminent, clarification should be sought as early as possible as to whether a living will can still be issued. If there is a risk that the patient's capacity to give consent could be called into question afterwards, current capacity to give consent should be confirmed by a medical specialist's certificate. This statement can either be attached to the living will or included in its text.

13.3.3.3 Age of Majority

In addition to the capacity to give consent, the legislator has also made the patient's age of majority (18 years) a requirement for a binding living will. For technical reasons, this is understandable, since the legal institution of the living will was incorporated into the guardianship law section of the civil law, and guardianship law only covers persons of full age anyway (see Sec. 1896 (1) s. 1 BGB). Since, on the other hand, living wills are essentially to be regarded as an expression of the right of personality, a lower age limit could also have been established. The age limit applying to capacity to make a will, for example, is 16 (see Sec. 2229 (1) BGB).

13.3.4 Specific Content of the Living Will

It is the patient's own responsibility to determine the contents of their living will. In principle, every conceivable wish can be expressed with regard to future medical treatment, especially with regard to limitations of treatment. The refusal of possible therapeutic interventions is always binding, since the physician may only carry out medical interventions with the patient's consent.

The decisive factor is that the instructions of a living will identify as clearly as possible the situation in which they are to be implemented. The law speaks of provisions for "certain" examinations, curative treatments or medical interventions (Sec. 1901a (1), s. 1 BGB). General statements such as "I do not want medical apparatus", "I want to die peacefully" or "I wish for a dignified death" are not sufficient. Even the phrase "Once I suffer from dementia, I do not want life-sustaining measures", is—according to the justification of the law—not sufficient to be binding "because it does not contain a sufficiently precise decision on treatment in a specific situation of illness" (Deutscher Bundestag 2008a, 15).

Consulting a physician and/or a lawyer is therefore recommended in order to inform oneself about possible applications or appropriate phraseology. Suggestions can be found, for example, in information leaflets published by the Federal Ministry of Justice, the state justice authorities or in forms available in bookshops or from patient organizations and hospice associations.

13.3.5   Examination and Implementation of the Living Will

When the patient requires treatment and are themselves no longer able to give consent, several legal regulations must be observed with regard to the review and implementation of the living will.

13.3.5.1   Existence of a Medical Indication

The medical determination of whether a certain measure is medically indicated or not is of fundamental importance for medical treatment in case of serious illness or at the end of life (cf. Sec. 1901b (1) BGB). By establishing the indication, the doctor sets the course for further treatment. If there is no indication for a certain medical intervention, then there is also no need to worry about the patient's wishes, and the living will then has no significance. "Only if the physician offers a life-prolonging or life-preserving treatment is the consent of the guardian... required at all" (Federal Court of Justice 2003, Sec. 64). The patient has no right to the implementation of therapies that are not medically indicated (Deutscher Bundestag 2008a, 7).

13.3.5.2   Need for Legal Representation

Since the patient is no longer capable of making decisions themselves when their advance directive is to be applied, the physician needs a legal representative of the patient as a partner in dialogue when implementing a living will. However, some authors believe that legal representation of the patient is not absolutely necessary if the living will of the patient as such is clear. The German Medical Association also shares this view, although it concedes that the law does not explicitly answer this question (Bundesärztekammer 2010, 879). The basis of this position is Sec. 630d (2) s. 1 BGB, according to which in the case of patients who are incapable of giving consent, the consent of an authorized person must be obtained "unless a living will in accordance with Sec. 1901a (1) s. 1 permits or prohibits the measure".

However, this view is not convincing. The legal provision describing the communication process between the physician and the patient's representative to determine the patient's wishes (Sec. 1901b BGB) does not limit it to "unclear" or "dubious" cases. The procedure ordered there can only be carried out if the patient has a representative. The mere existence of a living will does not permit the conclusion that the currently pending situation can be clarified by a precise advance directive of the patient. The evaluation and interpretation of the advance directive is not the primary responsibility of the physician, but is the responsibility of the patient's legal representative. While the physician has to determine the indication, it is the responsibility of the patient (or their representative) to decide in free self-determination whether or not to accept the proposed treatment (see above). A patient's legal representative should therefore examine what the patient has decided in their advance directive, even in seemingly 'obvious' cases.

The attending physician should also consider that the risk of misjudging the patient's wishes is theirs alone if a patient's representative has not participated in the process of decision making.

13.3.5.3   Conversation Between the Patient's Representative and the Physician; Decision of the Patient's Representative

When the doctor has established the medical indication for treatment and a written living will is available, it must first be established whether there are any signs of a revocation of the living will. If this is not the case, the patient's legal representative and the physician determine the patient's wishes in an extended dialogue process and check whether the patient's decisions are in accordance with their current life and treatment situation (Sec. 1901a (1), s. 1 BGB). Close relatives and other people trusted by the patient should be given the opportunity to express their opinion (Sec. 1901b (2) BGB).

If the patient's instructions do not accord with the current life and treatment situation, there is no direct binding effect, as defined by Sec. 1901a (1) or (2) BGB. The patient's written statements are then to be taken into account in determining their presumed wishes in respect of treatment (Sec. 1901a (2) s. 1 BGB) (see below).

The decision as to whether the patient's statement is sufficiently 'specific' and applies to the current life and treatment situation is the responsibility of their representative (cf. Sec. 1901a (1) s. 1 and (5) BGB). Because of the conversation with the attending physician and the involvement of close relatives or confidants, however, this will not be a 'lone' decision for the patient's representative. The dialogue procedure ensures that the decision is supported by the broadest possible factual basis.

13.3.5.4   Consensus Between the Patient's Representative and the Physician

If there is consensus between the patient's representative and the treating physician that the patient has made a determination that applies to the situation currently to be decided, the patient's instructions are implemented without the need for court approval (Sec. 1904 (4) BGB). If, for example, the patient has renounced the supply of a feeding tube, this form of artificial feeding will not be applied. The patient will then die within a few days as a result of their decision, while other medically indicated forms of treatment and nursing will be maintained.

If, after reviewing the living will, there is no consensus on the patient's wishes between the patient's representative and the physician, interruption of treatment intended by the patient's representative requires the approval of the Court of Protection (pursuant to Sec. 1904 (2) BGB). The criterion for the court's approval is the wishes of the patient (Sec. 1904 (3) BGB). The essential task of the court is to examine whether the available factual evidence is sufficient to identify a specific wish by the patient. The wish of the patient thus determined is binding. If the court is convinced that the decision of the patient's representative corresponds to the patient's wishes, it must grant permission (Deutscher Bundestag 2008a, 18). If the wish of the patient cannot be ascertained or cannot be ascertained with sufficient reliability, then the principle prevails that in case of doubt a decision must be made in favour of life (see below).

13.4   Procedure in the Absence of a Living Will

The German legislator has also regulated the standards according to which a decision is to be made if there is no living will or a defective living will:

> If there is no living will, or if the determinations of a living will do not correspond to the current life and treatment situation, the guardian must determine the wishes with regard to treatment or the presumed will of the person under guardianship, and decide on this basis whether he consents to or prohibits a medical treatment pursuant to paragraph (1). (Sec. 1901a (2) s. 1 BGB).

13.4.1   Treatment Wishes

'Treatment wishes' are all specific expressions of the patient's wishes relating to the current treatment situation, which in the absence of written form cannot claim any direct binding force as a living will. Furthermore, all concrete treatment-related oral or written statements made by minors or persons who are not clearly capable of giving their consent, as well as oral statements made by adults, are also considered 'treatment wishes', since these statements provide the legal representative with the exact decision to be made but do not meet the legal requirements of a living will (majority, ability to give consent, written form).

To be distinguished from this are 'general treatment requests', which do not provide a specific decision for the current situation. These are basically indistinguishable from other general previous oral or written statements that, in the opinion of the legislature, provide clues to determining the 'presumed will' (see Sec. 1901a (2) s. 2 BGB).

13.4.2   Presumed Will

The second source for the patient's representative's decision is the 'presumed will'. There is very little information in legal documents about what is meant by 'presumed will'. Essentially, the information is limited to a reference to the case law of the Federal Court of Justice (Deutscher Bundestag 2008a, 11, 15, 19).

13.4.2.1 Decision-Making Guidelines for the Patient's Representative

The concept of 'presumed will' gives rise to misunderstandings and must therefore to some extent be considered misleading. For in cases in which the patient has not made a decision themselves either by means of a living will or by means of a specific treatment-related statement, their wishes cannot really be at issue. A patient who is no longer able to give consent at the time of treatment can no longer form or express a wish regarding the pending decision due to their illness. Nevertheless, 'presumed will' are often presented as a manifestation of the right of self-determination. It resembles a personal decision that can be attributed to the patient, and from this perspective it then claims to be binding.

In reality, however, it is not a real wish of the patient, in contrast to a concrete oral wish for treatment originating from the patient themselves, but a decision-making criterion for the patient's legal representative. We are dealing here with a substitutional decision that should be based on the patient's general opinions and values. The guardian or representative "ultimately establishes a thesis of how the patient would have decided in the specific situation if he could still decide about himself" (Bundesgerichtshof 2014, Sec. 33).

13.4.2.2 'Concrete Indications'

According to the law, the presumed will "must be ascertained on the basis of concrete indications" (Sec. 1901a (2) s. 2 BGB). These "concrete indications" are not to be confused with concrete specifications by the patient concerning the current treatment situation, since these would already either be directly binding as a living will or—in oral form—would have to be considered as treatment wishes in the narrower sense. When looking for "concrete indications" of the presumed will, only statements, beliefs and values which do not directly refer to the current treatment decision can be taken into account. It is therefore advisable for the patient's representative to examine very carefully any possible sources of a particular attitude on the patient's part, and to concentrate on establishing a real foundation of facts for their own decision. In many cases this is unlikely to lead to success if a restrictive approach is taken.

13.4.2.3 Criteria

As decisive criteria for determining the presumed will, the law mentions in particular "previous oral or written statements, ethical or religious convictions and other personal values" of the person under guardianship (Sec. 1901a (2) s. 3 BGB). It thus reflects the essential criteria of the Federal Court of Justice's case law on presumed will (Deutscher Bundestag 2008a, 15).

"Previous oral or written statements" which do not refer to the specific treatment situation (see above), hardly offer firm ground for an assumption that the person concerned would make a specific decision in the current situation. The "moral or religious conviction" as such will also contribute little to the current decision-making process. There is hardly any religious community in which binding attitudes determine the necessity of taking or refraining from individual treatment measures. Even if such norms existed, the wishes of this individual patient might deviate from the general ideas of their religious community. Finally, "other personal values" of the patient may help to shed light on the patient's character and general views, but hardly provide more than vague hints as to how the patient would decide in the current situation.

In order to avoid having to apply these rather unspecific criteria in the first place, cancer patients in particular should inform themselves about imminent treatment steps and alternatives for treatment, and should make appropriate decisions. In many cases the further course of treatment can be predicted quite clearly, so that the drafting of a living will would be an appropriate solution.

13.4.2.4 Binding Effect

With regard to the binding effect, the law does not differentiate between "treatment wishes" and "presumed will". The presumed will does not have the same binding effect as a living will (Sec. 1901 (1) s. 2 BGB). The guardian should merely come to their own decision "on the basis" of the presumed will (Sec. 1901 (2) s. 1 BGB).

Wishes for treatment that have only been expressed orally, but which contain clear instructions regarding a specific treatment, cannot be ignored by the patient's representative. Unless there are special circumstances that force the guardian or representative to make a different decision, specific oral treatment wishes must be respected. Treatment wishes in the narrower sense are therefore highly binding.

There is a difference between general wishes for treatment and the "concrete indications" that are supposed to substantiate a "presumed will". Since the information to be taken into account does not reflect the concrete situation of the decision (see above), it is usually not very binding for the patient's legal representative. One can therefore only follow the "presumed will" if a particularly high degree of certainty about the patient's decision preference can be obtained. A mere "prevailing" probability that the patient would have refrained from medically indicated life-prolonging measures should not be sufficient to terminate treatment.

13.4.2.5 Review and Implementation

The procedure for determining the "presumed will" of the patient follows the same rules as those for dealing with a written living will, cf. Sec. 1901b, 1904 (4) BGB (see above). As a result, if the treating physician and the patient's representative agree, even decisions to refrain from treatment on the basis of the "presumed will" do not require the approval of the Court of Protection. Bearing in mind the frequently uncertain factual basis of the "presumed will", this absence of judicial control must be regarded critically.

13.4.3 Procedure Without Indications of the "Presumed Will" of the Patient

Finally, the question arises as to what should happen if a patient who is unable to make a decision has neither drafted a living will nor expressed treatment wishes, and where there is also insufficient specific evidence to determine a presumed will. Since the legislator has not addressed this problem, the principles developed so far in case law and literature remain valid. According to the case law of the Federal Court of Justice, the patient's representative must consider the "well-being" of the patient (Bundesgerichtshof 2003, Sec. 51; 2016s. 56). This is in accordance with the general principle of decision making in the Law of Guardianship (see Sec. 1901 (2) s. 3 BGB). In the absence of expressions of wishes or recognizable wishes, therefore, a harm/benefit assessment oriented towards the well-being of the patient must be carried out, in which reference is usually made to the principle of *in dubio pro vita* (Deutscher Bundestag 2008a, 16; 2008b, 4; Bundesgerichtshof 2016, Sec. 56).

In the absence of legal regulation of these cases, the procedural steps described above (discussion between the patient's representative and the physician; if necessary, approval by the Court of Protection) are not directly applicable. However, the same procedure is recommended. If, after hearing close relatives and other confidants of the patient, there are no clear indications of the patient's presumed will, there should be an attempt to reach consensus on further treatment based on the patient's well-being. "If nothing is known about the patient's preferences, representatives and the physician may assume that the patient would agree to the medically indicated measures" (Bundesärztekammer 2010, A879). If differences remain between the patient's representative and the physician, the Court of Protection must be involved (Sec. 1904 (2) BGB).

13.5 Representation of the Patient

Particularly in the case of cancer, patients are often able to give consent right up to the final stage of the disease. For most treatment options, the patients themselves can therefore be questioned. In addition, the course of the disease can often be predicted quite specifically, so that corresponding advance directives can be made in a living will.

On the other hand, with every illness there is also the danger of a surprising and unforeseeable escalation. The only way to provide for such situations is to determine in advance who should decide on the treatment or its refusal in the place of the patient when they are no longer able to consent.

13.5.1 Power of Attorney

Irrespective of whether they have made a living will, cancer patients should always authorize a trusted person to represent them in the event of their inability to make a decision ("power of attorney"). In Germany, the power of attorney for medical care is not specifically regulated by law, but represents a subcategory of a general power of attorney as defined by Sec. 167 BGB. In practice, it is always given in writing. "Semi-official" text forms provided by the Federal Ministry of Justice or the state Ministries of Justice may be used.

Above all, it is important that the person granting the power of attorney talks to the authorized representative about their wishes, so that the latter can observe and implement these wishes in their decisions later on.

13.5.2 Guardianship Directive

In the absence of a trusted person, a power of attorney should not be granted. However, a person may make suggestions for the selection of a guardian or their wishes regarding care in a "guardianship directive" (see Sec. 1901c (1) BGB). As far as the future guardian is concerned, it will rather be a matter of information as to which person among relatives or acquaintances ought *not* to be appointed as a guardian. If a person is considered a guardian (from the point of view of the patient concerned), this person should be appointed as a legal representative by the patient.

It should be noted that information in a guardianship directive is not really binding on the court. However, the wishes of the person concerned are to be taken into account, as far as this is reasonable and practicable.

13.5.3 Guardian

If the patient has not taken any precautionary measures themselves, the Court of Protection can appoint a legal representative *ex officio*: the guardian (see Sec. 1896 (1) s. 1 BGB). According to the requirements of Sec. 1897 BGB, persons who have been nominated by the patient themselves are primarily considered as guardians (Sec. 1897 (4) s. 1 BGB). Accordingly, the spouse, children, parents, life partners and other persons with family or personal ties are to be taken into account in particular (Sec. 1897 (5) BGB). Only if no other suitable person is available a professional guardian will be appointed (Sec. 1897 (6) BGB).

13.5.4 General Prevention of Abuse

In principle, there is a risk of abuse in all cases of representation, especially if the person represented is no longer able to exercise their rights. It is therefore also a task of the Court of Protection to enforce the welfare of the patient by means of general abuse control.

The Court of Protection has the power to take measures necessary for the welfare of the patient. This power is not limited by the statutory provisions on living wills. Anyone—the physician, a relative or another person—may suggest that the court review the activities of the representative (the guardian or the appointed representative) (see Deutscher Bundestag 2008a, 19; 2008b, 4).

If the patient has a guardian, the court may at any time limit the guardian's powers or replace them with a more suitable person (see Sec. 2008b (1) s. 1 BGB) if the guardian's actions do not correspond to the well-being of the person concerned.

Also, if the patient has given a power of attorney, the Court of Protection can intervene if necessary. It can order the appointment of a "supervising" or "control" guardian (Sec. 1896 (3) BGB). If the authorized representative does not respect the wishes or disregards the well-being of the patient, the supervising guardian can ultimately revoke the power of attorney on behalf of the patient.

These options can be seen as a form of social control. On the one hand, they should not be overestimated, but on the other hand, they form a reasonable complement to the rather limited legal mechanisms of protection in the application of living wills. A living will is, in itself, nothing more than a written document. Only if the persons who are involved in the use of this document handle it in a responsible way can the wishes of the patient ultimately be realized.

13.6   Conclusion

Patients with cancer can use living wills to assert their self-determination with regard to medical treatment even if they will no longer be able to make decisions by themselves. Due to the usually considerable period of time between diagnosis and inability to make a decision, a living will can often still be written by cancer patients. The patient's determinations regarding their future treatment, in particular the decision to refrain from medical treatment, are binding on the physician if they are formulated in sufficiently specific terms. In addition, the patient should appoint a trusted person as their authorized representative.

German law is based on the patient's own initiative and personal responsibility. Only in the case of conflict, when differences of opinion arise between the patient's legal representative and the treating physician, the actions of the patient's representative need to be approved by the Court of Protection.

Despite these options for binding advance directives, a certain degree of insecurity may remain for most patients. "Security of planning at the end of life" cannot be guaranteed for anyone. It may therefore be worth considering not only taking precautions respecting treatment in a state of incapacity, but also—if it corresponds to one's own religious beliefs—regarding preparation for life after death. Despite all medical progress, cancer often confronts those affected very clearly with the limits of existence. In this situation, not only the confidence of being able to realize one's own ideas about treatment, but also the perspective that death does not have the last word, may provide some relief for the patient.

References

Beckmann R (2009) Patientenverfügungen: Entscheidungswege nach der gesetzlichen Regelung. MedR 27:582–586

Beckmann R (2018) Indikation und „Therapiezieländerung". MedR 36:556–562

Bundesärztekammer (2010) Empfehlungen der Bundesärztekammer und der Zentralen Ethikkommission bei der Bundesärztekammer zum Umgang mit Vorsorgevollmacht und Patientenverfügung in der ärztlichen Praxis. DÄBl 107:A877–882

Bundesärztekammer (2011) Grundsätze der Bundesärztekammer zur ärztlichen Sterbebegleitung. DÄBl 108:A 346–348

Bundesgerichtshof (2003) Urteil vom 17.03.2003, Az. XII ZB 2/03. https://openjur.de/u/66395.html

Bundesgerichtshof (2014) Urteil vom 17.09.2014, Az. XII ZB 202/13. https://openjur.de/u/740963.html

Bundesgerichtshof (2016) Urteil vom 06.07.2016, Az. XII ZB 61/16. https://openjur.de/u/894368.html

Deutscher Bundestag (2008a) Entwurf eines Dritten Gesetzes zur Änderung des Betreuungsrechts. BT-Drs. 16/8442

Deutscher Bundestag (2008b) Beschlussempfehlung und Bericht, BT-Drs. 16/13314

Duttge G (2006) Das österreichische Patientenverfügungsgesetz: Schreckensbild oder Vorbild? ZfL 15:81–87

Enquete-Kommission des Deutschen Bundestages (2004) Zwischenbericht Patientenverfügungen. BT-Drs. 15/3700

Mayo Clinic Staff (2018) Living wills and advance directives for medical decisions (Dec. 2018). https://www.mayoclinic.org/healthy-lifestyle/consumer-health/in-depth/living-wills/art-20046303. Accessed 30 Dec 2019

Österreichisches Patientenverfügungsgesetz (öPatVG) https://www.ris.bka.gv.at/GeltendeFassung.wxe?Abfrage=Bundesnormen&Gesetzesnummer=20004723. Accessed 30 Dec 2019

Raspe H (2015) Die medizinische Indikation und ihre Regulierung in Zeiten der evidenzbasierten Medizin. In: Dörries A, Lipp V (eds) Medizinische Indikation, Stuttgart 94–112

Euthanasia and Assisted Suicide: Realization or Abandonment of Self-determination?

14

Axel W. Bauer

14.1 Limits and Dissolution in Politics and Science

In 2017, the author of this chapter published (in German) a book entitled *Abolition of Normative Boundaries* (Bauer 2017). In this chapter, normative boundaries at the end of life and the processes of their abolition will be discussed from the perspective of a medical ethicist. The views expressed by the author are not those of *the* medical ethicist par excellence, but those of an individual whose point of view is characterized by the conservative 'pro-life' position. Other medical ethicists would presumably set out the opposite view, especially if they belong to the liberal 'pro-choice' faction within the discipline. At the beginning of every morality, even ethically reflected morality, there is an ultimate axiom that cannot be taken away without causing the entire thought building to collapse (Engelhardt 2012).

People have been dealing with the issue of borders and politically enforced topographical, demographic and social openness in Europe, especially in Germany, since at least the autumn of 2015. Just as more than two decades ago, when—with the advent of the internet—the word 'networking' was suddenly on everyone's lips until it became an oft-used, popular metaphor, the issue of *boundaries* and their dissolution currently has the potential to become a new interdisciplinary focus of reflection and discourse.

But while *network* and *networking* have acquired more positive connotations, the status of *boundaries* is quite different. The protagonists of abolition of moral boundaries use, with a greater or lesser degree of subtlety, the still effective horror vison of the Iron Curtain between East and West, especially as represented by the death strip between the former German Democratic Republic (GDR) and the former

A. W. Bauer (✉)
History, Philosophy, and Ethics in Medicine, Medical Faculty Mannheim, Heidelberg University, Ludolf-Krehl-Strasse 13-17, 68167 Mannheim, Germany
e-mail: axel.bauer@medma.uni-heidelberg.de

© Springer Nature Switzerland AG 2021
A. W. Bauer et al. (eds.), *Ethical Challenges in Cancer Diagnosis and Therapy*,
Recent Results in Cancer Research 218,
https://doi.org/10.1007/978-3-030-63749-1_14

Federal Republic of Germany (FRG), with the result that borders in general take on the appearance of repulsive, constricting and fatal facilities. The hero of stories narrated with suggestive force in this context is always someone who—like US President Ronald Reagan (1911–2004) on 12 June 1987 in front of the Brandenburg Gate in Berlin—demands in a rhetorically brilliant way: "Mr Gorbachev, tear down this wall!"

However, boundaries do not always have to be viewed from the perspective of someone who wants to demolish them. After all, boundaries often have a protective function, such as a hedge in the front garden or the medieval city wall defending the city from outside attack. In morality, we can create normative limits in order to distinguish *good* from *bad*. However, such boundaries have been in dispute in modern pluralistic societies for many years. An almost normative abolition has been set in motion in life sciences, specifically in relation to the beginning and the end of human life.

It is noticeable that in the *front stage* context—in the sense used by sociologist Erving Goffman (1922–1982)—it is above all noble and positively connoted concepts such as *ethics of healing* or *respect for self-determination* that are obsessively positioned at the heart of the debate. But *backstage,* in the interest of biological research, the focus is often on leaving it as late as possible to start protecting human life, and under the pressure of demographic and supposed economic necessities, ending this protection early. Medical ethics and bioethics, which in the literal sense of the words ought to be the ethics of healing or living things per se, are being gradually transformed before our very eyes into disciplines that too often bring death, the untimely appearance of which is to be justified by means of moral philosophy.

14.2 The Publicly Conveyed Illusion of 'Self-determined' Death

Nowhere can this fatal development be followed more exactly than in the field of euthanasia, particularly with the current issue of assisted suicide. We should therefore take a look at the normative loss of limits concerning euthanasia. In the last 25 years there has been an increasing tendency to emphasize the self-determination of patients. This tragedy of this development is that it is euthanasia that seems to be the prime target of self-determination (Bauer 2009a, 169–180; Bauer 2016). Indeed, the right to self-determination has recently begun to be identified with a right to the self-determined time of death. Constantly reiterated stereotypes about self-determined dying or dying with dignity are irritating, seeking as they do to persuade us that we have tremendous latitude when we are dying, and that an unplanned death is ultimately undignified (Bauer 2013).

Legal scholars and medical ethicists claim that suicide is an expression of personal autonomy, and therefore at least a fundamentally respectable form of human action. But is that really true? Autonomy in the meaning of Immanuel Kant (1724–

1804), as the capacity of the rational man to give himself rational moral laws to act upon (not arbitrary ones), has its irreducible reason in the physical existence of the human being. It is therefore the consequence and not the cause of our biological constitution. Hence, on this physical basis the legitimate scope of human self-determination is actually limited to this area. Manfred Wetzel has pointed out the obvious logical weaknesses in Kant's unrestricted prohibition of suicide as an obligation to support life: for the maxim underlying suicide, it does make a difference whether it postulates 'at will' or, for example, 'in the case of years of painful incurable illness'. Only the maxim 'at will' would create a transcendental-philosophical self-contradiction (Wetzel 2004, 390–391).

Although man is capable of killing himself, he cannot simply rely on self-determination to legitimize this step. An actor who intentionally and irreversibly destroys the physical structure that makes his freedom of action possible is in the first place acting in a morally unjustifiable way, even though his motivation for suicide may be emotionally understandable. Moreover, plausibility on the one hand and moral endorsement on the other are two different approaches to this problem, as well as to other ethical issues. Not everything that is somehow understandable can be morally approved for this reason alone.

14.3 Assisted Suicide as a Subject of Legal Policy in Germany

Since suicide itself is not a criminal offence, assisted suicide in general was not unlawful in Germany until December 2015, due to the principle of accessoriness in the Criminal Code. Neither abetting (Section 26 StGB) nor aiding (Section 27 StGB) were (are) illegal. Even a 'death helper' acting in his own financial interest, who benefited from the suicide, could (can) procure the means of action, abet the person and otherwise support them without being prosecuted. As late as 2011, 93% of Germans still mistakenly believed that aiding and abetting suicide were illegal (Bauer 2015a).

In November 2015, however, the Federal Parliament (*Bundestag*) passed a new Section 217 German Criminal Code (*Strafgesetzbuch*, StGB). This section reads as follows:

Section 217 StGB

(1) Every person who, with intent to facilitate the suicide of another person, businesslike grants, provides or conveys this person the opportunity to do so, is punishable by imprisonment for up to three years or by a restitution fine.
(2) A secondary participant (abetter or aider) will not be prosecuted if he is not doing business and is either a relative of the other person referred to in subsection (1) or close to them.

According to this regulation it is supporting suicide *businesslike* that is criminalized. Unlike *commercial activity* where there is an intention to make a financial profit, businesslike activity can also be said to exist when someone intends to make the repetition of similar acts the subject of their professional activity (Winkelmeier and Bauer 2018). Section 217 of the Criminal Code under paragraph 1 penalizes the promotion of suicide as a business activity. However, according to paragraph 2, an abetter or aider of the new offence will remain unpunished if the secondary participant is not acting businesslike and if he or she is either a relative of or close to the suicidal person.

It remains unclear why the authors of the bill, by attributing fundamentally "altruistic motives", "deep pity" and "compassion" to relatives and people close to the suicidal person, justified their impunity. Even "dependents of health care professionals", thus above all doctors, are not to be charged "in an individual case" with the offence in Section 217 paragraph 1 StGB, because they would typically not be acting businesslike (Brand et al. 2015). Which specific methods of "suicide escort" will be allowed for legal medical suicide assistance is not explained, since at least so far, the Narcotic Drugs Act (*Betäubungsmittelgesetz*, BtMG) has not been changed. The gift of sodium pentobarbital, which can be prescribed in Switzerland, is only permitted in Germany for euthanizing animals (Bauer 2018).

The law raises more problems than it can solve. How should one, especially when doctors are involved, distinguish a choice of conscience in 'exceptional cases' from regular, 'business-type' action? It would be necessary to clarify each case in court, probing with what intention and what "awareness of regularity" the suicide helper may have acted. In the Federal Parliament debate on 2 July 2015, the lead author of the new law emphasized that only actions that were "designed for repetition" should be threatened with criminal prosecution. Dealing with 'mortal tourism' to Switzerland may also be difficult. Suicide assistance that is organized "as a business" is now a criminal offence under German law. This means that a person could be punished in Germany if they were a participant in this mortal tourism, such as supporting a suicide in Zurich just by driving their grandfather there in a car.

But there is an exception: relatives or "related" persons will not face prosecution as instigators or assistants according to Section 217 paragraph 2 StGB, provided they themselves do not act "in a businesslike manner". At the internet address www.sthd.ch, the branch of the Association for Euthanasia Germany (StHD) that is based in Zurich has already established itself as a publisher. In principle, the new Section 217 (StGB) should prevent people from being "directly or indirectly marginalized" by organizing suicide-related offers of suicide. But a direct or indirect urge to commit suicide is most likely to occur in families: a seriously ill person will listen attentively if their daughter or a close friend talks about a possible trip to Switzerland (Kamann 2015).

It should also not be overlooked that there are forces in the medical profession who are looking for a legal vacuum that may give them the opportunity to provide patients with a lethal poison for suicide—and perhaps to do even more. The general mood in the district and regional medical associations does not reflect an unanimous belief on the part of doctors that suicide assistance is not one of their professional tasks. Rather, there are efforts in some quarters to undermine the position of the German Medical Association by a sort of silent opposition.

It is therefore no coincidence that the wording of Section 16 of the Professional Code of the State Medical Association of Westphalia-Lippe deviates from the (Model) Professional Code of the German Medical Association. The original sentence "Doctors *must not* help to commit suicide" appears here in a relativized form as "Doctors *should not* help to commit suicide". The Bavarian State Medical Association went still further: in Section 16 of the revised version of the Professional Code for the Physicians of Bavaria, the two sentences from the model Professional Code of the German Medical Association containing a prohibition on suicide assistance do not appear at all. Thus, the Bavarian Professional Code does not rule out medical participation in suicide. The State Medical Association of Baden-Wurttemberg made the same choice in its changed Professional Code. Thus, both in Bavaria and in Baden-Wurttemberg, there would be sufficient physicians who want to provide assisted suicide in a "non-businesslike" way. This represents a new departure in the history of medicine, a deliberate breach of the tradition of the Hippocratic Oath which has been cultivated for more than 2400 years and which categorically excludes any participation in the killing or suicide of a patient (Bauer 1995, 2009b).

14.4 Dangers of Section 217 StGB Concerning the Preservation of Life

From the initial debate on a ban on organized participation in suicide, a discussion about the statutory organization of assisted suicide was launched during the year 2015. It was no longer about the restriction, but about the impunity of this act, especially for relatives and doctors. As it ended up with only businesslike assisted suicide being banned, the legislator suggested that non-business and privately rendered euthanasia should be considered acceptable and legitimized by the state.

In the view of its initiators, businesslike dealings within the meaning of Section 217 paragraph 1 Criminal Code apply only to those who make the granting, procuring or brokering of the opportunity to commit suicide a permanent or recurring part of their activity, regardless of intention to make a profit and regardless of any connection with an economic or professional activity. However, it is also crucial for the definition of an offence that the suicide helper is pursuing specific self-interests, typically directed at the execution of suicide, and that their inclusion thus calls into question the "autonomous" decision of the person willing to die.

Thus, the legal back door, already in sight, is likely to become a gateway for physicians and relatives. If no self-interest is recognizable and provable by the prosecution, assistance with suicide may go unpunished if it is committed in a "non-businesslike" way. But even if only 50,000 of the approximately 365,000

working physicians in Germany each helped one single patient per half-year 'out of
life' in this disinterested manner, there would be 100,000 legal physician-assisted
suicides a year, which would currently—since there are about 868,000 deaths
annually in Germany—account for a total of 11.5% of all deaths.

A physician who participates in the suicide of a patient must at least have the
required pharmacological and technical know-how, so that the euthanasia does not
fail, resulting in a severely disabled patient. This knowledge is not yet on the
curriculum at medical faculties and universities. Those who otherwise systematically appropriate it are apparently intent on applying this 'art' in practice to repetition. That would be "businesslike" action.

14.5   The Unconstitutionality of Section 217 StGB

The Federal President of Germany signed the law on 3 December 2015 and it
entered into force on 10 December 2015 (Bauer 2015b). The Hamburg-based
Euthanasia Germany (StHD) considered the new Section 217 StGB unconstitutional; four members of the association then raised—among other appellants—a
constitutional complaint to the Federal Constitutional Court.

The Federal Constitutional Court rejected the adoption of the interim injunction
against the law by its decision of 21 December 2015. The reason was that a
provisional continued application of Section 217 StGB until a decision on the main
issue would only lead to a further postponement of the intended form of assisted
suicide, which could still be implemented if the constitutional complaint were
successful. For this reason, the occurrence of irreversible consequences was not to
be feared (Bundesverfassungsgericht 2015, Rn. 16).

On 26 February 2020, the Federal Constitutional Court announced its final
verdict. Since then, the ban on promoting suicide on a commercial basis has been
considered unconstitutional (Bundesverfassungsgericht 2020). Not only did the
court thus annul the poorly thought-out and inadequately crafted Section 217 of the
Criminal Code, which would in itself have been respectable. It also postulated—by
virtue of its supreme judicial authority and without the need to do so—a new
individual right to suicide and to outside support, citing the right to self-
determination and human dignity. It suggested appropriate safeguarding measures
by the legislature, such as the introduction of requirements on information and time
lapse before assisted suicide, which are already familiar from the advice provision
in Section 218a of the Criminal Code in the case of abortion. In the opinion of the
Federal Constitutional Court, the right to suicide also means the admissibility of
suicide assistance is not dependent on material criteria such as the presence of an
(incurable) illness like cancer.

This judgement paves the way for a society in which human dignity and the right
to self-determination will serve to legitimize the—allegedly—voluntary suicide of
desperate people with the help of third parties and to gloss over this final act as the
ultimate expression of civil liberty. The Federal Constitutional Court has certainly

done no service to the supporters of the preservation of life. However, those who in 2015, against all warnings, thought they had to introduce Section 217 of the Criminal Code, must be asked whether they themselves provided the occasion for the verdict of 26 February 2020. Unfortunately, being well-meaning is often the opposite of doing well.

14.6 The Doctors in Awe of Life League and Their Goals

In spring 2016, the Doctors in Awe of Life initiative was founded in Cologne, drawing attention to itself with an image of Albert Schweitzer (1875–1965). The first signatories to this medical league, including the author, said in their appeal that the doctor must always be on the side of life; he should never change to the side of death. The statement continues:

> There must never be an interaction between the doctor and the patient whose goal is that the patient is subsequently dead. After the adoption of the new Section 217 StGB an attempt is made to exert pressure on physicians to enter into such interactions within the framework of a suicide support. However, the law does not allow this. Such behaviour would also be incompatible with the medical ethos of the Hippocratic tradition and would in the long run deeply shatter the relationship between physicians and patients. Therefore, we demand that the clear statement in Section 16 of the (Model-) Professional Code of the German Medical Association that physicians are not allowed to support suicide, must be included in the professional codes of all 17 State Medical Associations.

Doctors are the preservers of life. They must not be a danger to the lives of their patients. To assist a suffering person with suicide contravenes the 2400-year-old medical ethos of the Hippocratic Oath. Every person who is mentally or physically ill needs expert medical help and genuine compassionate care, as well as the assurance that the doctor will do anything to cure the illness or, if this is not possible, alleviate the patient's suffering. The desire for assistance with suicide springs primarily not from fear of unquenchable pain, but from the fear of being a burden on others, being at the mercy of losing control or being alone.

Patients who wish to commit suicide usually do not expect their death to be induced promptly. Mostly, the desire for assisted suicide is a cry for help and is temporary in nature. In nearly 90% of cases, its basis is a mental illness. Due to medical advances and social ties, medicine is today able to care for seriously ill and dying people in such a way that they do not have to suffer unbearably, but feel well cared for. It is in the nature of man that at the end of life, to a great extent we are dependent on our fellow human beings. The limitation of our autonomy or self-determination is not caused by that human condition. Assisted suicide requires that a human being's life is judged to be unworthy by a third party, namely by the person assisting. But herein the limit to euthanasia has already been exceeded.

14.7   The Situation in Swiss Retirement Homes

In Switzerland, meanwhile, the pressure on old people's homes and hospitals to open their doors to suicide helpers is growing (Switzerland 2016). In 2014, the organization Exit assisted 60 elderly people in old people's homes to commit suicide. Most institutions, however, are resisting letting euthanasia organizations in. In the canton of Bern, no institution is required to admit suicide assistants, nor in the cantons of Basel-City and Valais. Eduard Haeni, director of the Municipal Retirement Home Bern (Burgerspittel), welcomed this rule: "If a person wants to end her life in an old-age institution, this is on the one hand a personal decision. But on the other hand, it also touches many other people." In addition to family members, fellow inmates and employees would be affected. Witnessing the suicide of a resident would be a great burden for all these people, argues Christian Streit, the Managing Director of the Senesuisse group of 350 retirement facilities (Diener-Morscher 2016). In the canton of Ticino, in March 2016 the parliament clearly and unambiguously stated that there was no right to suicide assistance in health care facilities (Ticino 2016).

In 2015, around 1,300 people committed suicide in Switzerland using the organizations Dignitas, Exit or Eternal Spirit. This can be seen from the figures published by the three Swiss euthanasia associations. In addition to its steady membership growth, Exit attributed the further increase in death attendance of about 30% primarily to the significant aging of society. The average age of the suicides was 77.4 years. According to Exit, there were already bottlenecks at the rented 'death studios' as well as in the training of new suicide attendants, due to high demand. Even the controversial euthanasia society Eternal Spirit, that had procured two Scots—who were afraid of being alone—a deadly poison cocktail, complained about a lack of space (Assisted Suicide 2016). Neighbours had obtained a court ruling that the organization was not allowed to continue operating in a residential district because the mental burden was unbearable, and it should seek premises in the industrial district (Zaslawski 2016). Temporarily, the organization wanted to give its 'customers' their deadly drugs in camper vans. The cost of a suicide escort is also significant at Eternal Spirit: foreigners pay 10,000 Swiss francs (CHF), Swiss citizens pay CHF 3,000.

The cash flow of the euthanasia associations is enlightening, with each organization claiming to be cost-effective and operating without profit. The organizations can set their own prices. Exit offers the cheapest services: suicide support costs between CHF 900 and 3,500, depending on how long the person has been a member of the organization. After three years' membership death is free. Exit now numbers 100,000 paying members (annual fee: CHF 45), whose average age is 67. All members must have Swiss nationality. 995 people ended their lives with Exit in 2015. 222 people died supported by Dignitas, with suicide tourism playing a major role: about 75% of those wishing to die came from Germany, Britain and France. The organization has about 7,100 members, and charges a registration fee of CHF

200 and an annual membership fee of CHF 80. For a 'suicide escort' Dignitas charges CHF 7,000. An additional fee of CHF 3,500 has to be paid, if a funeral is to be arranged (Switzerland 2016).

14.8 The Development of Euthanasia in the Netherlands and Belgium

In the Netherlands, where homicide upon request is allowed, 15 people died every day in 2015 due to euthanasia, according to data from the Euthanasia Regional Review Committees (RTE). From 2006 to 2015, the number of cases shot up by almost 300% to 5,516 people per year (Regionale Toetsingscommissies Euthanasie 2016). "Ten times more people die in the Netherlands through euthanasia than in traffic," said Eugen Brysch, chairman of the German Foundation for Patient Protection on the occasion of the World Conference of Euthanasia Advocates in Amsterdam. In Belgium, too, the number had increased five-fold from 429 to 2,021 over the same period. Brysch sees the example of the two Benelux countries as a dire warning: "Obviously killing is contagious" (Tyrolean Newspaper 2016).

The deadly drugs for suicide can be ordered—albeit illegally—via the so-called China or Mexico routes. A few days later they are delivered by the postman, usually wrapped in a birthday card as a camouflage. Dealers' addresses and mobile phone numbers are no secret in the Netherlands. In 2016, there were plans to offer the deadly drugs—called 'last-will pills' legally on the open market. Potential suicides would have the drugs at home and could even end their lives without the help of a doctor. Not least, this raises ethical and legal questions on how far the right to self-determination should go.

In 2001, the Netherlands was the first country in the world to provide euthanasia. So far, however, only doctors are allowed to perform euthanasia, and that only in patients who are suffering in a hopeless and unbearable way. In addition, a second and independent physician must agree to such a request. However, some doctors reject euthanasia for moral reasons. In addition, physicians have complained in the past about the mental stress associated with suicide support. They actually want to save lives, but on the other hand feel they ought to give deadly infusions to patients.

Now, the process is to be reformed so that doctors may play only a minor role in future. In November 2015, the Dutch Voluntary End of Life Association (NVVE), the country's most influential lobbying organization, presented various proposals. "Doctors have become judges on euthanasia issues in the current system," claimed Robert Schurink, the director of NVVE. Some patients would like to end their lives, but have a family doctor who cannot or will not fulfil their wishes. "With new regulation, more autonomy could be created so that the individual can decide for himself," Schurink explained (NVVE 2015).

How exactly delivery of the 'last-will pills' could work is still unclear. It is conceivable, for example, that in future they could be issued under strict specifications by special institutions. Doctors would not inevitably be necessary. Even today, organizations such as the NVVE or De Einder provide information on how to obtain the deadly drugs abroad. While suicide assistance is a crime in the Netherlands, advice on it is not. If the NVVE had its way, aid would be lawful in the future, for example, exonerating relatives who help with suicide.

The medical ethicist Professor Theo Boer of the Protestant Theological University in Groningen has said that in fact the deadly pills are already available today. Boer does not fundamentally reject more autonomy or the free availability of deadly medicines. However, he urges extreme caution over relieving doctors of responsibility: "Decisions about life and death must be under control," Boer says. NVVE Director Schurink also wants to exclude certain possibilities, such as drugs getting into the hands of criminals, or being taken by the mentally ill, or by people who are bereaved or suffering from a broken heart. The experience of recent years had shown that liberal but controlled euthanasia does not lead to abuse, Schurink argues. Now, supposedly, it is ready for change and adjustment (Dürr 2016).

14.9   Demographic Ageing and Thanatopolitics

The predicted demographic ageing of the population in most Western countries means that in the foreseeable future, more people will experience a much longer retirement than their parents or grandparents, even if the retirement age is raised to 67 or even 70. As we grow older, more and more expensive diseases attack us, especially cancer. People who keep physically fit for a long time may not experience the illnesses that struck their parents at 75 until the age of 80 or 85. However, they will not be spared these illnesses. This also increases the costs of illness and care during the last phase of life. It would be an illusion to believe that in the near future we will die overnight, not just later, but even in a 'healthy' state—except through (assisted) suicide.

What would happen to old and sick people in 2030, if politicians succeeded in convincing them that a voluntary departure from a fulfilled life was a virtue, even a social obligation? Today we are already familiar with those euphemistic terms with which academic medical ethicists like to gloss over unpleasant facts. So there is a significant semantic difference between 'active help to die' and 'homicide on request'. The first term sounds like a humane act, the second a punishable offence against life. However, both expressions mean one and the same thing.

A situation in which only relatives—and possibly family doctors—would be permitted to assist suicide, protected by the Criminal Code, would in itself be life-threatening for people in need of care. But we have to acknowledge that our society is ageing. Between 1950 and 1970, almost twice as many children were born each year in Germany than in the present. The more than 25 million people, well over a quarter of all citizens of the country, who are now between 50 and 70 years old, will be society's senior citizens in the 2030s. The problem of expensive pensions, medical and nursing costs will then escalate.

In this situation, alleged 'self-determined' suicide of older people would come into effect at the right moment, because in the years after 2025 there will be fewer and fewer young people earning the pensions for the ever-growing generation of seniors. With pensions in 20 years' time unfortunately relatively well below their current level, the question must be asked whether the conspicuous political tolerance for participating in suicide will in future refer only to seriously ill patients in the terminal stages of cancer, as the argument—pompously—mostly goes.

In Aldous Huxley's (1894–1963) novel *Brave New World,* published in 1932, people end their lives before they become seriously ill and before the restoration of their health would cost a lot of money. Huxley set his narrative in the year 2540. We have to realize that in the meanwhile we have come dangerously close to this sobering corporate design. It is amazing how the then 38-year-old author predicted, nearly 90 years ago, a technically perfected civilization of inhumane horror. Was he too optimistic when he postponed this scenario till some 600 years into the future? He probably underestimated the speed of development.

In 1978, in his book *Modern Death. The end of humanity,* Swedish author Carl-Henning Wijkmark (1934–2020) made a (fictitious) medical ethicist claim that many men and women who—as doctors or as relatives—have experienced long-term care and the care of 'hopeless cases', felt a deep desire not to have to suffer in the same way themselves later. Wijkmark's novella described a futuristic scenario playing out in the 1990s, with a symposium of senior Swedish politicians and scholars addressing the problem of too many old and sick people in times of threatened prosperity. From the retrospective of the year 2020, the book seems both almost prophetic and oppressive (Wijkmark 2001; Rehder 2014).

14.10 Neither Superfluous nor Pointless: On the Critical Range of Sustainable Moral Norms

Ethical discourses have culture-specific features, and the resulting assessments are changeable. Discussions about medical ethics are not purely ethical debates, but rather debates about hidden interests. Uncovering these interests and analyzing how they interweave with ethical decision making is an essential task (Maio 2001, 80).

The independence of ethical analysis is difficult to achieve in real life (Bauer 2002). We are influenced by numerous concrete interests of our own. In individual cases, it can hardly be proven positively, because we never know all of our fellow human beings' interests, not even our own preferences, down to the last detail. Concrete moral norms, on which the individual—and society as a whole—has to make a conscious decision, but which cannot be deductively derived from rational considerations, will as a rule be moderately anti-naturalistic and will therefore always encounter a certain social resistance. Pro-naturalistic norms would be superfluous, because what they prescribe would happen anyway, while extremely anti-naturalistic norms would be pointless, because what they require would be biologically impossible. Hence there is neither a moral requirement 'You should breathe' nor a moral requirement 'You should not breathe', because demanding the first would be superfluous and demanding the second would be pointless. In the more or less wide range between 'no longer superfluous' and 'not yet senseless', however, there is scope for concrete moral thinking and acting, through which those rules must be created for which our evolutionary development has not defined a mandatory behaviour (Schmitz and Bauer 2000). If the moral rules set by man are moderately anti-naturalistic, they will, within certain limits, always be exceeded in practice.

But it is precisely this that shows not the failure of a moral system, but on the contrary its functioning. Moral systems always followed by everyone involved would either be superfluous (because too pro-naturalistic), or else they would be the inhumane rules of a dictatorial police state. We cannot want both in a democracy. Morality is always a good thing as long as it does not affect us personally and make claims that are against our wishes. This is implicitly the currently popular maxim for solving ethical problems.

14.11 Conclusion

At a time when the discipline of ethics is seen as merely a methodological and scientific, even a value-neutral keyboard of state-compliant morality and thus as an instrument for obtaining political legitimacy, the continuous relativization of binding values caused by the polyphonic chorus of carefully selected exponents of contradictory ethical positions seems very convenient for the politically responsible elites. If it is possible to brand the opponents of suicide involvement an allegedly antiquated fringe group of 'conservative hardliners' and to position them outside the social mainstream, then in Europe, the traffic lights for the 'free ride to death' will irrevocably turn green.

If citizens have had much less freedom in their lives than they had hoped for in their youth and had been promised, in an illusory way, in order to keep up their spirits and efficiency for decades, then this freedom should now be theirs, or should at least be granted as 'self-determined dying'. And modest as many citizens have become with regard to political freedoms in the post-democracy era, they appear to be willing to welcome the temptingly presented offer of a 'self-chosen' farewell to earthly existence. What luck for the powerful who rule a population that can be manipulated so quietly and exemplarily to an early death. But woe to the country and its citizens who relentlessly indulge these rulers and their siren sounds!

With suicide, a person actually takes away their freedom of decision for ever. Suicide irrevocably brings the end of every freedom of action. As trivial as this knowledge may be, it makes us think about it whenever we address 'self-determination' at the end of life. Let us question the psychological, social and economic interests behind the organized death policy and let us no longer be distracted by euphemisms about 'autonomy'.

References

Assisted Suicide (2016) Schweiz macht ernst mit Altersfreitod für Ausländer. Die Angst vor getrennten Altersheimen trieb schottische Pensionisten in den Suizid. IMABE Bioethik aktuell, February 2016. http://www.imabe.org/index.php?id=2152. Accessed 10 Dec 2019

Bauer AW (1995) Der Hippokratische Eid. Medizinhistorische Neuinterpretation eines (un) bekannten Textes im Kontext der Professionalisierung des griechischen Arztes. Zeitschrift für medizinische Ethik 41:141–148

Bauer AW (2002) Ethik oder Moral - was brauchen Ärzte wirklich? Überlegungen zu den konzeptionellen Schwierigkeiten des Unterrichtsfaches „Ethik in der Medizin". In: Groß D (ed) Ethik in der Medizin in Lehre, Klinik und Forschung. Königshausen & Neumann, Würzburg, pp 19–36

Bauer AW (2009a) Grenzen der Selbstbestimmung am Lebensende. Die Patientenverfügung als Patentlösung? Zeitschrift für medizinische Ethik 55:169–182

Bauer AW (2009b) Hippokrates' Albtraum. Rheinischer Merkur 64(12):4

Bauer AW (2013) Todes Helfer. Warum der Staat mit dem neuen Paragraphen 217 StGB die Mitwirkung am Suizid fördern will. In: Krause Landt A (ed) Wir sollen sterben wollen. Warum die Mitwirkung am Suizid verboten werden muss. Manuscriptum, Waltrop, Leipzig, pp 93–169

Bauer AW (2015a) Notausgang assistierter Suizid? Die Thanatopolitik in Deutschland vor dem Hintergrund des demografischen Wandels. In: Hoffmann TS, Knaup M (eds) Was heißt: In Würde sterben? Wider die Normalisierung des Tötens. Springer VS, Wiesbaden 2015, pp 49–78

Bauer AW (2015b) Verrat am Lebensschutz. Der neue § 217 StGB als Einstieg in den assistierten Suizid. Der Durchblick 88:16–17

Bauer AW (2016) Der Autonomiebegriff im bioethischen Diskurs der 1990er Jahre. Imago Hominis 23:199–211

Bauer AW (2017) Normative Entgrenzung. Themen und Dilemmata der Medizin- und Bioethik in Deutschland. Springer VS, Wiesbaden

Bauer AW (2018) Tod auf Rezept? Irrwege bei der Sterbehilfe. Katholisches Sonntagsblatt 166:28–29

Brand M, Griese K, Vogler K et al (2015) Entwurf eines Gesetzes zur Strafbarkeit der geschäftsmäßigen Förderung der Selbsttötung. Deutscher Bundestag, 18. Wahlperiode, Drucksache 18/5373 of 1 July 2015. http://dipbt.bundestag.de/doc/btd/18/053/1805373.pdf. Accessed 10 Dec 2019

Bundesverfassungsgericht (2015) Beschluss vom 21.12.2015 - Az. 2 BvR 2347/15. https://www.bundesverfassungsgericht.de/SharedDocs/Entscheidungen/DE/2015/12/rk20151221_2bvr234715.html. Accessed 10 Dec 2019

Bundesverfassungsgericht (2020) Verbot der geschäftsmäßigen Förderung der Selbsttötung verfassungswidrig. Pressemitteilung Nr. 12/2020 vom 26. Februar 2020. Urteil vom 26. Februar 2020—2 BvR 2347/15, 2 BvR 651/16, 2 BvR 1261/16, 2 BvR 1593/16, 2 BvR 2354/16, 2 BvR 2527/16. https://www.bundesverfassungsgericht.de/SharedDocs/Pressemitteilungen/DE/2020/bvg20-012.html. Accessed 26 Feb 2020

Diener-Morscher E (2016) Immer mehr Berner Heime erlauben den Freitod. BZ – Berner Zeitung, 25 April 2016. http://www.bernerzeitung.ch/region/kanton-bern/immer-mehr-heime-erlauben-den-freitod/story/17631357. Accessed 10 Dec 2019

Dürr B (2016) Niederländer erwägen Legalisierung von Todespillen http://www.spiegel.de/gesundheit/psychologie/niederlande-debatte-ueber-legalisierung-von-todespillen-a-1065819.html. Accessed 10 Dec 2019

Engelhardt Jr HT (2012) Bioethik „after morality": Entmoralisierung und Deflation der traditionellen Moralität und Bioethik. Preprints and working papers of the centre for advanced study in bioethics, 39. https://www.uni-muenster.de/imperia/md/content/kfg-normenbegruendung/intern/publikationen/_fellows/39_engelhardt_-_bioethik_after_morality.pdf. Accessed 10 Dec 2019

Huxley A (1932) Brave New World. A Novel. Chatto & Windus, London

Kamann M (2015) Das sind die vier Möglichkeiten bei der Sterbehilfe. Im Bundestag nehmen die verschiedenen Gesetzentwürfe zur Suizidhilfe Gestalt an. http://www.welt.de/142227868. Accessed 10 Dec 2019

Maio G (2001) Ärztliche Ethik als Politikum. Zur französischen Diskussion um das Humanexperiment nach 1945. Medizinhistorisches J 36:35–80

NVVE (2015) Nederlandse Vereniging voor een Vrijwillig Levenseinde. https://www.nvve.nl/. Accessed 10 Dec 2019

Regionale Toetsingscommissies Euthanasie (2016) Jaarsverslag 2015 van de regionale toetsingscommissies euthanasie. Press Report of 26 April 2016. https://www.euthanasiecommissie. nl/binaries/euthanasiecommissie/documenten/persberichten/2016/april/26/persbericht-jaarverslag-van-de-regionale-toetsingscommissies-euthanasie-2015/persbericht-rte-jaarverslag-2015.pdf. Accessed 10 Dec 2019

Rehder S (2014) „Wir sollen sterben wollen". Warum Ärzte keine Suizidhilfe leisten dürfen und sich viele dennoch für den „Freitod" erwärmen. Ein Gespräch mit dem Medizinethiker Axel W. Bauer. Published 23 April 2014. *Die Tagespost* 47:3

Schmitz D, Bauer AW (2000) Intuition oder Evolution? Ein skeptischer Blick auf die prinzipienbasierte Bioethik. Zeitschrift für medizinische Ethik 46:13–22

Switzerland (2016) Druck auf Altersheime für Suizidbeihilfe wächst. In den Niederlanden sterben täglich 15 Menschen durch Tötung auf Verlangen. IMABE Bioethik aktuell, May 2016. http://www.imabe.org/index.php?id=2295. Accessed 10 Dec 2019

Ticino (2016) Kein Recht auf Sterbehilfe. Published 24 March 2016. https://www.medinside.ch/de/post/tessin-kein-recht-auf-sterbehilfe. Accessed 10 Dec 2019

Tyrolean Newspaper (2016) Patientenschützer warnen vor Ausbreitung der aktiven Sterbehilfe. Tiroler Tageszeitung online, 12 May 2016. http://www.tt.com/home/11492113-91/patientensch%C3%BCtzer-warnen-vor-ausbreitung-aktiver-sterbehilfe.csp. Accessed 10 Dec 2019

Wetzel M (2004) Praktisch-politische Philosophie, 1: Allgemeine Grundlagen. Königshausen & Neumann, Würzburg

Wijkmark CH (2001) Der moderne Tod. Vom Ende der Humanität. Matthes & Seitz, Berlin

Winkelmeier LP, Bauer AW (2018) Das 2013 gescheiterte deutsche Gesetzgebungsverfahren zum assistierten Suizid. Imago Hominis 25:205–214

Zaslawski V (2016) Wo Sterben nicht genehm ist. Suizidhilfe im Wohnquartier. Neue Zürcher Zeitung, 11 February 2016. http://www.nzz.ch/schweiz/keine-frage-der-ethik-1.18693240. Accessed 10 Dec 2019

Routine Oncology Treatment and Its Human Deficits

15

Ralf-Dieter Hofheinz

Shortly after taking up his post as President of the World Medical Association in 2018, Leonid Eidelman (*1952) warned of a "pandemic of physician burnout". The *Deutsches Ärzteblatt* (German Medical Journal) quoted Eidelman as saying that "Physician burnout is a symptom of a larger problem—a healthcare system that increasingly overworks doctors and undervalues their health needs". Nearly 50% of the world's ten million physicians, Eidelman added, have symptoms of burnout (Weltärztebund 2018). However, these alarming figures have barely given rise to any wide public debate in Germany. There are doubtless many causes behind this phenomenon. A major issue in modern medicine is the growth in bureaucratization, "technologization" and "SOP-ization" that has the potential to subtly alienate doctors from patients and thus prevent a more personalised, creative and/or more time-intensive approach to interaction with patients.

This article takes stock of the current literature on this phenomenon in medical oncology. It starts by presenting data on the prevalence of (self-reported) burnout and job satisfaction in oncologists, followed by a discussion highlighting the consequences for doctors' health, patient–doctor interaction and the healthcare system. The third section of the article describes interventions that can be implemented at an individual or organisational level to increase resilience and optimise work conditions. Given the variety of healthcare systems and cultural differences across the world, one *caveat* is required: this article focuses primarily on working conditions and situations in Western healthcare systems.

R.-D. Hofheinz (✉)
Interdisziplinäres Tumorzentrum, TagesTherapieZentrum, Medical Faculty Mannheim,
Heidelberg University, Theodor-Kutzer Ufer 1-3, 68167 Mannheim, Germany
e-mail: ralf.hofheinz@umm.de

© Springer Nature Switzerland AG 2021
A. W. Bauer et al. (eds.), *Ethical Challenges in Cancer Diagnosis and Therapy*,
Recent Results in Cancer Research 218,
https://doi.org/10.1007/978-3-030-63749-1_15

15.1   Job Satisfaction and Burnout in Oncology

We start by considering working conditions for hospital-based doctors in Germany generally as stated by the 2019 *Marburger Bund Monitor*, the results of which were presented in January 2020 (Korzilius 2020). Three quarters of the 6,500 doctors who took part in this survey reported that their health was affected by their work setting. 15% of survey participants had already received medical or psychotherapeutic help for this reason. These forms of distress have led to a steady trend towards part-time working (2013: 15%, 2019: 26%). Full-time workers reported that they worked on average 56.5 h per week, with 25% of survey participants reporting at least 10 h overtime per week. The huge increase in administrative tasks in everyday work is evidenced by the fact that 35% of doctors spent at least four hours a day on bureaucratic tasks (by comparison, the figure was 8% in 2013).

The distress described appears to be a particular problem for younger doctors. A data-based survey of German doctors and nursing staff aged ≤ 35 captured their working conditions and health status (Raspe et al. 2020). Data was obtained from a total of 855 doctors (60.4% female). Weekly working hours were far greater than those of nursing staff (>48 h per week: 71% versus 10%, p < 0.01). Over 70% of young hospital-based doctors reported symptoms of burnout. 22% of doctors and 15% of nursing staff said that they had already taken medication for work-related stress. Nursing staff were more often affected by verbal and physical aggression from patients than medical staff. 84% of nursing staff and 70% of doctors reported more than four verbal attacks from patients per year. 74% of nursing staff and 34% of doctors reported that they had been subjected to more than four physical attacks per year. Participants in this survey had very high levels of psychosocial work-related distress and were more likely to over-engage compared with national and international studies. This distress was associated with impaired health and a significant increase in burnout risk. Doctors approved the following measures to improve working conditions: reducing mandatory documentation (88%), optimising of individual clinical training (86%) and reducing the impact of budgetary considerations on professional decision-making (86%).

Before presenting data on burnout prevalence in oncology, we need to provide a brief definition of this syndrome. However, there are no generally accepted diagnostic criteria, and "burnout syndrome" is not listed as a diagnosis in the *Diagnostic and Statistical Manual of Mental Disorders* (DSM-5). The definition of burnout covers a range of psychological problems and disorders, particularly around work-related stress. The world's most frequently used burnout questionnaire, the *Maslach Burnout Inventory* (MBI), defines "burnout syndrome" in terms of three dimensions (Maslach et al. 1986). (i) *Emotional Exhaustion*, resulting from being emotionally overextended or physically exhausted (stress dimension); (ii) *Depersonalisation*, i.e., creation of an increasing distance between, for example, doctor and patient with increasing indifference, cynicism, etc.; (iii) *Low Personal Accomplishment,* i.e., feeling you are not achieving any success despite being overloaded. The discrepancy between requirements and actual accomplishments is experienced as personal inefficacy.

Lifetime prevalence of self-reported burnout in German in the general population was investigated in the representative *Study of Adult Health in Germany (DEGS1)* and found to be 4.2%. 12-month prevalence was 1.5%. (Maske et al. 2016). Women were at a higher risk than men (5.2% versus 3.3%). Prevalence was found to be highest in DEGS1 in subjects aged between 40 and 59 and subjects with medium to high socio-economic status. Another interesting aspect of this analysis was that around 70% of subjects diagnosed with burnout syndrome within the previous 12 months also met the criteria for a DSM-IV mental disorder (principally somatoform, affective and anxiety disorders).

Table 15.1 lists some key data and studies used to list prevalence in oncology clinicians. The *2020 Medscape National Burnout and Suicide Report*, which was based on data collected from a total of 15,180 physicians using an online questionnaire in summer 2019, gives a burnout rate of 42% in oncologists (Medscape 2020). The principal causes reported by all participants are bureaucracy (55%), overtime (33%), lack of respect from supervisors and/or colleagues (32%) and increasing computerisation of operating procedures (30%). The main compensation mechanisms for burnout were reported as: isolation (45%), physical training (45%), talking to friends and/or relatives (42%). However, consumption of junk food (33%)

Table 15.1 Selected burnout prevalence studies, expanded and modified in accordance with Murali et al. 2018 (q.v. for older references)

Author	Region	Years	N	Population	Questionnaire	Burnout rate (%)
Whippen	USA	1990	598	Oncologists	Study-specific	56
Allegra	USA	2003	1740	Oncologists	Study-specific	62
Glasberg	Brazil	2004/5	102	Oncologists	MBI	69
Blanchard	France	2010	204	Haemato-oncologists	MBI	44
Roth	International	2010	410	Paediatric oncologists	MBI	38
Mordant	Europe	2010	404	Oncology surgeons (assistants)		25
Shanafelt	USA	2012/13	1490	Oncologists	MBI	45
Rath	USA	2013	436	Gynaecological oncologists	MBI	32
Eelen	Flanders	2012/13	70	Oncology physicians	MBI	≈50
Shanafelt	USA	2013	1345	surgeons (assistants)	MBI	34
Leung	Australasia	2013	220	Radiotherapists	MBI	37
Banerjee	Europe	2013/14	737	Oncologists < 40	MBI	71
Lazarescu	France	2013/14	239	Radiotherapists	MBI	70
Mampuya	Japan	2015/16	87	Radiotherapists	MBI	21
Paiva	Brazil	2016/17	227	Oncology physicians	MBI	58
Osborn	USA	2017/18	125	Radiotherapists (assistants)	Study-specific	47
Medscape	USA	2019	n/a	Oncologists	N/a	42

or "binge eating" (20%) and consumption of alcohol (24%) are also in the top 10. Around one sixth of participants said that they suffered periods of depression, and one in four had had suicidal thoughts or had attempted suicide. Two thirds of participants said that they were unwilling to seek professional help for burnout or suicidal thoughts.

Similar results had been found a few years previously in a survey conducted exclusively with members of the American Society of Clinical Oncology (ASCO) (Shanafelt et al. 2014). 1,490 oncologists reported working an average of 57.6 h per week in this study. 44.7% suffered from burnout on the emotional exhaustion and/or depersonalisation domain. There was a significant correlation between burnout rates and hours spent in direct patient contact. Age was also a major demographic risk factor in burnout: younger respondents had a significantly higher burnout risk; each year older reduced the risk of burnout by approximately 4–5% (i.e., statistically, an oncologist 10 years older had a 40–50% lower risk). Despite the data, the majority of oncologists were satisfied with their career (83%) and chosen specialism (81%), i.e., they stated that they would be willing to become a doctor or oncologist again. The authors emphasise that this level of job satisfaction is extremely high compared with other specialist disciplines. The data overall suggests that a high burnout rate is not necessarily associated with a low level of job satisfaction.

Another more recent study also reports high levels of job satisfaction in oncology professionals (Raphael et al. 2019). This global survey (excluding the USA) evaluated data from 1,115 doctors from 42 countries who reported on their job satisfaction on a scale of 1 (unsatisfying) to 10 (satisfying) on a questionnaire. 20% of respondents reported low job satisfaction, 51% moderate, and 29% high job satisfaction. Doctors with low job satisfaction were significantly younger and/or had fewer years in clinical practice. The five most commonly stated reasons for low satisfaction were (i) high clinical workload with consultations with many patients (70%), (ii) little time for reading or continuing personal development (40%), shortages of (iii) oncologists (32%) or (iv) nursing staff (21%) and (v) limited availability of new therapies (25%). The data from this analysis is comparable overall with data on the situation in the USA. Just 20% of oncologists reported low job satisfaction.

The prevalence of emotional exhaustion, depersonalisation and reduced personal accomplishment is significantly higher among doctors compared with other oncology staff, according to a Belgian study (Eelen et al. 2014). In this study, 51.2% of oncologists suffered from emotional exhaustion, 31.8% from depersonalisation and 6.8% from low personal accomplishment. Burnout risk was higher than in other comparator professional groups (social workers, psychologists, nurses), according to the authors due to the high workloads, the large patient numbers under their care and constant time pressure. Specialist nurses reported low personal accomplishment in particular, but had fewer problems in the domains of emotional exhaustion and depersonalisation. The authors suggest that intensive contact with patients which can be a source of high occupational satisfaction may provide a certain amount of protection against burnout. Being part of a tight-knit multidisciplinary team may also have a protective effect.

A study of 261 German oncologists using the *Stress questionnaire of physicians and nurses* showed that structural conditions make oncologists' work more difficult and cause (Hipp et al. 2015). This survey of members of the *Arbeitsgemeinschaft Internistische Onkologie* (AIO; a working group of the German Cancer Society) on stress in physicians revealed that structural conditions such as time pressure, administrative overload or lack of time for patients' concerns generate the highest levels of stress in oncologists under 50. Structural changes to the German healthcare system over the last few decades such as the significant reduction in clinic bed numbers, shortening of inpatient stays and increase in outpatient treatment are resulting in an intensification of work and stress for medics. Particularly high stress levels were reported by female oncologists in this study. Their quality of life was correspondingly significantly lower.

The observation that younger oncologists in particular show signs of burnout is also reflected in a large pan-European study by the *European Society for Medical Oncology* (ESMO) (Banerjee et al. 2017). This study determined the prevalence of burnout using the MBI and examined relevant work-related and lifestyle factors. This study found that 71% of young oncologists under 40 had clear signs of burnout. 50% were affected in the depersonalisation sub-domain, 45% in emotional exhaustion and 35% in reduced personal accomplishment. Depersonalisation was significantly more common in men than in women. Reduced personal accomplishment was found to be particularly high in the group aged 26–30. Working in European regions, lack of a good work–life balance, no access to support services, living alone and inadequate vacation time were identified as independent risk factors for burnout syndrome.

An Italian study by the AIOM questioned 201 oncologists under 40 (Dieci et al. 2018). The prevalence of men and women reporting emotional exhaustion at least several times a week varied between 37 and 52% with no gender differentiation. Job satisfaction differed depending on the specific aspect measured. Satisfaction with interaction with supervisors (hospital management, older colleagues/tutors) was considered poor by 44–73% of respondents. 80% of respondents, however, said interaction with younger colleagues was at least satisfying. In this survey, too, more than 80% of respondents reported high satisfaction with genuinely medical activities, i.e., interaction with patients, forming empathy and clinical skills.

As mentioned at the outset, job satisfaction and burnout rates and their causes will be perceived differently across different healthcare systems, cultures and countries. The studies that we have selected here can only be seen as individual examples. A very good summary of the overall burnout phenomenon in oncology, independently of the factors cited above, is provided by a recently published meta-analysis that analyses data from 26 individual surveys on physician burnout in oncology (all measured using the MBI) from different cultures and countries (Yates and Samuel 2019). The data was gathered from a total of 5,768 oncologists between 1995 and 2017. The authors report a prevalence of 32% (95% confidence interval [CI] 28–37%) for emotional exhaustion, 24% for depersonalisation (95% CI 17%–32%) and 37% (28–49%) for low personal accomplishment. In this study, factors associated with higher levels of physician burnout were grouped into demographic factors, individual factors (psychological and private life) and work factors.

With respect to demographic factors, the authors describe an association with partnership status: oncologists who were married or living in stable relationships were less likely to suffer burnout. Younger people in this analysis were also at a higher risk of burnout. With respect to individual factors, the authors stress that higher levels of burnout are associated with reduced psychological resilience and use of anxiolytics, with the direction of causality clearly open to question. The data basis is largest for work-related factors: some of the studies analysed reported an association between burnout and number of patient visits or direct patient contact and contact with severely ill and dying patients; the number of overtime hours worked and excessively high requirements, as well as poor work–life balance were also associated with higher levels of burnout. Overall, however, given that the results were not clear and conclusive in every respect, the authors called for further studies into the association between work and burnout risk.

15.2   Consequences for Doctors' Health, Patient–Doctor Interaction and the Healthcare System

The potential consequences of the changes referred to at the outset as a "burnout pandemic" for doctors' health, interaction with patients and indeed for healthcare systems are far-reaching. Conservative estimates put the costs of physician burnout to the US healthcare system at $ 4.6 billion (Han et al. 2019). These included in particular costs related to physician turnover and reduced working hours attributable to burnout. At organisational level, this means an annual cost due to turnover associated with burnout of $ 7,600 per employed doctor.

With respect to individual consequences of burnout, as already noted above, compensation mechanisms such as medication with tranquilisers (up to 20%) or excessive alcohol consumption (up to 25%) or poor eating habits (consumption of junk food and "binge eating", each up to 30%) are reported by a large percentage of doctors with burnout symptoms—with all the consequences for their physical and mental health (Hlubocky et al. 2020). For example, burnout and depression— although separate entities—co-occur here and need to be rigorously differentiated (McFarland et al. 2019). Suicide risk is around 1.4 times higher than for the normal population for male doctors and 2.3 times higher for females. It is striking that these suicides in doctors are far less likely to have been preceded by mental disease than in the normal population (McFarland et al. 2019). As already set out above, the majority of doctors suffering from burnout are unwilling to present to a therapist with their symptoms (Medscape 2020).

Burnout was repeatedly associated with sub-optimal patient care and self-reported treatment errors (references in Hlubocky et al. 2020). A large number of studies also provide evidence that poor (health) status or burnout of healthcare professionals negatively correlates with treatment satisfaction and safety of patients. In a systematic review, Hall et al. (2016) report that in 22 out of 27 studies (81.5%) which analysed both the health of "healthcare professionals" (i.e., medical and nursing staff) and patient safety, a correlation was identified, in sub-aspects at least, between poor health status (including depression, anxiety, despair, stress at work) and poorer patient safety. The majority of studies also identified a clear association between doctor/nurse burnout and treatment errors (21 out of 30 studies, equivalent to 70%).

In a systematic review, Dewa et al. (2017) studied the correlation between doctors' burnout and quality of medical care in general. Patient safety and patient satisfaction/quality of communication by doctors were measured as care parameters. Just twelve articles met the eligibility requirements for the analysis. A significant association between burnout and medical errors was described consistently in all four articles that investigated this association. There were also four studies that evaluated the correlation between burnout and patient satisfaction/quality of care. A significant negative correlation was identified in three of the studies. Depersonalisation in particular correlated with low patient satisfaction in those studies that allowed correlation with individual MBI sub-domains. It is plausible to apply this data to the conditions in medical oncology. However, just one of the 12 articles studied in this systematic review is based on a study with 125 Southern European oncologists (Travado et al. 2005).

This suggests that there is still little data on treatment satisfaction/doctor–patient interaction in oncology, in particular synchronous questionnaires administered to patients and their oncologists. In the years since then two large surveys have been published that describe how patients view the attention that doctors pay to their concerns and worries.

The outcome of a German survey conducted at AIO centres is that communication does not meet the needs of patients in many respects (Tauchert et al. 2015). Around 2,000 patients completed a questionnaire consisting of 17 questions with information regarding their physical, psychological and social discomfort. The same questionnaire was then completed by the patients for a second time with respect to the attention that was paid to these issues in doctor–patient consultations. Median age of patients was 61, and 60% of patients were female. The principal cancers were breast cancer (n = 442), colon cancer (n = 246) and lymphoma (n = 123). The main distressing factor (severe/very severe) reported by patients was "what is going to happen" (35%) followed by "physical weakness" (28%), "fears and worries" (24%) and "tiredness and lack of concentration" (23.1%). Cancer and treatment-associated symptoms, such as "nausea and vomiting" (6%), "diarrhoea" (6%) or "pain" (11%), were considerably less frequently reported as severe/very severe distressing factors. With respect to satisfaction with doctor–patient communication, patients were very satisfied with respect to "pain" and "nausea/vomiting". Lowest satisfaction rates were reported for "sexual life" (40%) and "fears and worries" (49%) and "social problems" (51%). The authors emphasise that the patients' burdens have undergone a major shift over the previous year compared with older surveys but doctor–patient communication does not appear to have adjusted to this and patients express considerable dissatisfaction in this regard.

A similarly sized survey of patients with breast cancer (82%) and colon cancer at 17 community cancer centres in the USA recently had similar results (Smith et al. 2019). The authors used questionnaires to examine the prevalence of pain, fatigue and distress, as well as subjective satisfaction with the opportunity to discuss these symptoms with the therapists. A total of 2,487 questionnaires were completed. Prevalence of the three symptoms was as follows: pain 61%, fatigue 74% and distress 46%. Of the 2,487 patients, 76, 78 and 59% reported talking to doctors about pain, fatigue and distress, respectively. 70, 61 and 54% of patients reported receiving advice during these discussions. Of those patients actually experiencing each symptom, just 58% reported getting the help that they wanted for pain, 40% for fatigue, and 45% for distress. Multivariate analyses revealed particularly poor results for patients who had received curative treatment earlier. In their conclusion, the authors of this large-scale study state that around 30–50% of patients with cancer in the setting of US community cancer centres did not report discussing, getting advice, or receiving desired help for any of the three main symptoms.

Both of these large-scale surveys suggest very clearly that patients' perceptions are that distressing symptoms are not addressed, or not adequately addressed in routine oncological treatment, even in specialist institutions. In the German study, patient satisfaction with communication/help with typical cancer or cancer treatment-related symptoms is still relatively high in this respect, although the psychosocial problems that now appear to account for most cancer patients' distress are also not adequately addressed during doctor–patient consultations, according to this study. In the US study, which focuses on two types of cancer and three symptoms, there are also severe shortfalls in patient satisfaction with the attention given to and care provided to their physical symptoms.

Although a causal relationship between these shortfalls in oncologist advice and treatment and the psychological and physical stress of the treating oncologists cannot of course be proven, it would appear plausible that there is a connection. As already mentioned, synchronous surveys of patients and their therapists would be useful, perhaps also as a "pre-/post-evaluation" following individual or structural interventions (at organisational level) to improve treating staff's resilience.

15.3 Moving from Burnout to Resilience

In principle, both individual interventions and "structural" interventions (i.e., those implemented at organisational level) can be used to improve resilience or prevent and improve physician burnout. Naturally, these interventions must reflect each specialism's particular needs in addition to generally optimising individual resilience or cross-organisational processes. A meta-analysis published in 2016 provided a systematic review of the prevention and reduction of physician burnout (West et al. 2016). It analysed 15 randomised studies including 716 doctors and 37 cohort studies including 2,914 physicians. Three of the randomised studies investigated structural interventions and 12 individual interventions (such as stress management or "self-care" training, working in small groups and communication training). The cohort studies covered both types of intervention at roughly the same ratio. None of the 52 studies investigated simultaneous individual and structural interventions. The MBI was used in all of the randomised studies. The success rate for the intervention was generally measured immediately it ended. Only one third of the prospective studies report long-term outcomes. 34 of the 37 cohort studies also used the MBI and just four reported long-term effects of each type of intervention.

The meta-analysis shows that overall burnout decreased from 54 to 44% ($p < 0.0001$) regardless of study type (randomised versus cohort) and regardless of which doctors were participating (training or practising). A continuous variable analysis of the individual burnout dimensions revealed significant improvements in the depersonalisation domain and the emotional exhaustion domain. With respect to emotional exhaustion, there was no difference between study type, participating doctors or individual/structural intervention. Interventions based on mindfulness-based stress reduction or stress management were significantly better at reducing emotional exhaustion than other interventions. Analysis by categories, i.e., the impact of the interventions on "high" emotional exhaustion, showed a significant decrease from 38 to 24%. There were no significant differences between study type and type of intervention; intervention success was significantly higher in practising doctors than in doctors in training.

A continuous variable analysis of the outcome of interventions with respect to depersonalisation also showed a significant improvement. As with emotional exhaustion, there were no differences by study type, participants or type of intervention. Interventions for reducing stress were also more useful than others in this analysis. Although the rate of decrease in high depersonalisation was significant, it only decreased from 38 to 34%. There were no differences by sub-groups in this analysis.

In summary, this very detailed analysis demonstrates that interventions are effective in preventing and reducing burnout. The roughly 20–30% relative risk reduction in overall burnout and emotional exhaustion was numerically larger than in depersonalisation (12%). It is not clear as yet which type of intervention (individual or structural) is best suited for each individual target group or burnout dimension nor can any reliable statement be made as to the sustainability of an individual intervention since long-term effects are only reported in a small number of studies. Interventions for (mindfulness-based) stress reduction were particularly beneficial for certain individual aspects as described.

The *American Society of Clinical Oncology* discussed the problem of burnout in oncology doctors at a round table in May 2019 and recently published its findings and recommendations (Hlubocky et al. 2020). This article notes that improvements in reducing burnout are needed at both structural and individual level but states that there are still too few dedicated studies in oncology. Helpful interventions at organisational level according to the editorial panel include relieving oncologists of administrative tasks and improving work culture, for example, with respect to cooperation and workplace civility and respect. Interventions at individual level such as cognitive behavioural therapy-based measures, optimising communication skills and dealing with stress are also recommended. The ASCO Working Group's main recommendations are (i) improving clinical education by including burnout prevention in the oncology training curriculum, or developing a package of measures for professional skills training (such as communication, ethical decision-making, etc.); (ii) introducing or rolling out assessment, and establishing doctors' wellbeing and burnout as quality metrics for oncology practices; (iii) funding more research.

15.4   Conclusion

Oncology has changed dramatically in recent years. Huge progress has been made on drug treatments, surgical interventions and radiotherapy, alongside a steady increase in interdisciplinary approaches. Findings in the field of molecular biology and the ability to access even "whole genome" tumour analyses in short timeframes (through, for example, Molecular Tumour Boards) are transforming clinical practice. At the same time, the workload is increasing with the rise in bureaucratic procedures, more documentation and quality assurance such as certification and patients' justifiably higher expectations for the new opportunities promised by "modern oncology". Scratch the surface, however, and we see a large and growing number of oncologists with symptoms of burnout, often associated with unhealthy living and dissatisfied patients whose main symptoms are not (adequately) addressed during doctor–patient consultations. The implications for the healthcare system—not only in terms of funding—have received insufficient attention to date, and there is an urgent need to implement structural and individual interventions to improve these issues. This side of "modern oncology"—we might call it the "dark side"—urgently needs to be brought to the public's attention and a wide public debate initiated.

References

Banerjee S, Califano R, Corral J et al (2017) Professional burnout in European young oncologists: Results of the European Society for Medical Oncology (ESMO) young oncologists committee burnout survey. Ann Oncol 28:1590–1596

Blanchard P, Truchot D, Albiges-Sauvin L et al (2010) Prevalance and causes of burnout amongst oncology residents: A comprehensive nationwide cross-sectional study. Eur J Cancer 46: 2708–2715

Dieci MV, Massari F, Giusti R et al (2018) Gender influence on professional satisfaction and gender issue pereption among young oncologists. A survey of the Young Oncologists Working Group of the Italian Association of Medical Oncology (AIOM). ESMO Open 3:e000389

Dewa CS, Loong D, Bonato S, Trojanowski L (2017) The relationship between physician burnout and quality of healthcare in terms of safety and acceptability: a systematic review. BMJ Open 7:e015141

Eelen S, Bauwens S, Baillon C et al (2014) The prevalence of burnout among oncology professionals: oncologists are at risk of developing burnout. Psycho-Oncology 23:1415–1422

Hall LH, Johnson J, Watt I, Tsipa A, O'Connor DB (2016) Healthcare staff wellbeing, burnout, and patient safety: a systematic review. PLoS ONE 11:e0159015

Han S, Shanafelt TD, Sinsky CA et al (2019) Estimating the attributable cost of physician burnout in the United States. Ann Intern Med 170:784–790

Hipp M, Pilz L, Al-Batran SE et al (2015) Workload and quality of life of medical doctors in the field of oncology in Germany–a survey of the working group quality of life of the AIO for the study group of internal oncology. Oncol Res Treat 38:154–159

Hlubocky FJ, Taylor LP, Marron JM et al (2020).A call to action: Ethics committee roundtable recommendations for addressing burnout and moral distress in oncology. JCO Oncol Practice 16:191–199

Korzilius H (2020) MB-Monitor 2019: Ärzte fühlen sich überlastet. Dtsch Arztebl 117:B168-169

Lazarescu I, Dubray B, Joulakian MB et al (2018) Prevalence of burnout, depression and job satisfaction among french senior and resident radiation oncologists. Cancer Radiotherapie 22:784–789

Maslach C, Jackson SE, Leiter MP (1986) The Maslach Burnout Inventory Manual. Consulting Psychologists Press, Palo Alto

Maske UE, Riedel-Heller SG, Seiffert I et al (2016) Häufigkeit und psychiatrische Komorbiditäten von selbstberichtetem diagnostiziertem Burnout-Syndrom. Psychiat Prax 43:18–24

McFarland DC, Hlubocky F, Susaimanickam B et al (2019) Adressing depression, burnout, and suicide in oncology physicians. Am Soc Clin Oncol Educ Book 39:590–598

Medscape (2020) Medscape National Physician Burnout & Suicide Report 2020: The Generational Divide (Page 5/29). https://www.medscape.com/slideshow/2020-lifestyle-burnout-6012460#5. Accessed 7 Jul 2020

Murali K, Makker V, Lynch J, Banerjee S (2018) From burnout to resilience: An update for oncologists. Am Soc Clin Oncol Educ Book 38:862–872

Osborn VW, Doke K, Griffith KA et al (2019) A survey of female radiation oncology residents' experiences to inform change. Int J Radiat Oncol Biol Phys 104:999–1008

Paiva CE, Martins BP, Ribeiro Paiva BS (2018) Doctor, are you healthy? A cress-sectional investigation of oncologist burnout, depression, and anxiety and an investigation of their associated factors. BMC Cancer 18:1044

Raphael MJ, Fundytus A, Hopman WM et al (2019) Medical oncology job satisfaction: Results of a global survey. Sem Oncol 46:73–82

Raspe M, Koch P, Zilezinski M et al (2020) Arbeitsbedingungen und Gesundheitszustand junger Ärzte und professionell Pflegender in deutschen Krankenhäuser. Bundesgesundheitsblatt Gesundheitsforschung Gesundheitsschutz 63:113–121

Shanafelt TD, Gradishar WJ, Kosty, et al (2014) Burnout and career satisfaction among US oncologists. J Clin Oncol 32:678–686

Smith TG, Troeschel AN, Castro KM et al (2019) Perceptions of Patients With Breast and Colon Cancer of the Management of Cancer-Related Pain, Fatigue, and Emotional Distress in Community Oncology. J Clin Oncol 37:1666–1676

Tauchert FK, Bankstahl UK, Winkler EC et al (2015) Changing symptom burden in cancer patients: Does physician-patient communication cover physical, psychological, and social discomfort? A Survey among 2009 German patients. J Clin Oncol 33 (suppl; abstr. e17717)

Travado L, Grassi L, Gil F et al (2005) Physician-patient communication among Southern
    European cancer physicians: the influence of psychosocial orientation and burnout.
    Psychooncology 14:661–670
Yates M, Samuel V (2019) Burnout in oncologists and associated factors: A systematic literature
    review and metaanalysis. Eur J Cancer Care 28:e13094
Weltärztebund (2018) Warnung vor "Burnout-Pandemie." Dtsch Arztebl 115:A1844
West C, Dyrbye LN, Erwin P, Shanafelt TD (2016) Interventions to prevent and reduce physician
    burnout: a systematic review and meta-analysis. Lancet 388:2272–2281

Experiencing Cancer. An Ethnographic Study on Illness and Disease

16

Christine Holmberg

16.1 Introduction

In 1972, Richard Nixon (1913–1994), the 37th President of the United States of America, declared a "war on cancer", something that led to various studies on the use of language, particularly the metaphors of war, associated with cancer in the twentieth century (Mathews et al. 2015). The metaphors used in the context of cancer suggest that urgent and drastic measures are needed immediately to conquer the enemy. Cancer is considered a "dread disease" (Patterson 1987). The language used reveals, however, that cancer is more than a disease; it is a cultural trope that stands for uncontrolled growth, invasion, otherness, damage or things being "eaten away" (Mathews et al. 2015; Potts and Semino 2019). It has been portrayed as *the* disease of the twentieth century, a symbol also of the uncontrollable growth of big cities and lifestyles of excess.

Cancer is as much associated with a dreadful death as it is with hopes of biomedical treatments and cure (Good 2001). As Potts and Semino (2019) have recently shown, however, these negative metaphors remain in the public sphere, despite—they argue—the tremendous advances that have been made in the prevention and treatment of cancer; something that gives them cause for concern:

> Overall, the choice of an extremely common illness as a metaphor for a wide range of alleged evils can therefore be described not just as generally insensitive for people affected by cancer but also as reinforcing a view of the disease that may exacerbate anxiety, distress, pessimism and even stigma. (Potts and Semino 2019, 93)

C. Holmberg (✉)
Medical School Brandenburg Theodor Fontane, Institute of Social
Medicine and Epidemiology, Hochstrasse 15, 14770 Brandenburg/Havel, Germany
e-mail: christine.holmberg@mhb-fontane.de

© Springer Nature Switzerland AG 2021
A. W. Bauer et al. (eds.), *Ethical Challenges in Cancer Diagnosis and Therapy*,
Recent Results in Cancer Research 218,
https://doi.org/10.1007/978-3-030-63749-1_16

Cancer, the authors contend, is so fitting and remains popular as a metaphor because it represents a shared cultural experience that everyone can relate to. Sontag (1978) was among the first to study cancer as a metaphor. While investigating her personal experience of cancer, she highlighted the stigma associated with having the disease precisely because of the metaphors used in the public sphere. Sontag's plea was part of a larger movement aimed at bringing the experience of having cancer into the public realm and de-stigmatizing those affected (Klawiter 2008; Lerner 2001). It was made at a time when cancer treatments were changing dramatically, with systemic-medical approaches such as chemotherapy coming to the fore. It also led to a movement that is today known as 'survivorship', and to the dissemination of heroic stories of those who live with, or who overcome, cancer. The grand narrative of cancer that is portrayed is to a large degree painted along the story line of breast cancer (Aronowitz 2007; Lerner 2001), the most 'public' cancer to date. Breast cancer is the most common cancer in women, both in Germany and worldwide (International Agency for Research on Cancer 2019; Robert Koch Institute 2018). Early detection of the disease to improve health outcomes for women became the mantra of the twentieth century (Klawiter 2002). It began with the increased possibilities of surgery in the late nineteenth century, when surgical excision of the tumour, as radically and as early as possible, was the method of choice, introduced and promoted by the surgeon William Stewart Halsted (1852–1922). Radiation and finally chemotherapy became important additions to the treatment of cancer in the course of the twentieth century (Fisher 1999; Lerner 2001).

These changes in medicine also made it necessary to change women's behaviours. Women needed to know that they should consult a physician with signs of cancer. Marketing campaigns were launched to educate women to understand that breast cancer was not necessarily a death sentence and that appropriate treatments at the right time would change the course of the disease. In the course of the twentieth century, marketing campaigns changed from messages that guided women to recognize symptoms to those that encouraged them to proactively search for breast cancer in the body (Klawiter 2002) through mammograms and breast self-examination (Aronowitz 2001). In order for such campaigns to be successful, de-stigmatizating the disease was necessary, as was the discourse of hope (Delvecchio Good et al. 1990) in oncology.

Physicians' associations and citizen movements such as the women's movement and patient advocacy groups worked hand in hand to change the public face of cancer more generally, and breast cancer specifically (Klawiter 2008; Lerner 2001). The silence that historically surrounded a cancer diagnosis (Gordon 1990), its 'unspeakability', had to disappear in order for women to be prepared to undergo long-lasting and debilitating treatments to 'conquer' the disease. The silence that historically surrounded cancer could be felt in medical consultations where physicans usually sought words not including the 'C-word' to describe a diagnosis, and it was present in women's social interactions and everyday lives. Women rarely shared their diagnosis or disabilities experienced from the cancer with others.

Particularly with the advent of chemotherapy, the active participation of patients in their treatment became necessary. Disclosure of the diagnosis became important, as was the need for patients to understand the importance of treatments in order to 'survive' the disease. Crucially, the patient needed to know the diagnosis in order to engage them in the 'fight' against the disease (Aronowitz 2007). These changes in treatments led to changes in societal perceptions of and dealings with cancer (Cantor 2009; Klawiter 2004; Proctor 2018).

The hope narrative remains the master narrative for oncological treatments and research, fuelled today by precision medicine and its promise of targeted therapies, increased longevity and fewer side-effects. The race for a cure, the pink ribbon movement and the stories of survivors all fill the tabloids to raise awareness of and money for research (Sulik 2011). The 'war on cancer' requires individuals diagnosed with cancer to have the will to fight this war together with their physicians and the research industry. Enmeshed in this is a culture of hope or a 'biotechnical embrace' that engages patients and carers in dealing with the disease (Good 2001; McMullin 2016). Today, precision medicine, together with the 'big data' promise, is the hook for research money and the foundation of society's hope that this disease will finally be mastered. The science driving this hope has led to increased technological possibilities of diagnosis, including the continued differentiation of ever-more detailed characterizations of tumours, leading to the massing together of a whole array of diseases under the symbolic and value-laden label of cancer.

On the flip side of this is the *experience* of the disease: women suffering from breast cancer. It is this suffering that is shaped and structured by the master narratives and the public stories of hope, heroism and defeat. In the following, I will highlight how such hope and war discourses have shaped the experience of breast cancer for women diagnosed with the disease in Germany over the course of the last 20 years. To do so, I will draw on materials from an ethnographic study of how women diagnosed through early detection, such as mammograms, experientially become cancer patients (Holmberg 2005, 2014). I will also draw on an interview study of the experience of having, or overcoming, breast cancer (Blödt et al. 2018), collected for a German-language website that shares experiences of illness with the wider public (www.krankheitserfahrungen.de (Engler et al. 2016; Herxheimer and Ziebland 2008; Lucius-Hoene et al. 2015; Ziebland and McPherson 2006). Most quotes used in this chapter from women who talk about their breast cancer experiences are derived from the website and can be found in German under http://krankheitserfahrungen.de/module/brustkrebs. The chapter also draws on other published work on cancer experiences.

16.2 Experiencing Breast Cancer

Kleinmann and Seemann (2000) suggest that personal experiences of illness are framed by and deeply entrenched in cultural representations and social experiences. How then do such master narratives and collective experiences of survivorship shape the experience of illness?

16.2.1 The Diagnosis

As I have described in previous work, becoming a breast cancer patient is enacted through a speech act by a physician, which forms the culmination of a diagnostic process (Holmberg 2005, 2010, 2014). The diagnostic process may begin with some bodily signs considered out of the ordinary by the woman herself, such as a lump in the breast, an inverted nipple or some sense of difference in how the breast feels.

> It was really by accident. I was in the sauna with my friends and my nipple inverted. I asked the others if they were experiencing the same thing. "No" they answered, "you should go to the doctor. Something isn't right". So I went and the doctor sent me on to do a mammogram. (5 years after cancer diagnosis)

The above woman's diagnosis took place in 2008, when she was 68 years old. Like many other women talking about the time of diagnosis, she felt dissociated from herself in this first phase of the diagnosis. She described it as thinking that the physician was really talking about someone else; it was not she who had cancer. The idea of being a cancer patient and identifying as someone who has or has had cancer, often only comes after the sociological role of the cancer patient in the clinic (Holmberg 2005).

The processes through which a cancer diagnosis is made can be very diverse. Sometimes a woman may be told by a doctor about a suspicion arising during a regular check-up with the gynaecologist or a routine mammography screening, others may feel a lump or other strange sensation in the breast that leads them to visit a gynaecologist. As a 38-year-old mother of two explained: "Cancer came into my life on December fifth, entirely unexpected".

> I had an event from work the evening before. …. The next morning I go to my gynaecologist. …. No one in my family has had cancer. I had read that if you breastfeed you are at decreased risk, so I was never worried about breast cancer. Well, I went for the check-up and my OB-GYN examined my breast. She did an ultrasound and I realized she is serious. She tried to calm me and said that [it] may not mean anything but she really wanted it checked. She organized a mammogram and I cried. I thought, "This is incredible. I wanted to do some chores". I did them automatically, went home and cried and cried. (1 year after diagnosis; 37 years old at diagnosis)

Diagnosis is the moment where illness and disease meet, argues the sociologist Jutel (2009). In anthropology, illness is distinguished from disease in order to differentiate varying conceptualizations of sickness and diverse medical systems across cultures. *Disease* is the realm of medicine that classifies bodily states into the normal and the abnormal through biomedical diagnostic technologies, while *illness* is understood as the individual's subjective bodily experience of being unwell. The connection between illness and disease is the symptom, and it is the symptom reported by patients to medical doctors that leads to a search for the underlying bodily pathologies and— hopefully—to a diagnosis that will guide treatment decisions. This historical approach has, however, long been overtaken. Illness and disease are interconnected in a society's cultural system (Young 1982). The interconnection of illness and disease in contemporary society, when and how they may converge and how bodily signs and symptomatization processes come to be an illness experience, are only slowly becoming the focus of research (Brandner et al. 2014; Offersen et al. 2018).

Following Jain (2013) and McMullin (2016), Offersen et al. consider cancer a "'total social fact' [that is] present in most aspects of social life" (Offersen et al. 2018)—through its widespread metaphors and public media narratives. It therefore structures people's health behaviours and experiences long before an actual cancer diagnosis. Fear of cancer and the importance of early detection are part of people's tacit knowledge, and are common themes in the "cancer mythologies" (ibid.) of the Global North. These mythologies necessarily consist of an understanding of cancer as a deadly disease of the individual, for which individual health behaviours may be responsible, or may help to improve both the onset and progression of the disease.

Particularly with breast cancer, cultural knowledge and shared social experiences are already present, even before diagnosis. The fear of breast cancer is a common and shared experience of many women living in the Global North (Holmberg et al. 2015; Press et al. 2000). It is, furthermore, generally not a feeling of illness or malaise that initiates the process of diagnosis, but rather early detection when the disease itself is still asymptomatic.

> The diagnosis is a shock. A shock in which one feels helpless and unable to do anything. This feeling can come back anytime, for many years to come. You supposedly can handle your everyday life, but you never feel safe from that feeling of shock returning. (9 years after diagnosis; aged 40 at diagnosis)

This shock, I argue, is a necessary prerequisite for becoming experientially **ill** with cancer. It is necessary to be willing to undergo long-lasting and debilitating treatments. The diagnostic process, as well as the cultural knowledge and experience of cancer, leads to an experience of shock that is similar to a traumatic event, which for some leads to a long-lasting loss of self-belief and more importantly a loss of faith in their own body (Holmberg 2014). A cancer diagnosis thus provokes ontological uncertainty. Furthermore, the embodied, subjective experience of feeling unwell—of illness—is initiated and enacted through the doctor's speech act (Holmberg 2005, 2014) of diagnosis, and it is very often described in terms of out-of-body sensations or feelings of total estrangement, of disassociated states of mind (Jenkins 1996, 2003).

Women thus experience breast cancer as a disease first through the trauma of diagnosis, leading to a sense of disconnect and bewilderment, of total otherness. The normal is inverted to become strange, and this initiates the transformation that a woman diagnosed with breast cancer undergoes. This is an interesting and very radical process, one that several scholars have referred to in terms of liminality (Blows et al. 2012; Dauphin et al. 2020; Holmberg 2005; Rees 2017). The anthropologist Turner (1964), writing about ritual processes, characterized liminality as "betwixt and between", and described it as a necessary stage in the transformation of an individual from one social state or role to another.

Jutel (2009) has argued that a diagnosis, as a sociological category, connects illness and disease and is important for the adoption of a social sick role. This is a category that allows the patient to become part of the medical system, to receive treatment and be recognized institutionally as a cancer patient, and to access particular benefits from the social security system. With breast cancer, however, these categorizations are often independent of the subjective feeling of being ill. Diagnosing is a messy business in which stories and experiences are translated into potential biomedical categories. The ambiguities and uncertainties of diagnosis, of the relation between professional and lay conceptions of disease and illness, the triggers that bring an individual to consult the professional medical system, are all enmeshed in what ultimately becomes an illness experience (Brandner et al. 2014, 2017). In the case of breast cancer, the institutional role of cancer patient is often taken up before the experiential feeling of being ill and the embodied restrictions that come with it in terms of fulfilling everyday tasks.

The advent of increasingly high-resolution imaging techniques and novel laboratory technologies to investigate the human body are contributing to an ever-widening gap between the experience of feeling ill and being diagnosed as diseased (Kühlein et al. 2013). In contrast to descriptions from women experiencing breast cancer in the nineteenth century, who report feeling unusually tired or having swollen arms as symptoms that led them to consult a doctor, women today describe feelings of nausea or tiredness, being unable to complete everyday tasks, or swollen arms as effects of the treatments (Aronowitz 2007). The triggers for consulting a physician today appear long before the debilitating effects of the disease: it may be a check-up or a lump in the breast that initiates the diagnostic process. In many countries of the Global North, the underlying threat of cancer is a constant possibility and worry (Press et al. 2000). Offersen et al. have analyzed this omnipresence of what they call "cancer mythologies" (2018) in the Global North, which structure health behaviours long before the potentiality of a deadly disease turns into a given diagnosis. The trauma, the shock of diagnosis, which in reality is the shock that something that was a potentiality has become reality, is thus a necessary part of the cancer trajectory—albeit one that is regularly missing from the master narratives of cancer.

> What is important to me is to make officials aware of the systemic care gap we have in cancer care. Women who receive the diagnosis experience a shock. That is not taken care of, neither medically nor therapeutically. You may go to a psychooncologist and get a little help. But that receiving a cancer diagnosis is a long-term traumatic event, which often has long-lasting effects on our lives is never talked about. Women are not explained that their feelings of hopelessness or fear may return years later, triggered by tiny events. Or the massive fears that some women experience every time they go to a follow-up mammogram after the treatment phase. This massive fear is not talked about, and should not be talked about it seems. I miss this. I think this is given too little attention during this whole treatment phase. Where can women go if—years after the treatment—they suddenly experience the loss of their femininity due to hormone therapies or other issues linked to their cancer diagnosis? (9 years after diagnosis; diagnosed at age 40)

Today there exists a vast body of research literature on the experience of cancer, including the long-term effects and the liminal phases involved (Campbell-Enns and

Woodgate 2017; Holmberg 2005, 2014; Kerr et al. 2018). The research, however, has yet to inform health care delivery and policy makers responsible for structuring and organizing (cancer) care.

16.2.2 Experiencing Treatments

Following the shock of diagnosis, the physical transformation into a cancer patient is completed during the treatment phase of the disease, which is often associated with experiences of fatigue, pain and nausea. The everyday world of the patient is radically transformed. The precise treatments depend on the extent and type of the cancer. In addition to the removal of the actual tumour tissue, treatments aim to reduce the risk of recurrence and spread of the disease to other parts of the body. The diagnostic process and the treatment phase are interrelated, with ongoing uncertainty for the patient regarding the spread of the disease, the effectiveness of the chosen therapies and decision-making regarding the course of action (Blödt et al. 2018).

Many women experience emotional distress (Mehnert et al. 2014; Mehnert and Koch 2007) during and after the initial treatment phase. Furthermore, the different treatments all have their own challenges that must be coped with. Losing a breast through surgery is, for instance, sometimes experienced as a loss of femininity. The scar, the missing breast or the 'fake' breast are also all constant reminders of the disease, which many women try to hide in public and some also in their private environment. Some women avoid looking at themselves naked in the mirror, others hide the scar from their husbands and families. Others still might start massaging their scar tissue as a way of re-engaging with their alienated body and re-connecting with the breast. For many women the deformation of the breast through surgery presents a challenge and often requires careful re-invention of their identity. Some use photography or body painting as a means of re-appropriating their body and as part of their individual healing journey (Kirschning 2001; Kirschning and Clar 2017).

Chemotherapy seems to be the most feared treatment because of its potential to cause nausea, hair loss and fatigue (see http://krankheitserfahrungen.de/module/brustkrebs for the range of experiences women talk about in relation to chemotherapy). The woman's estranged body is further alienated by the toxins that are released into the body to kill the (remaining) cancer cells. Radiotherapy also presents a challenge for some. Many report that at the beginning of a treatment phase, it is not knowing what may come next that is the most worrying. The liminal phase of the diagnosis, characterized by the social extraction and isolation of the individual, becomes an embodied experience of fragility and the alienation of sensation. However, it is also a time of bonding with other patients in hospital wards or during the chemotherapy sessions, as well as with the nursing and therapeutic staff.

[The chemotherapy room] was made rather nicely. It was a small space, maximum one to four women in the room, maximum five chairs of which three were usually occupied. The chairs were recliners, very comfortable. We had a TV and you could get a soup or something to drink. There was always a nurse looking out after us. I joked that it was like my living room. We had good contact among the women. They even organized a Christmas party for us there. We could also always contact the nurse in between from home. I appreciated that. I have to say it went well for me. (3 years after her diagnosis; 55 years old at diagnosis)

Radiotherapy for many is less burdensome than chemotherapy, but it adds to the physical changes through scars, hair loss, fatigue, nausea and feelings of sunburn or 'elephant skin'. As a former breast cancer patient who was diagnosed at age 68 said, five years after her diagnosis and treatment:

I was tired from the x-rays. How shall I explain, I was exhausted. You need time to recuperate. One really isn't efficient and capable. ... The spot on my breast still feels weird. The tissue is not supplied with blood. This will stay.

The strange feeling of parts of the body and the alienation of the taken-for-granted 'being in the world' can remain for a long time.

16.2.3 Returning to One's Life: "I just Want It to Be Normal"

As a result of treatments, the women have a changed body, one that feels and maybe looks different, and with this their 'being in the world' changes. The urge to heal, to regain a sense of self and be in control, and the urgent wish to return to 'normal life' that patients talk about during the treatment phase all confirm treatment as a liminal phase. How profound and long-lasting such a transformation and novel state of being are depends on the person's age at diagnosis and what life brings them after cancer (Kerr et al. 2018). Nevertheless, the wish to return to 'normal' as far as is possible is voiced by many.

I want everything to be normal again. That's why I had my breast reconstruction right after treatments (Holmberg 2005)

Many women with breast cancer do indeed have a chance to return to 'normal', and this, I would argue, marks the end of the ritual process. However, it does not lead to the normal that was there before but to a new normality, one in which they have to re-integrate into their former lives, re-appropriate their bodies, find ways to handle the continued tiredness and/or generally find ways to live with what lies behind them. Society offers a new social role of 'breast cancer survivor', a heroic role that suggests closure and success.

Some, even as long-term survival increases, must deal with the reality that they will not return to normal (or 'survive'), but must rather prepare themselves for the palliative phase and ultimately death—though how long this phase will be is impossible to know. Six years after her initial diagnosis, which she received at the age of 47, this woman shared her experience of prolonged uncertainty and palliative, rather than curative, treatment:

It took me a year to recover from the chemotherapy treatment. Another year later they accidentally found bone metastasis around my shoulder. The subsequent diagnostics brought to light the fact that my whole body was full of bone metastasis and my ovaries seemed suspicious. So they took them out. During the operation they realized that my whole belly and belly tissue were full of metastasis. I refused the hardcore chemotherapy at that point. I refuse everything that reduces my quality of life even in the slightest way. So I now receive tablets that I can handle without any side-effects. Then one year later they worried that I might have liver, lung and brain metastases. This remains unresolved. When they found the bone metastasis, they gave me a life expectancy of 20 to 25 months. I am way beyond that. I take my tablets. The growths don't really care, they continue to grow, just a bit slower they say.

Even for those who do experience successful treatments, however, life after cancer, the new normal, does not mark a definitive conclusion of the cancer journey, let alone the heroic survivor or transformation narrative. Observations in a clinic where women come for follow-up appointments and their yearly check-ups reveal a picture of women who are worried and afraid (Holmberg 2005). They report symptoms that would, to others, be part of normal experience, but they worry that these may be a sign of the cancer returning. They ask for tests and seek reassurance from the physicians. Others avoid the medical system altogether and remain fearful and cautious. Regaining trust in their body and allowing the body to recede into the background again, so that they can walk confidently through life, is what these women strive for. Some do so by becoming members of new biosocial communities (Rabinow and Rose 2006). Some go to breast cancer self-help groups. Others leave the treatment phase behind and work to forget what they have been through.

16.3 Discussion and Conclusion

Cancer remains an inherently uncertain disease, despite ever-improving predictive tools. In fact, these tools bring cancer and the fears associated with it into social life long before an actual diagnosis. Offersen et al. (2018) contend that the significance of the disease burden of cancer worldwide makes it an essential cultural matter, with culturally specific everyday-life manifestations. An ethnographic lens on the disease allows an understanding of the cultural assumptions underlying the biomedical disease concept of cancer. This in turn sheds light on the inherently tacit influence of such cultural assumptions on individuals' experiences, most importantly the profound impact current modes of cancer diagnosis have on the experience of being in the world (Holmberg 2005; Lock and Gordon 1988). Such a view also shows how the biomedical categorization of diseases of the mind, in contrast to diseases of the body, cannot be upheld when we investigate disease through the lens of illness experiences (Good 2012; Kleinman 1989). As medical surveillance and diagnostics progress to the point where the gap between disease conceptions and illness experience (Kühlein et al. 2013) is becoming ever wider, this requires dissemination among the lay public of both cognitive knowledge of cancer and an understanding of the affective dimensions of the disease, in order to ensure that people seek health care as considered appropriate (Offersen et al. 2018) and that they accept debilitating treatments as necessary. Finally, the ethnographic lens can also highlight how supposedly subjective illness experiences, as described above, are not only personally relevant to the afflicted individual and her social networks, but have social and political significance, and are embedded within particular social and political structures that shape, but are also shaped by, individuals' experiences.

Politically, the structuring of our understanding of disease as something that happens in an individual body, whose causes lie in the individual and for which healing necessarily also takes place in the individual body (McMullin 2016), guides the focus both of how research priorities are set and how health care structures are enacted to allow for the best possible care under these assumptions. This biomedical disease concept allows for a narrow focus on diseased tissue and what treatments may be used to remove it, and for this particular goal, optimal structures can be provided. The broader implications this has for the individual, however, and for other theories of the causes of cancer that lie outside the individual's body, remain hidden and neglected. The public narratives on the fight—the war—against cancer reinforce the focus on the individual body, as cancer patients become soldiers. These metaphors may cause suffering and feelings of disempowerment for those who are afflicted because they don't have the right weapons to fight the war (Hendricks et al. 2018). More importantly, these metaphors and the associated 'survivor' metaphor leads to patients feeling responsible if they lose the war.

Cancer, the dread disease, is at the same time a cultural trope and the crystallization of what contemporary culture in the Global North stands for: an orientation towards the future through a manipulation of the present, guided by predictions of the future (Beck et al. 2014; Beck 2016; Giddens 2013). Both the war against, and the associated hope discourses around, cancer focus on grasping the disease through early detection, making it manageable and controllable. From the perspective of those afflicted with the disease, shock and trauma as well as long-term changes to one's life remain. Understanding the suffering associated with these conceptions of disease as a necessary part of the process could help us to improve health care services for those afflicted.

References

Aronowitz RA (2001) Do not delay: breast cancer and time, 1900–1970. *Milbank* Q 79:355–86, III https://doi.org/10.1111/1468-0009.00212

Aronowitz RA (2007) Unnatural history: Breast cancer and American society. Cambridge University Press, Cambridge

Beck U (2016) Risikogesellschaft: Auf dem Weg in eine andere, Moderne edn. Suhrkamp, Berlin

Beck U, Giddens A, Lash S (2014) Reflexive Modernisierung: Eine Kontroverse, 6th edn. Suhrkamp, Berlin

Bell K (2012) Remaking the self: trauma, teachable moments, and the biopolitics of cancer survivorship. Cult Med Psychiatry 36:584–600. https://doi.org/10.1007/s11013-012-9276-9

Blödt S, Kaiser M, Adam Y, Adami S, Schultze M, Müller-Nordhorn J, Holmberg C (2018) Understanding the role of health information in patients' experiences: secondary analysis of qualitative narrative interviews with people diagnosed with cancer in Germany. BMJ Open 8: e019576. https://doi.org/10.1136/bmjopen-2017-019576

Blows E, Bird L, Seymour J, Cox K (2012) Liminality as a framework for understanding the experience of cancer survivorship: a literature review. J Adv Nurs 68:2155–2164. https://doi. org/10.1111/j.1365-2648.2012.05995.x

Brandner S, Müller-Nordhorn J, Stritter W, Fotopoulou C, Sehouli J, Holmberg C (2014) Symptomization and triggering processes: ovarian cancer patients' narratives on pre-diagnostic sensation experiences and the initiation of healthcare seeking. Soc Sci Med 119:123–130. https://doi.org/10.1016/j.socscimed.2014.08.022

Brandner S, Stritter W, Müller-Nordhorn J, Fotopoulou C, Sehouli J, Holmberg C (2017) Taking responsibility. Anthropol Act. https://doi.org/10.3167/aia.2017.240107

Campbell-Enns HJ, Woodgate RL (2017) The psychosocial experiences of women with breast cancer across the lifespan: a systematic review. Psychooncology 26:1711–1721. https://doi.org/ 10.1002/pon.4281

Cantor D (2009) Choosing to live: cancer education, movies, and the conversion narrative in America, 1921–1960. Lit Med 28:278–332

Dauphin S, van Wolputte S, Jansen L, de Burghgraeve T, Buntinx F, van den Akker M (2020) Using liminality and subjunctivity to better understand how patients with cancer experience uncertainty throughout their illness trajectory. Qual Health Res 30:356–365. https://doi.org/10. 1177/1049732319880542

Delvecchio Good MJ, Good BJ, Schaffer C, Lind SE (1990) American oncology and the discourse on hope. Cult Med Psychiatr 14:59–79. https://doi.org/10.1007/BF00046704

Engler J, Adami S, Adam Y, Keller B, Repke T, Fügemann H, Lucius-Hoene G, Müller-Nordhorn J, Holmberg C (2016) Using others' experiences. Cancer patients' expectations and navigation of a website providing narratives on prostate, breast and colorectal cancer. Patient Educ Couns 99:1325–1332. https://doi.org/10.1016/j.pec.2016.03.015

Fisher B (1999) From Halsted to prevention and beyond: advances in the management of breast cancer during the twentieth century. Eur J Cancer 35:1963–1973. https://doi.org/10.1016/ s0959-8049(99)00217-8

Giddens A (2013) The consequences of modernity. Wiley, Oxford

Good MJ (2001) The biotechnical embrace. Cult Med Psychiatry 25:395–410. https://doi.org/10. 1023/A:1013097002487

Good BJ (2012) Medicine, rationality and experience. Cambridge University Press, Cambridge

Gordon DR (1990) Embodying illness, embodying cancer. Cult Med Psychiatr 14:275–297. https://doi.org/10.1007/BF00046665

Hendricks RK, Demjén Z, Semino E, Boroditsky L (2018) Emotional implications of metaphor: consequences of metaphor framing for mindset about cancer. Metaphor Symbol 33:267–279. https://doi.org/10.1080/10926488.2018.1549835

Herxheimer A, Ziebland S (2008) Das DIPEx-Projekt: Eine systematische Sammlung persönlicher Krankheitserfahrungen. Neurol Rehabil 14:24–30

Holmberg C (2005) Diagnose Brustkrebs: Eine ethnografische Studie über Krankheit und Krankheitserleben. Zugl.: Berlin, Humboldt-Univ., Diss., 2002. Kultur der Medizin, vol 13. Campus, Frankfurt

Holmberg C (2010) Klinisches Emplotment: Erfolgreiche Arzt-Patienten-Beziehungen?! In: Witt C (ed) Der gute Arzt aus interdisziplinärer Sicht: Ergebnisse eines Expertentreffens. KVC-Verl, Essen, pp 141–156

Holmberg C (2014) No one sees the fear: becoming diseased before becoming ill-being diagnosed with breast cancer. Cancer Nurs 37:175–183. https://doi.org/10.1097/NCC.0b013e318281395e

Holmberg C, Whitehouse K, Daly M, McCaskill-Stevens W (2015) Gaining control over breast cancer risk: transforming vulnerability, uncertainty, and the future through clinical trial

participation—a qualitative study. Sociol Health Illness 37:1373–1387. https://doi.org/10.
1111/1467-9566.12307

International Agency for Research on Cancer (2019) Cancer fact sheets: breasts. https://gco.iarc.fr/
today/data/factsheets/cancers/20-Breast-fact-sheet.pdf. Accessed 14 May 2020

Jain SL (2013) Malignant: how cancer becomes us. University of California Press, Berkeley

Jenkins JH (1996) Culture, emotion, and pychiatric disorder. In: Sargent CF, Johnson TM
(eds) Handbook of medical anthropology: contemporary theory and method. Greenwood Press,
Westport, pp 71–87

Jenkins JH (2003) Schizophrenia as a paradigm case for understanding fundamental human
processes. In: Jenkins JH, Barrett RJ, Harwood A (eds) Schizophrenia, culture, and
subjectivity: the edge of experience. Cambridge University Press, Cambridge, pp 29–61

Jutel A (2009) Sociology of diagnosis: a preliminary review. Sociol Health Illn 31:278–299.
https://doi.org/10.1111/j.1467-9566.2008.01152.x

Kerr A, Ross E, Jacques G, Cunningham-Burley S (2018) The sociology of cancer: a decade of
research. Sociol Health Illn 40:552–576. https://doi.org/10.1111/1467-9566.12662

Kirschning S (2001) Brustkrebs: Der Diagnoseprozess und die laute Sprachlosigkeit der Medizin.
Eine soziologische Untersuchung. VS Verlag für Sozialwissenschaften, Wiesbaden

Kirschning S, Clar C (2017) Partizipative Kunst und Gesundheit. Präv Gesundheitsf 12:41–53.
https://doi.org/10.1007/s11553-016-0554-1

Klawiter M (2002) Risk, prevention and the breast cancer continuum: the NCI, the FDA, health
activism and the pharmaceutical industry. Hist Technol 18:309–353. https://doi.org/10.1080/
0734151022000023785

Klawiter M (2004) Breast cancer in two regimes: the impact of social movements on illness
experience. Soc Health Illness 26:845–874. https://doi.org/10.1111/j.1467-9566.2004.421_1.x

Klawiter M (2008) The biopolitics of breast cancer: changing cultures of disease and activism.
University of Minnesota Press, Minneapolis

Kleinman A (1989) The illness narratives: suffering, healing, and the human condition. Basic
Books, New York

Kleinmann A, Seemann D (2000) Personal experience of illness. In: Albrecht G, Fitzpatrick R,
Scrimshaw S (eds) Handbook of social studies in health and medicine. SAGE Publications Ltd,
London, pp 230–242

Kühlein T, Freund T, Joos S (2013) Von der Kunst des Weglassens. Deutsches Ärzteblatt
110:2312–2314

Lerner BH (2001) The breast cancer wars: hope, fear, and the pursuit of a cure in twentieth-century
America. Oxford University Press, USA

Lock M, Gordon D (eds) (1988) Biomedicine examined. Springer, Netherlands, Dordrecht

Lucius-Hoene G, Breuning M, Palant A (2015) Patientenerfahrung als Ressource: die Website
www.krankheitserfahrungen.de. In: Amelung VE, Eble S, Hildebrandt H, Knieps F, Lägel R,
Ozegowski S, Schlenker R-U, Sjuts R, Althaus A (eds) Patientenorientierung: Schlüssel für
mehr Qualität. Medizinisch Wissenschaftliche Verlagsgesellschaft, Berlin

Mathews HF, Kampriani E, Burke NJ (2015) Anthropologies of cancer in transnational worlds.
Routledge, Abingdon

McMullin J (2016) Cancer. Annu Rev Anthropol 45:251–266. https://doi.org/10.1146/annurev-
anthro-102215-100217

Mehnert A, Koch U (2007) Prevalence of acute and post-traumatic stress disorder and comorbid
mental disorders in breast cancer patients during primary cancer care: a prospective study.
Psychooncology 16:181–188. https://doi.org/10.1002/PON.1057

Mehnert A, Brähler E, Faller H, Härter M, Keller M, Schulz H, Wegscheider K, Weis J,
Boehncke A, Hund B, Reuter K, Richard M, Sehner S, Sommerfeldt S, Szalai C, Wittchen
H-U, Koch U (2014) Four-week prevalence of mental disorders in patients with cancer across
major tumor entities. J Clin Oncol 32:3540–3546. https://doi.org/10.1200/JCO.2014.56.0086

Offersen SMH, Risør MB, Vedsted P, Andersen RS (2018) Cancer-before-cancer: Mythologies of
cancer in everyday life. MAT 5:30–52. https://doi.org/10.17157/mat.5.5.540

Patterson JT (1987) The dread disease: cancer and modern American culture. Harvard University Press, Cambridge

Potts A, Semino E (2019) Cancer as a metaphor. Metaphor Symbol 34:81–95. https://doi.org/10.1080/10926488.2019.1611723

Press N, Fishman JR, Koenig BA (2000) Collective fear, individualized risk: the social and cultural context of genetic testing for breast cancer. Nurs Ethics 7:237–249. https://doi.org/10.1177/096973300000700306

Proctor RN (2018) The Nazi War on Cancer. Princeton University Press, Princeton

Rabinow P, Rose N (2006) Biopower today. BioSocieties 1:195–217. https://doi.org/10.1017/S1745855206040014

Rees S (2017) Am I really gonna go sixty years without getting cancer again? Uncertainty and liminality in young women's accounts of living with a history of breast cancer. Health (London) 21:241–258. https://doi.org/10.1177/1363459316677628

Robert Koch Institute (2018) Breast. Cancer in Germany 2013/2014, vol 11. Robert-Koch-Inst; Ges. der Epidemiologischen Krebsreg, Deutschland, Berlin, pp 72–75

Sontag S (1978) Illness as metaphor. Farrar Straus and Giroux, New York

Sulik GA (2011) Pink ribbon blues: How breast cancer culture undermines women's health. Oxford University Press, New York, Oxford

Turner V (1964) Betwixt and between: the liminal period in rites de passage. In: Spiro ME (ed) Symposium in new approaches to the study of religion. University of Washington Press, Seattle, pp 4–20

Young A (1982) The anthropologies of illness and sickness. Annu Rev Anthropol 11:257–285. https://doi.org/10.1146/annurev.an.11.100182.001353

Ziebland S, McPherson A (2006) Making sense of qualitative data analysis: an introduction with illustrations from DIPEx (personal experiences of health and illness). Med Educ 40:405–414. https://doi.org/10.1111/j.1365-2929.2006.02467.x

Cancer and Life Beyond It: Patient Testimony as a Contribution to Subjective Evidence

17

Mariacarla Gadebusch Bondio and Ingo F. Herrmann

With an original text by Maria Cristina Montani.

17.1 Introduction

The narrative component of medicine has become the subject of debate surrounding methods employed in clinical research and decision making as well as the training of medical professionals (Zaharias 2018; Kalitzkus and Matthiessen 2009; Arntfield et al. 2013). During the advent of evidence-based medicine (EBM), the *British Medical Journal* devoted a series of five articles to the topic of 'narrative-based medicine', including the provocative term used by Trisha Greenhalgh and Brian Hurwitz as the title of their programmatic book a year earlier (Greenhalgh and Hurwitz 1998; Greenhalgh and Hurwitz 1999; Launer 1999; Elwyn and Gwyn 1999; Hudson Jones 1999; Greenhalgh 1999). Greenhalgh stresses the importance of the narrative dimension of medicine for medical professionals in bridging the gap between research and its application in practice:

> The dissonance we experience when trying to apply research findings to the clinical encounter often occurs when we abandon the narrative-interpretive paradigm and try to get by on 'evidence' alone. (Greenhalgh 1999: 323)

In medicine oriented to the EBM paradigm, one of the main challenges is how to take account of the uniqueness of individual patients. The supposed objectivity of empirical data is confounded when it comes to a person with their own medical

M. Gadebusch Bondio (✉) · I. F. Herrmann
Institute for Medical Humanities, Universitätsklinikum Bonn,
Venusberg-Campus 1, 53127 Bonn, Germany
e-mail: gadebusch.bondio@uni-bonn.de

I. F. Herrmann
Reflux-Center, Duesseldorferstr. 1, 40667 Meerbusch, Germany

© Springer Nature Switzerland AG 2021
A. W. Bauer et al. (eds.), *Ethical Challenges in Cancer Diagnosis and Therapy*,
Recent Results in Cancer Research 218,
https://doi.org/10.1007/978-3-030-63749-1_17

history in its particular context. Along with the philosopher Drew Leder, Greenhalgh emphasizes how the story about the 'person as ill', even where based on the best evidence, can end in absurdity (Leder 1990). This plea for a medicine based both on empirical evidence and narratives that take account of the complexity of the particular task at hand has garnered increasing support in recent years. The shared conviction here is that evidence in medicine cannot be understood monolithically. The 'objective evidence' that arises from strict empiricism alone (e.g., within the framework of randomized controlled trials) must be supplemented by 'subjective evidence' from individual patient experience:

> Narrative, phenomenological, and ethnographic research designs should be viewed as complementary rather than inferior to epidemiological evidence – though qualitative, like quantitative, research must be appraised for rigour and relevance. (Greenhalgh et al. 2015: 11)

This position has been boosted by new digital communication technologies. The DIPEx (Database of Individual Patient Experience) and *healthtalk.org* portals, established in 2000, are good examples of the increasing appreciation of patient experience. DIPEx is a charitably supported database that aims to capture patient experiences by category and use them for research. Qualitative, experience-based research should make it possible to combine best clinical evidence with patient experience. Its partner platform *Healthtalk* aims to inform patients and offer them orientation via the experiences of others. Systematically structured and alphabetically searchable pages contain videos of patients telling their stories. *Healthtalk* was founded in Oxford by GP Dr. Ann McPherson, CBE and Dr. Andrew Herxheimer after their own experiences of illness. As patients, they felt the urgent need for a better, autonomous exchange of information. The *Healthtalk* website is visited by more than 6 million people a year.

These initiatives, driven by social media, have created space for a patient-centered perspective within medicine. In principle, this is about the appreciation of the individual character of each patient, about the perception of the patient's personal history in a clinical context, in which the individual case has hitherto occupied the bottom rung in the hierarchy of evidence as determined by EBM. The upgrading of the patient experience, combined with an attempt to make it usable, is an important step towards augmenting and enriching medical practice that is otherwise based solely on objective evidence. The forms of patient expression disseminated on internet platforms are mainly video uploads and brief statements. Are these brief contributions addressing specific questions sufficient to enhance our understanding of the individual perspective of the patient and the experience of illness as such?

If subjective evidence can exist alongside objective evidence, how can it be generated? How can doctors experience, include and use the patient's perspective in a way that does not simply mean adhering to patients' express wishes as the required basis for therapeutic decisions?

Our conviction is that patient narratives are not only of great value for a medicine that wishes to understand the suffering of others (Greenhalgh 1999). They form the basis for what Miranda Fricker refers to as "hermeneutical justice" (Fricker

2007). In medicine, there is an intrinsic asymmetry to the doctor–patient relationship. The knowledge horizons and experience of those involved interact with each other in their respective professional and help-seeking positions, but clearly have different weights in the therapeutic process. The physician, thanks to the expertise derived from evidence-based knowledge and clinical experience, holds the power of interpretation. Toombs speaks of a "systematic distortion of meaning" (Toombs 1987: 221–222) in the doctor–patient relationship, resulting from the medical objectification of the progress of an illness.

> Thus, whereas the physician sees the patient's illness as a typical example of disease, the patient attends to the illness for its own sake. This is an explicitly different focus. Whenever one considers something as an example, it is not considered for its own sake, but only insofar as it exemplifies something other than the affair itself. (Toombs 1987: 223)

The experience of illness—and Toombs as a philosopher and patient speaks from his own experience (as a multiple sclerosis sufferer)—is paradigmatic of the "decisive gap" between the world of the subjective and immediate experience of illness and the objective view of the world of science. The "hermeneutic injustice" that arises from this corresponds to the tension between scientific expertise and subjective experience described by Miranda Fricker in relation to many other areas of society. In this classical relationship, objective evidence as an epistemic quantity stands above the subjective evidence arising from illness. Interpretive resources go hand in hand with the awareness that a life-threatening disease such as cancer, and the vulnerability associated with it, can only be meaningfully inscribed in one's own biography by the subject. If this linguistic act can be realized, the sick person takes authorial possession of their illness and thus of the power of interpretation. For those similarly affected, the nameability and narratability of the disease experience become evidence of patient empowerment, for they bring about a new weighting and distribution of the power of interpretation.

For medical ethics, the importance of patient narratives lies above all in the fact that the patient is in a unique position to reflect on and analyze aspects such as quality of life, the increased vulnerability and dependence resulting from their illness, the limits and shortcomings of medical treatments, and the challenges in communication between patient and doctors. Medical anthropology has long recognized the value of individual perception and narration of physical and/or psychological suffering, and has emphasized the expressiveness of illness narratives. Arthur Kleinman and Byron J. Good have pointed to the different dimensions of the concept of disease: illness (as the perception of the sick); sickness (as a general, non-medical description of a pathological condition); and disease (as a disease from the doctor's point of view) (Kleinman 1988; Good 1994; Currer and Stacey 1986). This classification and the associated approach contribute to a patient-centered understanding of illness. They offer physicians and caregivers the opportunity to deal with the multiple forms of expression by sick people (Lawton 2003; Shapiro 2011). Qualitative studies of the interactions between these dynamics, which focus on language as a medium for describing the experience of illness, have however only in recent years been recognized as a desideratum (Cepeda et al. 2008; Rosti 2017).

In what follows, we would like to focus on the story of a patient, Maria Cristina Montani (MCM), who fell ill with cancer in 2002. One of the present authors, Ingo F. Herrmann (IFH), attended this patient one year after the first surgical intervention and subsequent radiotherapy, and encouraged her to write a diary and document her experiences during the course of her protracted illness. Even now, after many years have passed and she has overcome cancer, he encourages her to continue writing. The other author, Mariacarla Gadebusch Bondio (MGB), has also been in contact with MCM since the creation of a joint book project, in which the translation of the autobiography (based on the diary) from Italian to German was accompanied by a commentary by both authors (Gadebusch Bondio et al. 2013).

The chosen methodological approach is phenomenological and is based on the phenomenology of illness approach (Carel 2016) developed by Havi Carel in relation to Merleau-Ponty (Wirth 2018). The disease experience of MCM is first condensed in its central dimensions, i.e., outlined by passages from her pathobiography. Thus the framework of her experience of illness is delineated as extending over several years. Finally, the patient's reflections on her current, post-cancer, situation are translated into English and published here for the first time. The passages and the reflections are available to the reader as original sources—whether in excerpts or in their entirety. Through these unique testimonies of illness, the experience of cancer is presented first hand and unmediated; it reveals itself, and can claim, as subjective evidence, to express actual lived and suffered existence in words (Carel 2012).

The close reading of this pathography focuses on three aspects: (i) the effect and power of her words; (ii) the process of change from wariness to awareness; and (iii) the maintenance of personal quality of life during and after cancer (Montani 2013; Gadebusch Bondio and Herrmann 2016).

17.2   The Sayable, the Said, and the Unsaid

Cancer is one of the chronic diseases whose experience can be accurately described with recourse to Karl Jaspers' concept of the "borderline situation" (Jaspers 1994: 56). For the chronically ill philosopher and physician, human beings find themselves in a borderline situation when they encounter death, suffering, struggle, especially the struggle for existence, and guilt. According to patient accounts, cancer radically amplifies the dependence and vulnerability of the human body, which is hostage to both the proliferating tumor cells and the medical apparatus used to destroy them (Kleinman [1988] 1997; Hydén 1997; Schuchardt 1991; Waller and Scheidt 2010; Lehmann 2007).

MCM was 37 years old when she became ill with an aggressive laryngeal carcinoma. In her autobiographical narrative, the first-person narrator becomes both the subject and object of the story. MCM opens her account by quoting the central passage from Hans Christian Andersen's fairy tale *The Little Mermaid*:

> You have the sweetest voice of any who dwell here in the depths of the sea, and you believe that you will be able to charm the prince with it also, but this voice you must give to me; the best thing you possess will I have for the price of my draught. My own blood must be mixed with it, that it may be as sharp as a two-edged sword.
>
> "But if you take away my voice," said the little mermaid, "what is left for me?"
>
> Your beautiful form, your graceful walk, and your expressive eyes; surely with these you can enchain a man's heart.
>
> H. Ch. Andersen, The Little Mermaid, http://hca.gilead.org.il/li_merma.html
>
> (Montani 2013: 19)

The mermaid, who is in love with a human being, makes a brutal pact with a witch. She will renounce her beautiful siren voice in order to be humanized, i.e. to exchange her fins for legs. The price for her humanization is highly ambivalent: after all, language and voice are among the distinctive characteristics of human beings. The witch's answer to the mermaid's question is perfidious: her elegant gait, "expressive eyes" and beautiful figure will be her characteristics. She will remain attractive to male eyes, even if she is dumb. Many elements of MCM's tale of suffering are condensed in this brief dialogue. At the end of her story, the reader may be astonished to see how closely the fairy tale and reality are interwoven.

MCM was a primary school teacher living with her husband and two young daughters in Rome when she noticed a slight hoarseness in October 2002. As the hoarseness increased and her voice did not return to normal, she became seriously worried. The decision to go to the doctor was followed by a devastating experience:

> The first visit to the specialist was traumatic. The hospital was a university hospital. The examination was performed by young medical doctors. Instead of trying to explain to me what the problem was, they discussed what to do among themselves.
>
> Finally, they suggested taking biopsies from my larynx a few days later.
>
> Inwardly, I decided not to go.
>
> (Montani 2013: 20)

MCM then went to a resident specialist, who also advised a biopsy. Her anxiety increased with the idea of being seriously ill. A second traumatic experience followed the extraction of the tissue sample.

> I was given the results of the biopsy by telephone. While I was alone, helping out in my parents' shop, I was told I had cancer of the larynx and I would have to undergo surgery. No one explained to me why and how. Strange behaviour! My family told me much later that they had been informed of the outcome of the examination while I was still in the operating theater. I was instructed to attend the clinic to be admitted that coming Saturday.
>
> (Montani 2013: 21)

Communication with the patient was patently inadequate right from the start: from the first examination to being informed of the suspected diagnosis and finally given the diagnosis by telephone. The family was informed of the preliminary result of the biopsy with the diagnosis of laryngeal carcinoma immediately after the examination and during the patient's post-anaesthesia. This tendency to 'protect' the patient from serious information at the family's request is still common in Italy. 'Gentle communication' ranges from euphemistic description to suggestion, or concealment to untruth. Studies have shown how, depending on the region and its different health care systems (e.g., the presence or absence of palliative institutions), the weight of traditional and religious ideas and the attitudes of doctors vary greatly (Surbone et al. 2004; Surbone 2003).

After the dramatic telephone call, MCM was deeply shocked and sought a third opinion from another specialist. The diagnosis and the need to surgically remove the tumor were confirmed.

> The specialist who examined me confirmed the diagnosis and said that I needed immediate surgery. Suddenly I was no longer afraid. I still only wanted this MONSTROSITY torn out as quickly as possible, which – once established – wanted to kill me. In the beginning, even before it comes true, the thought that you could be told "You're seriously ill, you have cancer" frightens you. But since it isn't yet certain, you're forced to wait for the results of the tests. You look for an answer in the eyes of those who do the tests. You don't find it. It is as if the face of a monster is staring at you from all sides. But when you finally know the diagnosis and know what to do, you think only of how to fight it, how to beat it.

(Montani 2013: 21–22)

The final diagnosis triggered her determination to act decisively. The first operation took place in October 2002. The patient was not informed about the type of surgery before the operation. She asked if the larynx might have to be removed. She was assured that this would not happen. When she woke after the operation, MCM could no longer speak. Half of her larynx had been removed and a tracheotomy performed. The opening in her neck and the plastic breathing tube plunged her into despair. She now had to be fed via a nasal probe. She had not been prepared for all this:

> When I arrived at the operating theater on that Monday, I was convinced that everything would turn out alright. I wasn't told exactly what surgery they wanted to perform, and I didn't ask questions, apart from the one about the possibility that my larynx might be removed. ... I was assured that I would keep my larynx.
>
> Before entering the operating theater, apart from my voice, I felt comfortable. (But now, after returning from the operating theatre, I was seriously ill).
>
> When I came back from the operating theatre, I felt utterly crushed. From my left finger I heard a beep, which followed me everywhere; even worse, I'd had a tracheotomy. I was shocked. I wasn't prepared for this new state of affairs. The plastic tube in the neck opening disturbed me deeply.

(Montani 2013: 22)

In this state, MCM asked to be discharged. She was allowed to go home, but nobody told her how to deal with her disabilities.

I didn't want to stay in that place any longer. I couldn't and didn't want to bear the look of pity from the nurses and other patients any longer. I longed for my daughters. I wanted to go home. The doctor who treated me took pity on me and allowed me to. He pulled the probe out of my nose and discharged me. The first problem that awaited me at home was that no one had shown me how to eat and drink with my disability. When I tried it alone, the food went into the larynx instead of the esophagus. I felt I was suffocating. Severe attacks of coughing, which after a short time caused me very severe abdominal pain, shook me so badly that I had to go to an emergency internist. We were now really adrift in the deepest of dark chasms. No one showed us the way out. When it came to my main problem, taking fluids, I was simply told that the food would provide enough fluid. This would prevent my body from drying out. It soon turned out that this was not true. I began to show symptoms typical of dehydration. Since I could not speak because of the tracheotomy, I had to write everything down.

(Montani 2013: 23–24)

Reduced to silence and without professional care, MCM and her family suddenly had to cope with everyday life. She began writing her diary.

There are a number of ethical implications to the history of this illness. All stages of the process, starting with the suspected diagnosis and the way it was communicated, the determination of the treatment and finally the (lack of) aftercare, are characterized throughout by inappropriate, inadequate or completely absent transmission of information. In the tension between the often untruthful 'said' and the 'unsaid', the patient's right to be informed is disregarded. The consequence is that she is deprived of the opportunity to decide for herself and her trust in the doctors involved diminishes. In her uncertainty, the patient becomes more and more sceptical and wary and begins a new search for specialists The first phase of MCM's experience of her illness is characterized by this tightrope act between the need for trust and mistrust.

17.3 From Wariness to Awareness

After this first phase, which culminates in the mutilating operation, there is radiation therapy with painful side effects (inflammation and suppuration of the neck wound combined with intolerance of the suture material). Finally, despite the radiotherapy, a fist-sized tumor metastasizes on the right side of her throat. The pain worsens considerably in August, the main holiday season in Italy, and the doctors who treated her are not available. In the absence of proper care, MCM becomes increasingly insecure. She travels to Paris with her husband and from there back to Rome with a recommendation. Fear grows under the increasing time pressure. Even at this point, the patient is left in the dark with inadequate and sometimes false information. Before a new surgical intervention, the opinions of the doctors consulted contradict each other. MCM therefore seeks out other specialists, while time pressure increases with the increasing pain. In this confusion, there seem to be no trustworthy doctors who can provide a transparent and considered basis for decision making. She urgently needs clear information about her future prospects and

treatment options. As she does not receive this, she must take on an additional fight
in which—as she notes at several points in her story—the smallest signs beyond
what has actually been said must be carefully deciphered. Guided by her increasing
concern, she acts and reacts to contradictory statements, careless remarks, ambi-
guity, lies or negative prognoses. She dares to question the authority of respected
specialists. Her vulnerability and the potential (albeit unintentional) harm done by
the doctor can be seen especially when she reflects on looks, gestures, spoken or
unspoken words and describes her own inner reactions to them.

In a conversation with one well-known specialist, any vestige of remaining hope
is destroyed:

> I had an appointment with a specialist at the University of A. …. We went in the hope of
> getting better news. It wasn't to be. The doctor had us make the long journey only to then
> tell me that the tumor had returned. It was inoperable. This was owing to the extensive
> radiation therapy over the previous months, which had severely damaged the tissue inside
> the neck. The tumor had infiltrated the carotid artery. He also told me that it was not worth
> looking for other surgeons. "No surgeon in the world would perform such an intervention."
> I had very little choice.

(Montani 2013: 29)

The reaction of the patient (and her relatives) to this radical verdict was not to
believe it, to defend herself, not to resign herself, to search again. The surgeon's
apodictic assertion would, in fact, turn out to be false. A turning point in this race
against time and the growth of the tumor came in the form of the first offer of help
that MCM perceived as honest because it was realistic. Without promising a cure
but also without excluding it, a surgical resection of the cervical metastasis was
considered and the reconstruction of the resulting defects planned. The possibility
of a targeted and jointly supported intervention arises. MCM feels she is at last in
good hands. Having been given up on by the previous specialists, the patient now
regains confidence. To achieve this, her first victory, she has had to trust in her own
survival instinct, help herself in her hour of need and doubt the expert opinions.
What she needed was a doctor who, in the sense of Jaspers' *Schicksalsgefährte*,
could act as comrade-in-arms and give her the self-determination she wanted, and
who was willing to try and battle the illness with her—or at least to offer her clarity
and honesty regarding her prospects of recovery (Jaspers 1947: 558).

The decision to undergo surgical reconstruction with the main objective of being
able to talk, drink and eat again was difficult for the patient at the beginning. MCM
was getting used to her condition, and after the emotional ups and downs, in which
the hope of survival had gradually faded, she had all but resigned herself to her fate.

> The doctor wanted to reconstruct the base of my neck, my throat and tongue so that I could
> speak again and improve my quality of life. There was no more time to lose since –
> according to the professor – experience had shown that a long period of silence changes the
> personality to such an extent that the desire and will to speak are extinguished. I changed
> my mind and accepted the plan that was presented to me. The surgical procedures that
> followed each other included trachea reassignment, treatment of the necrosis that occurred
> regularly after each procedure, and finally the restoration of my body until I could eat
> anything and not just semi-liquid food.

The reconstruction was successful:

He [the Professor] removed the silicone stent and the voice prosthesis (shunt valve) and asked me: "Please, try saying a long AAAAAA." I took a deep breath and closed the tracheostoma with my thumb. My new voice flew forth from my mouth. Unforced, with light breath, clear and warm, WONDERFUL.

I thought I was dreaming.

Thanks to those hands, I began to find my way back into my new normal life. I quickly became familiar with my new voice and immediately fell in love with it. I spoke without difficulty and without the need to pause frequently to catch my breath. It was a female voice. In the beginning, one small problem was that I was not able to pronounce consonants. T, S and P caused me particular problems. I trained by repeating words containing these two consonants in a loud voice with the help of a lexicon: *papera, topo, tappo* (very difficult), *patata*, etc.

(Montani 2013: 46–47)

The second stage of the illness did not end with this physical resurrection. In 2006, MCM decided to start a distance learning degree and planned to make the most of her hard-won new life.

By 2007, however, the pains had returned. Another metastasis was discovered at the base of the skull. A third operation was required. MCM sat waiting at the clinic:

The waiting time was very, very long and nerve-racking. I was tired and in pain. It was time for lunch. I decided to return to my room because I was too weak. They would call me again in the afternoon. Slowly, I moved through the corridors of the clinic and saw all the posters showing the procedures that usually took place in skull-base surgery. The pictures troubled me greatly. The captions to the pictures explained the possible risks.

(Montani 2013: 59)

In this state, MCM again encountered doctors who hurt and unsettled her with their scepticism and conflicting opinions, threatening to snuff out the last glimmer of hope.

After a brusque welcome, the assistant professor began to check my case notes. I understood immediately that he had doubts about the success of the upcoming surgery. He started to explain that the tumor had infiltrated the nasopharynx, that I would lose my hearing, and that the temporalis muscle would have to be moved to cover the resulting defect after the petrosectomy. In a moment of silence, he shook his head and drew a deep breath. Then he got up and on the way out said he'd be back soon. My family and I were lost for words. I didn't want to hear any more bad news.

(Montani 2013: 59)

The pronouncements and attitude of the assistant professor appeared contrary to the opinion of the professor who had proposed operating on the tumor. The apparent divergence in their assessment of treatment outcomes led MCM to the brink of despair. The situation illustrates both the lack of joint planning and consultation and the lack of collegiality on the part of the senior physician towards the head physician. A heated exchange took place in front of the patient on the way to the operating theatre, further exacerbating her plight. The memory of that moment makes MCM furious: she appeals to the professional ethos of the doctor and reiterates the medical duty to protect life and to behave according to the injunctions of the Hippocratic Oath:

> I was placed on the operating table …. The assistant professor from the day before was telling the professor that in his opinion the procedure was being pursued with a certain doggedness. … Finally the head professor's conviction saved my life in the face of the scepticism of those cowardly professionals, who hesitated to save a human life because of the risk of personal failure. They preferred to break the Hippocratic Oath they had taken before they were allowed to pursue their profession.

(Montani 2013: 55)

An eight-hour operation followed: resection of the entire petrosal (os petrosum), rerouting of the right facial nerve, resection of the tumor mass of the right skull base and the eustachian tube arriving in the nasopharynx, followed by the reconstruction of the resulting defect with fat tissue and temporalis muscle flap. The post-surgical consequences were hearing and equilibrium loss on the right side and paresis of the mandibular branch of the facial nerve. The surgery was followed by six months of chemo- and radiotherapy.

17.4   The Person Beyond Cancer

MCM's diary ends in 2009, with the threat to her life finally overcome. The story of her illness and survival has meant that she is restored to health but in her severely damaged body, she has to reshape her entire existence. The effort she has to make to maintain it is a feat of strength and determination. Mutilating operations, radio- and chemotherapy, the complete loss and then reconstruction of the female voice with tracheostoma have left their mark. Seen from the outside, the extent of the radical loss of organs and functions are barely visible, but they can be felt by the patient during every act of swallowing, while breathing, smelling, eating, drinking, tasting, hearing and speaking, and through disturbed balance, especially when walking in the darkness. The outwardly noticeable part is the tracheostoma, her pronunciation, which is not easy to understand for those who are not close to her and unfamiliar with the patterns of her vocalizations. Other markers can be concealed beneath hairstyles and clothing, through creative use of hands and arms in gestures that can be used to support speech and expression. Body language goes some way towards concealing the disability.

The continuation of the exchange with the patient gave us the opportunity to pose questions, to which she replied in writing. To begin with, we wanted to know what her new condition felt like. The answer was entitled "Self-portrait". It includes a detailed self-reflection that begins with the sentence:

> I sat down in front of the mirror this morning and carefully and attentively observed the image that was presented to me. A mask.

A deformed mask returned my gaze.

(Montani 2013: 92)

The description of the mask is followed by a razor-sharp analysis. The way that MCM chooses to reveal herself, her state and inner soul, is the exterior:

I look at myself and try to discover, with a Janus eye looking into the past, what is behind the mask. (Montani 2013: 93)

The eye directed towards the future sees a "woman marked by illness" who, despite everything, is happy in the awareness of having regained the possibility of life. After the diagnosis of a malignant tumor, after the radical removal of the tumor, and after the removal of metastases at the base of the skull, being tumor-free is a precarious condition, a perpetual uncertainty, which may or may not be confirmed at the annual PET-CT check-up. When asked how she felt about recording the experience of her illness, MCM gave this answer:

I experienced the writing of the book as a birth. By putting the pain down on paper, I have removed it from myself. When I now reread these pages, I do not feel pain, but empathy. It is as if my story belonged to another person. It helped me a lot to separate myself from what I had suffered in this way. The time of writing down was hard to bear. Or, to use the analogy of pregnancy, it was like the long and painful labour pains that end in the joy of birth.

(Montani 2013: 89)

The second question addressed to MCM related to the time that separates her life today from the experience of cancer. What is the effect of becoming older? We received her answer in August 2019.

The remainder of this article is Maria Cristina Montani's reply to the questions:

Circumcidenda ergo duo sunt, et futuri timor et veteris incommodi memoria; hoc ad me iam non pertinet, illud nondum.

Two elements must therefore be rooted out once for all; the fear of future suffering, and the recollection of past suffering.

L. A. Seneca, *ad Lucilium epistulae morales* Lib. IX, LXXVIII, xiv

(translated by Richard M Gummere, London Loeb Library 1970)

When I try to remember how I became the person I am today, I stand amazed at the very long distance that lies behind me with the infinite number of changes of course that I had to undergo on this tortuous path. To survive a disease that is still defined as incurable is not easy. But if this disease has inscribed body and mind indelibly, then it becomes even more difficult.

Seventeen years have passed since the day I was diagnosed with laryngeal carcinoma, 16 since the first relapse, 14 since the second relapse. In all these years I have tried to think as little as possible about my future and to live entirely in the present. My everyday life was characterized by examinations by specialists and medical treatments. I suffered from chronic fatigue and yet I tried with all my might to maintain my personal interests. As soon as it was possible for me, and my strength allowed it, I left the house and visited art exhibitions, visited the theater and cinema, or simply went for a walk to enjoy the beauties of my city. To this day, acquaintances still tell me that I'm never at home. I don't know if they say that to flatter me or if there's a hint of reproach there. What I do know is that these kinds of remarks irritate me. Especially because they have no idea of the willpower and effort it takes to persuade myself to return to life...

The impossibility of communicating orally made my repeated attempts to rise from the ashes of my first life more difficult. That life was basically extinguished by a medical judgement; a judgement that left little chance of survival. But my pugnacious, rebellious nature helped me in the most difficult moments of my life. I rebelled against my new condition of severe disability and sought ways never previously taken to return to life.

I still remember the astonished glances of the doctors when I told them that I had accompanied my children to a swimming pool, had climbed onto a water slide with the two of them in my arms, and ended in the centre of a small swimming pool. "You could have drowned, you have a tracheostoma," one of the doctors told me. This eventuality hadn't crossed my mind for a moment. Even today, although I'm aware of the danger, I get into the water because I only feel really free when I'm swimming. On the list of myriad deprivations which I am forced by the consequences of the tumor to endure, the impossibility of swimming or taking a shower are right at the top. In the pact that I had made with myself when I decided to live, and not merely survive, there was also a pact with the element of water. I do not fear the water, but it has to treat me with consideration. Since that day when I let myself be carried by the waves while my husband's arms cradled and swayed my body in the water and gave me the sensation of what it means to have blind trust in a human being, from that very moment I started to go into the water again. Of course, I take all precautions: I am always protected by the presence of my husband and wear a huge inflatable ring that keeps me on the surface. What a feeling of happiness I have in those moments! I move my legs free of the usual constrictions of weight and imagine myself swimming as I used to. I am not interested in the looks of passers-by, some curious, others sniggering. I let myself be carried by my thoughts, by the waves, and in these moments it becomes clear to me that I am truly happy. It is hard work ignoring indiscreet glances, crossing insurmountable barriers and taming uncontrollable fears.

The credit for this is not due to me alone. I was lucky to find a doctor who tried to heal body and mind, supported by a psychotherapist who helped me accept the new conditions of my body. Being 38 years old and standing there with visible scars on my neck, face and shoulders, no longer being able to speak normally, breathing through a hole in my throat and knowing that these conditions will accompany me forever is a bitter pill to swallow. The question was always the same: life or survival? Whether to allow the disease with all its consequences to take possession of my future life or to ignore it and its indelible memory? And all of this so as to take back the reins of my own life? I have chosen the second option. I wanted to start living again, even if it meant submitting to my new condition. But how was that supposed to work? I alone had to find my way out of the isolation I had created. The reason for this was my inability to accept the ostracization of a society which today derives its morality more from appearances than from being.

I began to cultivate my appearance more. I had resolved to recapture the femininity that had been stolen from me. This meant accepting myself again, emphasizing what I liked about myself, convincing myself that the glances that met me – as soon as I left the house – were marked by shared joy and not by pity. Only in this way was I able to tame the anger that gripped me in those moments. The desire to tear away the cloth covering my tracheostoma, to satisfy the curiosity of some people, was great. The instinct was often unstoppable, as was the desire to walk up to them and say, "this is a malignant cancer that has done this to me. Like you, I thought a long time ago that certain things could only happen to others."

Little by little I began to laugh at myself again, letting those moments when I would have liked to shout out my discomfort fall away. Now it might seem as if I am a misanthrope because I don't like crowds, the confusion caused by people who speak too loudly or make endless phone calls without regard to the people around them. I was also accused of being jealous: "You can't bear to hear others speak loudly or on the phone, because you can't do it yourself any more." Regardless of the fact that I consider this accusation totally unjust because I have never shared certain behaviours, even back then when I could still speak normally, today I nevertheless wonder whether there is some truth in that assertion. I know the answer. But to think the opposite at certain moments helps me to endure badly brought-up people more easily. How many strategies for bearing new things, how many disabilities had to be accepted. It was also necessary to keep my brain, my thoughts, under control. To overcome my concerns and fears, it was necessary to engage in new constructive activities.

I decided to use the free time forced onto me for activities that gave me moments of distraction. I began with photography, which, although it gave me extraordinary satisfaction, required the presence of a companion because I was afraid to go out alone. In fact, being deaf in my right ear, I have difficulty determining where sounds come from. I have serious problems making myself understood. If necessary, I could not have called for help. I decided to study and enrolled in the Beni Culturali faculty. I started reading again and memorizing poems. These new occupations have helped me to distance myself from the negative, pessimistic, angry thoughts seething in me. They still accompany and help me to this day.

Today I can say that I accept my condition almost completely.

I am no longer worried about provoking astonishment, looking like a rare specimen to be stared at out of curiosity. My new consciousness sometimes gives rise to situations that are very satisfying, even joyful. On other occasions it irritates me. It is what I call the Parable of Consciousness: while in the past I was busy searching for my future orientation, now that this path is predefined and I walk it with a certain joy, the thought arises in me that this state is irrevocable. That I will live with it until the end of my days. Often, as I look at others moving, being entertaining, joking, laughing, singing at the top of their voice, I find myself thinking that these possibilities have been lost forever. That I will always be forced to look for the quietest place when I enter a restaurant; that I will never make a telephone call again; that at concerts I attend I will never sing along again.

It is this sad certainty that sometimes spreads and darkens moments of happiness like a grey cloud. I can now live life normally: I organize dinners with my friends and although I know that I can neither talk nor eat with them, I do not want to forego the pleasure of their company. On these occasions this cloud appears for a moment and I push it away as best I can, but a touch of sadness always accompanies my hours of lightness. My resilience towards the power of events has its reward. Today I can call myself a normal person, but also a person who is special in a certain sense. Unfortunately, it is only through these sad and painful experiences that one is able to understand that life is to be lived in all its facets. The world should always be seen from different perspectives in order to enjoy its many blessings.

What I miss:
Speaking freely without closing the tracheostoma with my finger.
Looking at the mirror and seeing my face as it once was.
Being able to lift my right arm and keep my shoulders at the same height.
Hearing with my right ear.
Enjoying silence as I once could, before the humming in my ears began.
Eating a roll with salami while I read a book.
Swimming.
What I have:
I can talk.
I can look at myself in the mirror.
I can lift my right arm a little.
I can hear with my left ear.
I can *imagine* silence without humming in my ear.
I can eat.
I can swim with the inflatable ring.

References

Arntfield SL, Slesar K, Dickson J, Charon R (2013) Narrative Medicine as a means of training medical students toward residency competencies. Patient Educ Couns 91:280–286

Carel H (2012) Phenomenology as a resource for patients. J Med Philos 37(2):96–113. https://doi.org/10.1093/jmp/jhs008 (Epub 2012 Apr 2)

Carel H (2016) Phenomenology of illness. Oxford University Press, Oxford

Cepeda MS, Chapman CR, Miranda N, Sanchez R, Rodriguez CH, Restrepo AE et al (2008) Emotional disclosure through patient narrative may improve pain and well-being: results of a randomized controlled trial in patients with cancer pain. J Pain Symptom Manag 35:623–631

Currer C, Stacey M (eds) (1986) Concepts of health, illness, and disease. A comparative perspective. Providence, Oxford

Elwyn G, Gwyn R (1999) Stories we hear and stories we tell: analysing talk in clinical practice. BMJ (16 January):186–188

Fricker M (2007) Epistemic injustice. Power and the ethics of knowing. Oxford University Press, Oxford

Gadebusch Bondio M, Herrmann IF, Montani MC (2013) Innenansichten des Krankseins. Logos Verlag, Berlin

Gadebusch Bondio M, Herrmann IF (2016) Kranksein in Worte gefasst. In: Fischer P, Gadebusch Bondio M (ed) Literatur und Medizin – interdisziplinäre Beiträge für die Medical Humanities. Winter Verlag Heidelberg, pp 159–176

Good BJ (1994) Medicine, rationality and experience: an anthropological perspective. Cambridge University Press

Greenhalgh T, Hurwitz B (eds) (1998) Narrative based medicine: dialogue and discourse in clinical practice. BMJ Books, London

Greenhalgh T (1999) Narrative based medicine in an evidence-based world. BMJ 318:323–325

Greenhalgh T, Hurwitz B (1999) Narrative based medicine. Why study narrative? BMJ 318 (2 January):48–50

Greenhalgh T et al (2015) Six 'biases' against patients and carers in evidence-based medicine. BMC Med 13:200. https://doi.org/10.1186/s12916-015-0437-x

Hudson Johnes A (1999) Narrative in medical ethics. BMJ (23 January):253–256

Hydén LC (1997) Illness and narrative. SHI 19:48–69

Jaspers K (1997) Von der Wahrheit. 1st edn (1947). Pieper, München, Zürich

Jaspers K (1994) Philosophie, vol 1. Pieper, München

Kalitzkus V, Matthiessen PF (2009) Narrative-based medicine: potential, pitfalls, and practice. Permanente J 13(1):80–86

Kleinman A (1988) The illness narratives. Suffering, healing and the human condition. New York

Kleinman A (1997) The illness narrative. Suffering, healing and the human condition. New York (1988)

Lawton J (2003) Lay experiences of health and illness: past research and future agendas. SHI 25:23–40

Launer J (1999) A narrative approach to mental health in general practice. BMJ 318 (9 January): 117–119

Leder D (1990) Clinical interpretation: the hermeneutics of medicine. Theor Med 11:9–24

Lehmann A (2007) Reden über Erfahrung: Kulturwissenschaftliche Bewusstseinsanalyse des Erzählens. Berlin

Montani MC (2013) Wiederträumen können. In: Gadebusch Bondio M, Herrmann IF, Montani MC (2013) Innenansichten des Krankseins, pp 17–72

Rosti G (2017) Role of narrative-based medicine in proper patient assessment. Support Care Cancer 25(Suppl 1):S3–S6. https://doi.org/10.1007/s00520-017-3637-4

Schuchardt E (1991) Vom Gesund-Sein der Kranken: Forschungsergebnisse aus 500 Biographien der Weltliteratur zur Verarbeitung kritischer Lebensereignisse. In: Jork K, Kaufmann B, Lobo R, Schuchardt E (eds) Was macht den Menschen krank? 18 kritische Analysen. Basel, Boston, Berlin, pp 63–79

Shapiro J (2011) Illness narratives: reliability, authenticity and the empathic witness. Med Humanit 37(2):68–72

Surbone A (2003) Persisting differences in truth telling throughout the world. Support Care Cancer 12:143–146

Surbone A, Ritossa C, Spagnolo AG (2004) Evolution of truth-telling attitudes and practicies in Italy. Crit Rev Oncol Hematol 52:165–172

Toombs KS (1987) The meaning of illness: a phenomenological approach to the patient-physician relationship. J Med Philos 12:219–240

Waller N, Scheidt CE (2010) Erzählen als Prozess der (Wieder-) Herstellung von Selbstkohärenz. Überlegungen zur Verarbeitung traumatischer Erfahrungen. Z Psychosom Med Psychother 56.1:56–73

Wirth M (2018) Phenomenology and its relevance to medical humanities: the example of Hermann
    Schmitz's theory of feelings as half-things. Med Humanit. https://doi.org/10.1136/medhum-
    2018-011464 (11 Sept 2018)
Zaharias G (2018) What is narrative-based medicine? Narrative-based medicine 1. Can Fam
    Physician 64:176–180

Cancer in Literature: Between Phenomenology and Symbolism 18

Dietrich von Engelhardt

18.1 Context

The relationship between literature and medicine is complex, reciprocal and multi-dimensional, with a long tradition from ancient times to the present day (Binet and Pierre Vallery-Radot 1965; Carmichael and Ratzan 1991; Engelhardt 2018; Hoerni 2016; von Jagow and Steger 2005; Kaptein 2021; Manferlotti 2014). Literature and medicine are connected by similarities and reciprocal influences. Medicine itself combines art (*ars*) and science (*scientia*), natural sciences and humanities. Intuition, spontaneity and imagination are important for medical practice; surgery requires artistic skills; overcoming disease and producing health is a creative act; diagnosis, therapy and communication with patients transcend the logic of 'evidence-based medicine'; 'personalized medicine' and 'precision medicine' need empathy, fantasy, nonverbal and nonvocal capacities. Literature, as well as all the other arts, can be helpful in diagnosis and treatment (Downie 1994; Engelhardt 2018; Heimes 2017; Peschel 1980; Petzold and Orth 1985; Zifreund 1996). Aristotle (384–322 BCE) was convinced that tragedies can have a cathartic effect – very similar to physiological concepts of medicine – with purgation (*kátharsis*) of the emotions of pity or lamentation (*éleos*) and fear or fright (*phóbos*) provoked by the action on the stage. The effects of reading and writing have to be empirically evaluated, in order to differentiate specific dimensions of the patient's situation: relationship to time, to space and body, to social contacts, to self-image and worldview. However, literature always exceeds the ordinary therapeutic aims of medicine and psychotherapy. Franz Kafka (1883–1924) ascribes to literature the comprehensive function of being an "Axt für das gefrorene Meer in uns (axe for the frozen sea in us)" (Kafka 1999: 36).

D. von Engelhardt (✉)
Fichtestrasse 7, 76133 Karlsruhe, Germany
e-mail: dietrich.vonengelhardt@uni-luebeck.de

A. W. Bauer et al. (eds.), *Ethical Challenges in Cancer Diagnosis and Therapy*,
Recent Results in Cancer Research 218,
https://doi.org/10.1007/978-3-030-63749-1_18

The relationship between literature and medicine is at the same time marked by ontological differences in regard to the relationship to reality, tradition and progress or historical change, conceptual structure, phenomena, external causes and immanent dynamics. Physicians and especially psychiatrists have often emphasized the value of literary representations and interpretations. The psychiatrist and philosopher Karl Jaspers (1883–1969) was deeply convinced of the essential meaning of literature: "It is not mere chance therefore that poets have used symbols and figures of madness for the essence of human life in its highest and most horrible possibilities, in its greatness and decline. Thus Cervantes in *Don Quixote* and Ibsen in *Peer Gynt*, Dostoevski in *The Idiot*, Shakespeare in *Lear* and *Hamlet*." (Jaspers 1997: 786). The philosopher Georg Wilhelm Friedrich Hegel (1770–1831) underlines the specific advantage of art: "The hard shell of nature and the ordinary world make it more difficult for the spirit to penetrate through them to the Idea than works of art do" (Hegel 1975: 9). The Russian writer Fyodor Mikhailovich Dostoyevsky (1821–1881) underscores the higher reality of literary figures in comparison to figures of reality: "Authors for the most part attempt in their tales and novels to select and represent vividly and artistically types rarely met with in actual life in their entirety, though they are nevertheless almost more real than real life itself" (Dostoyevsky 1996: 4). Aldous Huxley (1894–1963) defines science as *nomothetic* or generalizing in the sense of establishing explanatory laws, whereas literature is *idiographic*: "Its concern is not regularities and explanatory laws, but with descriptions of appearances and the discerned qualities of objects perceived as wholes, with judgements, comparisons and discriminations, with 'inscapes' and essences" (Huxley 1963: 10).

Three types can be differentiated in the dialogue between medicine and literature: the *fictional function of medicine* as medicine's contribution to the understanding of literary texts; the *medical function of literature* as literature's stimulus in medicine and history of medicine; and the *genuine function of literarized medicine* as literary texts on literary topics influencing general views on disease and therapy, patient and physician. Eight dimensions of the world of medicine in the medium of literature deserve special attention: (1) pathophenomenology or the description of the disease; (2) aetiology or causality of disease; (3) diagnostics and therapy; (4) image of the physician; (5) subjectivity of the patient; (6) medical institution; (7) social reaction; and (8) symbolism.

Cancer is a central theme in reality, but also in literature as well as the other arts; historical documents testify to its ubiquitous nature. In its uncanny cruelty, cancer has repeatedly stimulated writers to representations and interpretations. Their interest has not only been in the phenomenology and aetiology of the disease, but also in the subjectivity of the sick person; not only in the physician and their therapy, but also in the social reactions and above all in the spiritual, cultural and symbolic meaning of this disease.

The number of literary texts on cancer is large, with particular intensity in stories and novels since the nineteenth century. Film adaptations based on literary models concerning cancer have also been made. In addition to literary examples, cancer has led to a wealth of so-called self-experience reports and narrative medicine. The boundary between art and reality is fluid in these texts, as is the transition to life assistance. Cancer has also received attention in poems, dramas and painting. In the play *Wit* (1995) by Margaret Edson (b. 1961), the young proactive oncologist Dr. Harvey Kelegian and the university professor of English Dr. Vivian Bearing, dying of ovarian cancer, illustrate exemplarily the opposition of objectivity and subjectivity in the disease and the interplay between rationality and emotion. Theology and philosophy, for their part, have developed essential concepts. A significant example in painting is Ferdinand Hodler's (1853–1918) series of drawings and paintings of his beloved Valentine Godé-Darel (1873–1915), who is dying of cancer. These works helped the painter to transform the thought of death into a powerful force (Hodler and Brüschweiler 1976).

18.2   Patient and Illness

The first documentation of the timeless elements of cancer – objective disease, subjective suffering, social situation, diagnosis, therapy, prognosis, honorary fee – is reported by Herodotus (490/480–430/420 BCE) in reference to Atossa (550–475 BCE), daughter of the Persian King Cyrus the Great (590/580–530 BCE) and wife of King Darius the Great (549–486 BCE). Atossa "developed a growth on her breast which subsequently burst and then spread further. While it was small, she hid it and did not tell anyone about it, out of shame, but later, when she was in pain, she sent for Democede and showed it to him" (Herodotus 2008: 224).

Literary examples reveal a complex picture of the patient's situation and how they cope with cancer and therapy, physicians and medical institutions, with relatives and friends, with the meaning of life and death, nature and culture.

After a fall, the high-ranking judge Ivan Ilyich Golovin in Lev N. Tolstoy's (1828–1910) novel *The Death of Ivan Ilyich* (1886) initially feels a dull pain on his left side, but it disappears quickly, leaving behind only a blue bruise; a little later he is disturbed by a strange taste in his mouth and an unpleasant pressure on the left side of his stomach. These sensations become stronger over time and increasingly affect his mood and behaviour. Ivan Ilyich closely follows the pain, its mode, intensity and duration, and begins to take increasing interest in other people's illnesses as well as in medicine. The pain becomes more and more unbearable, his appetite diminishes and turns into disgust for all food, his strength decreases. Illness and death are understood and accepted by him as his own destiny, all distractions and self-deceptions become obsolete, the illness forces him to "look at It, right in the eye, look at it and without doing anything endure inexpressible sufferings" (Tolstoy 2014: 79). Shortly before his death, in the nothingness that he feels coming towards him, Ivan Ilyich grasps a truth, a supporting substance; the pain disappears, the fear of death passes, a light appears to him: "'So that's it!' he suddenly said aloud. 'Such joy!'" (Tolstoy 2014: 110).

The reactions of patients to disease and death differ. In Thomas Wolfe's (1900–1938) novel *Of Time and the River* (1935) the old Gant, dying of cancer, tries in vain "to get some meaning out of that black, senseless fusion of pain and joy and agony, that web that had known all the hope and joy and wonder of a boy, the fury, passion, drunkenness, and wild desire of youth, the rich adventure and fulfilment of a man, and that had led him to this fatal and abominable end. But that fading, pain-sick mind, that darkened memory could draw no meaning and no comfort from its tragic meditation." (Wolfe 1935: 78). Body as well as spirit have decayed, but "the great hands of the stonecutter, on whose sinewy and bony substance there was so little that disease or death could waste, looked as powerful and living as ever" (Wolfe 1935: 78).

The cruel, unscrupulous, atheistic and materialistic captain Wolf Larsen of the sea schooner *Ghost* in Jack London's (1876–1916) *Sea-Wolf* (1904) is tortured by headaches and has to cope with his terrible suffering without any medical help. As diagnosis he himself suspects: "Something's gone with my brain. A cancer, a tumor, or something of that nature, – thing that devours and destroys" (London 1992: 311). Larsen goes blind, loses his hearing and his speech, becomes partially paralyzed, but retains his consciousness until the end – a victory of the spirit over the body. Despite all his physical weakness, his mental strength – "of a tremendous and excessive mental or spiritual strictness" – is preserved: "I can think more clearly than ever in my life before. Nothing to disturb me. Concentration is perfect. I am all here and more than here" (London 1992: 319).

Thomas Mann's (1875–1955) last story *The Black Swan* (1953) draws attention to the essence of hope, the biology of love, the power of youth and sadness of old age. Rosalie von Tümmler is 50 years old and at the same time still appears youthful, in terms of both her figure and her temperament. She increasingly suffers from "the extinction of her physical womanhood, to whose spasmodic progress she responded with repeated psychological resistance. It induced states of anxiety, emotional unrest, headaches, days of depression, and an irritability." (Mann 1961: 349). She thinks bleeding again is a sign of the new beginning of her femininity, and falls in love with a 24-year-old American. The truth is, however, that she has abdominal cancer, the consequences of which soon lead to her death. In her daughter Anna, born with a clubfoot and distanced from everything sensual, Rosalie finds a friendly, though not always understanding partner for the changes she faces. Before her end she wakes from unconsciousness and praises nature, in which she has been deceived:

> 'Anna, never say that Nature deceived me, that she is sardonic and cruel. Do not rail at her, as I do not. I am loth to go away – from you all, from life with its spring. But how should there be spring withouth death? Indeed, death is a great instrument of life, and if for me it borrowed the guise of resurrection, of the joy of love, that was not a lie, but goodness and mercy.' A little push, closer to her daughter, and a failing whisper: 'Nature – I have always loved her, and she – has been loving to her child.' Rosalie died a gentle death, regretted by all who knew her. (Mann 1961: 411)

The behaviour and attitudes of patients in Aleksandr I. Solzhenitsyn's (1918–2008) *Cancer Ward* (1968) are as varied as the types of cancer. Pavel Nikolayevich Rusanov comes in with a tumour on the right side of his neck, but does not want to admit his suffering and feels that his social position is insufficiently taken into account in the hospital. Oleg Filimonovich Kostoglotov fights against his stomach cancer and establishes private relationships with the doctor Vera Kornilyevna Gangart and the nurse Zoya. Sixteen-year-old Dyomka has to deal with cancer of one lower leg. Lively construction worker Yefrem Podduyev who has tongue cancer and cancer on his neck leaves neither himself nor his fellow men in any doubt about the malignant nature of his cancer. Twenty-six-year-old geologist Vadim Zatsyrko suffers from melanoblastoma and just wants to buy some time for his scientific work: "The real question is, what will I have time to achieve? I must have time to achieve something on this earth. I need three years. If they give me three years, I won't ask more than that. And I don't mean three years lying in the clinic. I mean three years in the field." (Solzhenitsyn 1971: 219). Asya, a young girl, is in despair at the thought of losing her right breast. She asks the young Dyomka, who is also suffering from cancer, to kiss her doomed right breast for the first and last time in her life: "You're the last one who can see it and kiss it. No one but you will ever kiss it!" (Solzhenitsyn 1971: 424).

Carson McCullers (1917–1967), in her novel *Clock Without Hands* (1961), follows the physical, psychological, social and mental development of the pharmacist Malone (? = I am alone) after his cancer. In the spring of 1953, Malone begins to feel weak and under attack; he diagnoses himself with "spring fever" (McCullers 1978: 2) and prescribes himself a tonic containing liver and iron. The doctor, whom he then visits, tells him the true diagnosis: leukaemia. His reactions are all the more characteristic since initially he is not greatly disabled by physical suffering. Malone seeks consolation in religion, and encouragement from friends and family, and at the same time feels constantly exposed to the relentless logic of time: "He was a man watching a clock without hands" (McCullers 1978: 28). The cancer makes him anxious, irritable and extremely sensitive: "The subjectivity of illness was so acute that Malone responded violently to whole areas of the most placid and objective concepts" (McCullers 1978: 65). His strength continues to ebb away, he is intermittently forced to go to hospital, he remains a victim of tantrums which fail to give him any relief. Towards the end he does not have to suffer, his tiredness increases, his bones feel heavy and he becomes particularly susceptible to sunrises.

Cancer can cause depression or a longing for the pleasures of life, suicidal tendencies or the affirmation of fate or indifference. In Isaac B. Singer's (1902–1991) narrative *The Witch* (1975), after suffering from cancer of the spleen, Lena Meitels only changes her appearance, not her mental state. She continues to read magazines and shallow novels and prefers to be left alone. "Lena waited for death, but death was apparently in no hurry to take her. Her heart went on beating, even if weakly and with hesitation. The other organs still went on functioning too, one way or another" (Singer 1975: 116). Lena's last request is to be turned to the wall after dying, and she dies alone. Kate Hegström, an American actress in Erich Maria Remarque's (1898–1970) *Arch of Triumph* (1945), is increasingly preparing for the end during the course of her cancer, is ready to say goodbye, but wants to take part one last time in a costume ball: "and I'll plunge into an orgy of sentimentality, and feel sorry for myself and take leave of all the wonderful superficialities of life, and from tomorrow on I'll read philosophers, write my will, and behave as befits my condition" (Remarque 1945: 247). The last picture she offers to her physician Dr. Ravic when she sails from France to the USA shows that she is already far removed from the earthly: "Slowly she went up the gangway. Her body swayed ever so slightly. Her figure, slimmer than all the others beside her, clear in its structure, almost without flesh, had the black elegance of certain death. Her face was bold as the head of an Egyptian bronze cat — only contour, breath, and eyes" (Remarque 1945: 300).

John Maxwell Coetzee's (b. 1940) *Age of Iron* (1990) takes the form of a long letter from Mrs Curren in South Africa to her daughter in the USA about her suffering from bone cancer and her difficult and lonely situation. She believes her cancer has a psychological and moral cause: "I have cancer from the accumulation of shame I have endured in my life. That is how cancer comes about: from self-loathing the body turns malignant and beginnst to eat away at itself" (Coetzee 1990: 132). Pills help only temporarily with the pain. During her coughing spasms she cannot keep any distance to herself: "There is no mind, there is no body, there is just I, a creature thrashing about, struggling for air, drowning" (Coetzee 1990: 121). She is thinking of suicide, but accepts the logic of nature or biology. "At one moment I think: Let me hurry to put an end to it, to this worthless life. At the next I think: But why should I bear the blame? Why should I be expected to rise above my times?" (Coetzee 1990: 107) An old homeless man, whom she let live in her home, assists her in her final days. "He took me in his arms and held me with mighty force, so that the breath went out of me in a rush. From that embrace there was no warmth to be had" (Coetzee 1990: 181).

In the realistic and poetic novel *A ordem natural das coisas* (*The natural order of things*, 1992) by the psychiatrist and writer António Lobo Antunes (b. 1942) Maria Antonia is informed by her nephew, an empathic and caring physician, that she is suffering from a brain tumour."'It's a brain tumor that can't be operated, next week we'll start cobalt treatments', and I patted his wrist, sorry to see him so grieved" (Antunes 2000: 259). She shows no verbal or nonverbal reactions: "I'm a quiet woman who has never appreciated gushiness or tears" (Antunes 2000: 259). The perception of her disease is connected with dreams and hallucinations. She rejects the cobalt therapy. Her own death and that of the other people in the novel correspond to the title of the novel: *The natural order of things* (Antunes 2000: 278).

18.3 Physician and Therapy

It is above all in cancer that medicine is confronted with its limits and physicians are challenged in their humanity beyond all diagnostic curative activities. Not only they, but also the medical institutions and their nursing staff are put to the test. The all too often few therapeutic possibilities, in turn, increase the psychological, social and cultural dimensions of the disease. In the history of medicine up to the nineteenth century, medical therapy has always meant assistance, not just treatment. Nurses and doctors must find their own response to cancer and reconcile their professional activity with their private lives. In addition, they have to cope with problems arising from the hierarchy of the hospital, from competition and envy, from the tension between the goals of care, cure and research.

In the literary world too, doctors have their own ideas about the causes of cancer. Opinions can differ widely and deviate not inconsiderably from established medicine in diagnosis and therapy. Graham Greene's (1904–1991) *Doctor Crombie* (1956) is deeply convinced of the sexual aetiology of cancer and in his educational lectures he tries to encourage the students at the grammar school to observe chastity. One of his former students, who has married four times, falls ill with lung cancer at the age of over 60 and recalls the former school doctor: "Of course the doctors attribute the disease to my heavy indulgence in cigarettes, but it amuses me all the same to believe with Doctor Crombie that it has been caused by excesses of a more agreeable nature" (Greene 2000: 135).

A mastectomy without any anaesthesia is reported in the story "Cancer" (1831) by Samuel Warren (1807–1877); Madam St.'s pain during the intervention is soothed by reading love letters from her absent husband, who at her request was not informed about the operation: "Her eyes continued riveted, in one long burning gaze of fondness, on the beloved handwriting of her husband; and she moved not a limb, nor uttered than an occasional sigh, during the whole of the protracted and painful operation" (Warren 1831: 49). Her concern about her husband's affection after the breast surgery is taken away by the kind and empathetic doctor: "'But, Doctor, my *husband*' – said she, suddenly, while a faint crimson mantled on her cheek; adding, falteringly, after a pause, 'I think St. will love me yet!'" (Warren 1831: 49–50).

Tolstoy's Ivan Ilyich consults doctors repeatedly and in vain. "Always the same. There'd be a small flash of hope, then a sea of despair would surge, and always pain, always pain, always despair, and always the same" (Tolstoy 2014: 98). A diagnosis of the disease is not communicated to him by the doctors, nor does Tolstoy mention it; the social and anthropological aspects of being ill seem more essential to him than any diagnostic classification. The doctors fail in their dealings with the sick and dying Ivan Ilyich. Their attitude is disinterested, they are pitiless in their encouraging words, they are only interested in fees and social recognition, the diagnosis is more important to them than the suffering of the sick person: "it wasn't a question of Ivan Ilyich's life but an argument between a floating kidney and the appendix" (Tolstoy 2014: 63).

In Thomas Mann's *The Black Swan*, the doctors have to realize that there is nothing more they can do. Dr Oberloskamp urges a definitive examination by the surgeon Professor Muthesius. The expert considers an immediate operation to be absolutely necessary; there is no doubt in his mind about the diagnosis of uterine cancer with metastasis in other areas:"But the picture that the opening of the abdominal cavity revealed, in the white light of the arc-lamps, to the doctors and nurses, was too terrible to permit any hope even of a temporary improvement. The time for that was long since past. Not only were all the pelvic organ already involved; the peritoneum too showed, to the naked eye alone, the murderous cell groups, all the glands of the lymphatic system were carcinomatously thickened, and there was no doubt that there were also foci of cancer cells in the liver" (Mann 1961: 408). Rosalie does not live much longer; the uremic coma spares her the pain, she gets pneumonia, which her heart cannot survive.

The doctors and their diagnostic-therapeutic reactions in Solzhenitsyn's *Cancer Ward* are described in detail. The doctors are therapists and researchers; their involvement with the patients can go beyond medical interest to problematic private relationships. Assistance, therapy and research must be balanced. The therapies in this novel consist of hormone therapy, radiation, surgery and treatment with colloid gold. Limits are seen and recognized, but professional engagement can also take on a life of its own. The operation on the brain tumour of the young Aubert in Jean-Edern Hallier's (1936–1997) *Le Premier qui dort réveille l'autre* (1977) is described precisely, along with the versatile talent of a good surgeon: "Le virtuose insiste, mêlant la brutalité à la plus extrême délicatesse (But the virtuoso does not let up, brutality is mixed with extreme delicacy)" (Hallier 1977: 15). Mrs Curren (Coetzee) does not expect to be cured of her cancer, but hopes for relief from her pains. "I have no illusions about my condition, doctor. It is not care I need, just help with the care" (Coetzee 1990: 168).

In science fiction, high hopes of therapeutic progress are repeatedly depicted. Freezing a cancer patient in Leonard Tushnet's (1908–1973) *In Re Glover* (1972) raises legal, medical and social problems about the determination of death, which are solved by the accidental thawing of the now really dead body. To escape the agony of cancer, the dictator 'Papa' Monzano in Kurt Vonnegut's (1922–2007) *Cat's Cradle* (1963), under the care of the former camp doctor in Auschwitz, Dr Schlichter von Koenigswald, puts an end to his life with a mysterious ice crystal; through a series of unfortunate circumstances, this suicide then triggers the icing over of the whole world. The fear of being sick with cancer can, however, also be exploited by doctors or quacks; Lady Delacour in *Belinda* (1801) by Maria Edgeworth (1767–1849), in the erroneous conviction that she suffers from cancer, is even prepared to have her breast removed, which – as in Warren's story "Cancer" (1831) – at that time still has to be done without anaesthesia.

Informing the patient is a recurring theme – as in real life, attitudes and conceptes in literature are controversial, both in the past and today. Repeatedly cited and discussed is Johann Wolfgang von Goethe's (1749–1832) statement: "Wofür ich Allah höchlich danke? Daß er Leiden und Wissen getrennt. Verzweifeln müßte jeder Kranke, Das Übel kennend, wie der Arzt es kennt (For what do I mightily thank Allah, that he suffering and knowledge separated. Every patient should despair, knowing the malady as the doctor knows it)" (Goethe 1967: 56). Autonomy of the patient is important, but in general, nobody must be informed against their will. Medicine has to mediate the well-being and the wishes of the patient.

In Remarque's *Arc de Triomphe*, Dr. Ravic, a German emigrant hiding in Paris before and during the Second World War, comes across an inoperable cancerous tumour in Kate Hegström during an abortion procedure. He conceals it from her, even when she questions him; the lie appears to him, in any case, as merely a postponement: "Was not everything postponement, merciful postponement, a bright flag which covered the remote, black, inexorably nearing gate?" (Remarque 1945: 70). But Kate Hegström suspects the truth and, on her return from Florence: "'Why didn't you tell me what was wrong with me?' she asked lightly, as if she were asking about the weather. He stared at her and did not answer. 'I could have stood it,' she said, and the ghost of an ironical smile with no reproach in it flitted across her face" (Remarque 1945: 208).

Ludmila Dontsova, the lead oncologist in Solzhenitsyn's *Cancer Ward*, does not want to take the suspicious symptoms of her own cancer seriously; she postpones the necessary examination and is only too happy to let her colleagues reassure her. "No, the patient shouldn't know everything. I always thought so and I still do. When the time comes for discussion, I shall leave the room" (Solzhenitsyn 1971: 480). Even in her own case she does not think much of information; she wants to be able to trust and does not want to know anything about the necessary steps: "The best thing would be if I knew nothing! I'm serious. You decide whether I'm go to hospital or not and I'll go, but I don't want to know in detail. If I'm to have an operation I would rather not know the diagnosis, otherwise I'll be thinking the whole time during the operation" (Solzhenitsyn 1971: 448).

McCullers' sick Malone hoped for positive information: "He had asked for the truth, but in asking, he had asked only for reassurance" (McCullers 1978: 68). The fact that the diagnosis is not associated with any therapeutic consequence deeply irritates him: "The trouble with Dr Hayden, he had never suggested any cures, nasty or otherwise, for that – leukemia. Name a man a fatal disease and not recommend the faintest cure – Malone's whole being was outraged" (McCullers 1978: 125). Malone sees several physicians, but no one can help him: their diagnoses remain the same – diagnostically and prognostically. Malone does not die in hospital, but at home, visited several times by Dr. Wesley, the doctor who looks after him, and his friend Richter Clane, and under the loving care of his wife. "But his livingness was leaving him, and in dying, living assumed order and a simplicity that Malone had never known before. The pulse, the vigor was not there and not wanted. The design alone emerged" (McCullers 1978: 261–262).

Marc in Françoise Sagan's (1935–2004) *The Corner Café* (1975) has no doubt after visiting the doctor that his death is imminent. However, he owes his knowledge more to himself than to the doctor: "And yet he had done all he could to force the doctor into this unaccustomed honesty, still unfashionable in Europe. He had certainly told him that he and his wife were separated, that his parents were senile, and that none of the children he might have fathered had any legal claim to him. It was no doubt because of these oversimplifications that he had received so formal a death sentence" (Sagan 1977: 142).

Compassion can produce extreme actions – on the part of patients, relatives and doctors alike. Euthanasia as an active termination of life by the doctor has been a topic of literature since the end of the nineteenth century. The Greek term *euthanasia*, coined by the Emperor Augustus (63BCE–14CE) designated not active termination of life, but the ideal of a gentle and honourable death (*felix vel honesta mors*). In Theodor Storm's (1817–1888) story *Ein Bekenntnis* (*A Confession,* 1887), Dr. Franz Jebe is moved to active euthanasia on his wife Elsi Füßli who is suffering from cancer. For a long time Jebe resists her repeated requests to save her from her hopeless and unbearable cancer, until in a last outcry she once again asks him for this act of pity. Shortly thereafter he learns from a medical journal about a new remedy that might have saved his wife; conscious of his failure, he now realizes the sanctity of life that places unassailable limits on medicine and, more generally, on any active ending of life. Jebe leaves home to expiate his scientific and medical misconduct and guilt in the fight against epidemics in East Africa (Storm 2016: 580–633).

Hospitals are settings for hope but often provoke disappointment and criticism. The institution shapes human suffering and social reactions to it; it can be a charitable framework for help in time of need, but also a place of anonymization, mechanization and degradation. The anger of the cancer-stricken men in Wolfe's *Of Time and the River* at the unknown power that has robbed them of their lives "suddenly took personal form in a blind resentment against doctors, nurses, interns, and the whole sinister and suave perfection of the hospital" (Wolfe 1935: 84). This resentment grows into hatred of the way in which dying is handled in the hospital: "It was an image of a death without man's ancient pains and old gaunt aging – an image of death drugged and stupefied out of its ancient terror and stern dignities – of a shameful death that went out softly, dully in anæsthetized oblivion, with the fading smell of chemicals on man's final breath. And the image of that death was hateful" (Wolfe 1935: 84). The sick child Aubert (Hallier) describes his stay in the modern clinic with the poetic and ambivalent verse "J'ai fait un pique-nique mélancolique dans une clinique de mathématiques" (Hallier 1977: 104).

18.4 Social Reactions

After all, cancer in the fictional medium is a special challenge for the environment – for relatives, friends, society, the state. The spectrum of reactions varies widely and can be divided into four principal types: (1) the healthy to the sick person: (2) the sick to the healthy person; (3) the sick to the sick person; and (4) the healthy to the healthy person with regard to illness and sick people.

Despite the deadly dangers that emanate from Wolf Larsen (London) even in his last days, the passengers threatened by them, Maud Brewster and Humphrey van Weyden, sympathize with and care for him, without receiving any gratitude in return. The attitudes of relatives and friends in Tolstoy's story *The Death of Ivan Ilyich* are disappointing. "This lie all around him and inside him more than anything poisoned the last days of Ivan Ilyich's life" (Tolstoy 2014: 86). Lie before illness and lie before death, as if dying was only Ivan Ilyich's business and not theirs as well, everyday obligations and social distractions are more important to them. Only the simple peasant boy Gerasim is prepared to take the right attitude: he understands his master's illness as a sign of his own frailty and his own future death. "Gerasim was the only one not to lie; everything showed he was the only one who understood what the matter was and didn't think it necessary to hide it, and simply felt pity for his wasted, feeble master. He even once said directly when Ivan was dismissing him: 'We'll all die. So why not take a little trouble?' He said this, conveying by it that he wasn't bothered by the work precisely because he was doing it for a dying man and hoped that in his time someone would do this work for him" (Tolstoy 2014: 58–59). Maria Antonia's friends (Antunes) often come to visit her, but in reality they are only concerned with their own problems: "They being worried about their own suffering, their own lives, wondering (for they were close to me in age) what form death would choose to haul them away, imploring 'Not cancer, for God's sake'" (Antunes 2000: 260).

After the amputation of a breast, the 28-year-old woman in Helen Yglesia's (1915–2008) *Semi-Private* (1972) feels devalued both as a patient and as a woman. Her husband greets her with the words "Well, baby, are you still going to divorce me?" (Yglesia 1972: 37). Helen Barton (Wolfe) suffers less from the care of her cancer-stricken father Gant than from the uncertainty of his end: "Do you know what it is to wait, wait, wait, year after year, and year after year, never knowing when he's going to die, to have him hang on by a thread until it seems you've lived forever – that there'll never be an end – that you'll never have a chance to live your own life – to have a moment's peace or rest or happiness yourself?" (Wolfe 1935: 13). Her brother Eugene hides the suffering of his father from the world when he is asked about his condition: "He's got some kind of kidney trouble, I think" (Wolfe 1935: 54). He himself feels a kind of hartred that comes "from the agony of heart and brain and nerves, the poisonous and morbid infection of our own lives, which a man dying of a loathsome disease awakes in us, and from the self-hate, the self-loathing that it makes us feel because of our terrible desire to escape him, to desert him, to blot out the horrible memory we have for him, utterly to forget him" (Wolfe 1935: 60).

The eleven-year-old Paul (Hallier) shares the fate of his brother Aubert, 17 months older, who is suffering from a brain tumour, until he reaches a form of self-abandonment: "Je fus même si éperdument Aubert, que je manquais souvent de basculer en lui au point de me perdre en son propre gouffre, irrésistiblement atteint par le vertige de son propre mal. (I was even so desperately Aubert, that I often almost fall into him to the point of losing myself in his own abyss, irresistibly affected by the vertigo of his own illness)" (Hallier 1977: 13). Paul must also acknowledge that the boundaries of individuality remain or cannot be overcome, a fact which: "Mais, aujourd'hui, je dois bien me résigner: ce mince corps inerte sanglé, les veines transpercées par les aiguilles des appareils de perfusion, est celui d'Aubert (But today, I must resign myself: this thin, inert, strapped body, the veins pierced by the needles of the infusion machines, is that of Aubert)" (Hallier 1977: 14).

Marylitz Tone realizes a specific act of social empathy in *Happy Onion* (1968) by Joyce Carol Oates (b. 1938). She becomes engaged to her lover Ly Cooper at his last concert; he is suffering from colon cancer and after his death in the intensive care unit, she accompanies him all the way to the autopsy. She considers herself married to him and wants to remember his face for the rest of her life. After the pathologist and his assistant have finished their work, she is certain that there is no longer any danger of forgetting. "She walked in her rapid bird-like manner, Ly's bride in black, his beautiful permanent darling" (Oates 1971/72: 475). Malone (McCullers) dies not in hospital but at home, cared for by his wife, who washes him once again in a profound ritual before his death."That night when Martha gave him his sponge bath, she bathed his feverished face and put cologne behind both his ears and pured more cologne in the basin. Then she washed his hairy chest and armpits in the scented water, and his legs and calloused feet. And finally, very gently, she washed his limp genitals" (McCullers 1978: 257).

Compassion can lead relatives and friends to hide the truth of the diagnosis, but at the same time create a feeling of loneliness in the sick person. In order to spare their mother, Robert and Kate in Jayne Anne Phillips (b. 1952) story *Souvenir* (1979) do not tell her the diagnosis of brain tumour. During their stay in hospital, mother and daughter visit a fairground and sit on a Ferris wheel. As the wheel reaches its highest point, the gentle lie turns out to be superfluous: "'I know exactly what's going on,' said her mother, 'I know what you didn't tell me.' The grey sky stretched above them, was inexorably in motion. Kate sat there calmly and swallowed; incessantly they fixed each other. She saw herself in her mother's brown eyes and felt as if she was slowly falling into them" (Phillipps 1979: 196). In her love for her daughter in the USA, Mrs Curren (Coetzee) relativizes the seriousness of her cancer, deceives her about the failure of the therapy: "My daughter is everything to me. I have not told her the truth, the whole truth about my condition. She knows I was sick, she knows I had an operation; she thinks it was successul and I am getting better" (Coetzee 1990: 66). The physical destruction of his wife Lena (Singer) causes social destruction for Mark Meitels – his passionate love for his ugly, vital student Bella, who magically claims to have caused his wife's death from cancer, forces him to give up his job and leave the city. "He was no longer Mark Meitels but some superstitious dupe driven by a compulsion or, as it might be described in Jewish terms, possessed by a dybbuk" (Singer 1975: 120).

Cancer can cause despair and suicide or ciminal acts against other people. Cancer can also be useful to disguise murder, as in Daphne Du Maurier's (1907–1989) novel *Rebecca* (1938). Although Rebecca was killed by her husband, the discovery of her inoperable disease, the prognosis of dying within a few months and her great fear of pain, suggested suicide and cleared her spouse of any suspicion. "When I go, Danny, I want to go quickly, like the stuffing out of a candle" (Du Maurier 1981: 358).

18.5   Symbolism

Cancer as a disease also appears repeatedly in idioms, proverbs, metaphors and symbols. Literature is neither reality nor science, even though there are contacts, overlaps and reciprocal influences. Literature gives meaning to facts, combines description with evaluation; the relationship between appearance and interpretation is characteristic of an epoch or an author, and is also shaped by the type of illness. Cancer refers to the centre of the living body, just as mental illness refers to the centre of consciousness. In sickness health can become understandable: *pathologia physiologiam illustrat* was how eighteenth-century physician and poet Albrecht von Haller (1708–1777) expressed this relationship.

Philosophy, theology and also the arts have developed interpretations of cancer that illuminate the peculiarity of the organism compared to inanimate nature and the world of the spirit, as well as the general connection between nature and culture, body and mind. Cancer and mental illness are among the diseases in which the broad spectrum between phenomenology and symbolism is manifested in a profound and moving way. Metaphors and symbols can be a danger (Sontag 1978) for patients, relatives and friends, but are at the same time a necessary aid for coping with illness and death. Life and human relationships need symbols.

Organs differ in their symbolic meanings. Marc in Sagan's *The Corner Café* is glad to be suffering from lung cancer and not colon cancer: "Thank God, his cancer was in the right place! Some cancers were ignominious: cancer of the colon, of the skin and other bits of one's inside. His was reserved for the élite: his would be a classic death, within three months, from lung cancer" (Sagan 1977: 143). Marc sees it just as positively that he is spared the misfortune of pathological diarrhoea or foreign diseases. To avoid dying of cancer, he causes a fatal car accident. Wolf Larsen's (*Sea-Wolf*) brain tumour can symbolically be related to a psychopathic and atavistic personality – a combination of Caliban (William Shakespeare) and Lucifer (John Milton) and a follower of Darwinism. His suffering is of a physical and at the same time spiritual nature; the tumour corresponds to a sadness "as deep-reaching as the roots of the race" (London 1992: 88). His strength was "terrible and compelling, like the rage of a lion or the wrath of a storm" (London 1992: 16).

The cancer of Mrs Curren (Coetzee) is placed in the context of the dangerous and destructive political situation during the apartheid regime in South Africa. Solzhenitsyn's *Cancer Ward* is a hospital and at the same time stands for Russia and even the world as a whole – with 'cancer' having a symbolic meaning. Life and death belong together as well as – in a specific and normative sense – medicine and literature.

Paul and Aubert's (Hallier) life partnership is above all a community of consciousness; their childlike play *The one who sleeps first, awakens the other* has the deeper meaning that the dying person is able to give truth to the living: "Il faut bien se survivre. En toutes choses le mort saisit le vif (One has to survive. In all areas the dead seize the living)" (1977: 163). The poetry of the symbols remains predominant in the portrayal of the medical world in this novel; before the eyes of the horrified surgeon, his assistants and the anaesthetist, the gelatinous tumour substance is transformed into a black bird that escapes from the opened skull: "Ainsi, l'oiseau de gliomes, autrement appelé le Simurgh, l'oiseau-Rock, venu de la nuit des temps, enfanté par la paroi déboîtée d'un crâne d'enfant, inouïe matrice cervicale, vient-il de se libérer (Thus, the glioma bird, otherwise known as the Simurgh, the Rock-bird, coming from the dawn of time, born through the dislocated wall of a child's skull, an unheard-of cervical womb, found its way out into the open air)" (Hallier 1977: 24).

Illness offers a chance, enables reflection on the essential issues of life, for which the healthy state of mind does not allow time or opportunity. The fatal disease of cancer confronts the pharmacist Malone (McCullers) with the existence of man and, above all, with his own existence and its finiteness. He conceives the value and help of literature in the hospital; above all he is fascinated by a book entitled *Illness to Death* (1849) whose author Søren Kierkegaard (1813–1855) is totally unknown to him; one sentence touches him immediately: "The greatest danger, that of losing one's own self, may pass off quietly as if it were nothing; every other loss, that of an arm, a leg, five dollars, a wife, etc., is sure to be noticed" (McCullers 1978:161). Mrs. Cullen's letter to her daughter (Coetzee) is her way of fighting against dying: "Death may indeed be the last great foe of writing, but writing is also the foe of death" (Coetzee 1990: 106). Ivan Ilyich's (Tolstoy) face becomes more beautiful and significant in death, bearing an expression of perfection, combined with a message: "reproach or reminder to the living" (Tolstoy 2014: 32). The philosopher Martin Heidegger (1889–1976) regarded this novel as an important example of the widespread way of dealing with death: "This evasive concealment in the face of death dominates everydayness so stubbornly that, in Being with one another, the 'neighbours' often still keep talking the 'dying person' into the belief that he will escape death and soon return to the tranquillized everydayness of the world of his concerns" (Heidegger 1962: 297).

Cancer can affect literary movements, philosophical currents and historical epochs. Friedrich von Hagedorn (1708–1754) speaks of "Aberglauben[s] Krebs, der viele Lehrer plagt (superstition of cancer, which plagues many teachers)" (Hagedorn 1757: 73). In his *Hesperus* (1795) Jean Paul (1763–1825) creates the metaphor "philosophisches Krebsgift (philosophical cancer poison)" (Jean Paul 1975: 1, 553) and makes the observation: "Der eifersüchtige Krebs auf der Brust ist nie ganz zu schneiden, wenn ich großen Heilkünstlern glauben soll (The jealous cancer on the breast can never be cut completely if I am to believe great healers)" (Jean Paul 1975: 2, 987–988).

18.6 Perspectives

Medicine in literature, or more broadly the connection of medicine and literature, has many dimensions and stimulates substantial debates on the nature of medicine, literature and reality. Health and disease are not merely medical facts; they are also vital themes in literature and art, philosophy, theology, sociology and psychology. In fact, these very disciplines remind medicine again and again of its 'anthropological' character, in the sense that medicine deals with the nature and destiny of human beings. Neither medicine nor the concepts of health and disease with which it deals can be properly understood by using the contrasting categories of natural sciences and human sciences as a framework. Medicine itself is a science and an art; and living with disease is also an art.

Culture is the cause of disease but culture is equally the product of disease. Culture shapes disease, diagnosis and treatment, the situation of the patient, the activity of the physician and social reactions. The dualism of body (*res extensa*) and mind (*res cogitans*) of René Descartes (1596–1650) consists in reality in four dimensions: subjectivity has the individual meaning (conscience of a single person) and the general meaning (culture); and objectivity also has the individual meaning (the body of a single person) and the general meaning (the world of nature). Besides the 'transcendent transcendence' of religion, an 'immanent transcendence' of culture exists, which can be experienced by listening to music, reading books or looking at paintings from antiquity to the present. Culture – meaning literature and all the arts – enables the acceptance of the limits of individual life, pain, disease and death. Beyond its real appearance, disease is always portrayed in literature as a painful symbol of the destruction of life, social reality and culture, but also as a consoling symbol of compassion and the victory that the spirit can achieve over the irrevocable finiteness of human existence.

The 'medical humanities' stands for the connection of natural sciences, humanities, literature and arts in medicine. Illness from this perspective is always understood as a physical, psychological, social and spiritual phenomenon – in other words as 'spiritual-socio-psycho-somatic'. Personalized medicine does not merely mean biological and genetic individuality, but it must also take into account the personality of the patient, their feelings, thoughts and living conditions. Evidence-based medicine cannot be limited to empirical-statistical evidence, but must also include immediate insight. Precision medicine must include – beyond objective accuracy – subjective accuracy on the part of the doctor and the patient. Medicine as 'medical humanities' is both human and humane – for the benefit and dignity of suffering, sick and dying men and women.

References

Antunes AL (2000) The natural order of things, in Portuguese 1992. Grove Press, New York
Binet L, Pierre Vallery-Radot P (1965) Médecine et littérature. Expansion Scientifique Française, Paris
Carmichael AG, Ratzan RM (eds) (1991) Medicine: a treasury of art and literature. Hugh Lauter Levin, New York
Coetzee JM (1990) Age of Iron. Secker & Warburg, London
Dostoyevsky FM (1996) The idiot, in Russian 1868. Wordsworth Editions, Ware, Hertfordhire
Downie RS (1994) The healing arts. Oxford Univ. Press, Oxford
Du Maurier D (1981) Rebecca. Pan Books, London
Edson M (1995) Wit. Faber and Faber, New York
Engelhardt Dv (2018) Medizin in der Literatur der Neuzeit. 5 vols. Matthes, Heidelberg
Engelhardt Dv (2018) Dimensionen der Bibliotherapie im historischen Kontext des heilsamen Lesens. Balint-Journal 19(4):109-115

Greene G (2000) Doctor Crombie, 1956. In: Collected stories. The Bodley Head & William Heinemann, London, pp 128–135

Hagedorn Fv (1757) Sämtliche poetische Werke, vol 2. Bohn, Hamburg

Hallier J-E (1977) Le premier qui dort réveille l'autre. Le Sagittaire, Paris

Hegel GWF (1975) Aesthetic. Lectures on fine art, in German 1830, vol 1. Clarendon, Oxford

Heidegger M (1962) Being and time, in German 1927. Harper and Row, New York 1962

Heimes S (2017) Lesen macht gesund. Die Heilkraft der Bibliotherapie. Vandenhoeck & Ruprecht, Göttingen

Hodler F, Brüschweiler J (1976) Ein Maler vor Liebe und Tod. Ferdinand Hodler und Valentine Godé-Darel. Ein Werkzyklus 1908-1915. Kunsthaus Zürich, Zürich

Hoerni B (2016) Cancer et littérature. His Sci Med 50:199–206

Huxley A (1963) Literature and science. Chatto & Windus, London

Jagow Bv, Steger F (2005) Literatur und Medizin: Ein Lexikon. Vandenhoeck und Ruprecht, Göttingen

Jaspers K (1997) General psychopathology, in German 1913, 1973, vol 2. Johns Hopkins UP, Baltimore

Jean Paul (1975) Hesperus, 1795. In: Werke, vol 1 and 2, Hanser, München

Kafka F (1999) Letter to Oskar Pollak, 27 January 1905. In: Briefe 1902-1912. Fischer, Frankfurt a. M., p 36

Kaptein AA (2021) Writing cancer. Support Care Cancer. https://doi.org/10.1007/s00520-020-05920-0

London J (1992) Sea-Wolf, 1904. Oxford University Press, Oxford

Manferlotti S (ed) (2014) La malattia come metafora nelle letterature dell'Occidente. Liguori editore, Napoli

Mann T (1961) The Black Swan, in German 1953. In: Stories of a Lifetime, vol 2. Mercury Books, London, pp 348–411

McCullers C (1978) Clock without hands. Barrie & Jenkins, London

Oates JC (1971/1972) Happy Onion, 1968. Antioch Rev 31(4):459–475

Peschel ER (ed) (1980) Medicine and literature. Neale Watson, New York

Phillips JA (1979) Souvenir. Black tickets. Delacorte Press, New York, pp 175–196

Remarque EM (1945) Arch of Triumph. Hutchinson & Co, London

Sagan F (1977) The Corner Café, in French 1975. In: Silken eyes. Delacorte Press/E. Friede, New York, pp 141–147

Singer IB (1975) The Witch. In: Passions and other stories. Farrar, Straus and Giroux, New York, pp 104–132

Solzhenitsyn A (1971) Cancer Ward, in Russian 1968. Penguin Books, Harmondsworth

Sontag S (1978) Illness as metaphor. Farrar, Straus and Giroux, New York

Storm T (2016) Ein Bekenntnis, 1887. In: Sämtliche Werke. Vol. 3. Novellen 1881–1888. Deutscher Klassiker Verlag, Frankfurt a. M., pp 580–633

Tolstoy L (2014) The Death of Ivan Ilyich, in Russian 1886. In: The Death of Ivan Ilyich and Confession. W. W. Norton & Company, New York, pp 25–112

Warren S (1831) Cancer, 1830. In: Passages from the Diary of a Late Physician. In: Harper & Brothers, New York, pp 44–50

Wolfe T (1935) Of Time and the River. Charles Scribner's Sons, New York

Yglesia H (1972) Semi-private. New Yorker 5(2):35–37

Zifreund W (ed) (1996) Therapien im Zusammenspiel der Künste. Attempto-Verlag, Tübingen